How Everyone Became Depressed

How Everyone Became Depressed

The Rise and Fall of the Nervous Breakdown

The Rise and Fall of the
Nervous Breakdown

EDWARD SHORTER, PhD, FRSC

OXFORD
UNIVERSITY PRESS

OXFORD
UNIVERSITY PRESS

Oxford University Press is a department of the University of Oxford.
It furthers the University's objective of excellence in research, scholarship,
and education by publishing worldwide.

Oxford New York

Auckland Cape Town Dar es Salaam Hong Kong Karachi
Kuala Lumpur Madrid Melbourne Mexico City Nairobi
New Delhi Shanghai Taipei Toronto

With offices in

Argentina Austria Brazil Chile Czech Republic France Greece
Guatemala Hungary Italy Japan Poland Portugal Singapore
South Korea Switzerland Thailand Turkey Ukraine Vietnam

Oxford is a registered trade mark of Oxford University Press in the UK and certain other
countries.

Published in the United States of America by
Oxford University Press
198 Madison Avenue, New York, NY 10016

© Edward Shorter 2013

Library of Congress Cataloging-in-Publication Data
Shorter, Edward.
How everyone became depressed : the rise and fall of the
nervous breakdown / Edward Shorter.
p. ; cm.
Includes bibliographical references and index.
ISBN 978–0–19–994808–6 (alk. paper)
I. Title.
[DNLM: 1. Depressive Disorder. 2. Affective Symptoms. 3. Stress, Psychological.
WM 171.5]
616.85′27—dc23
2012031859

3 5 7 9 8 6 4
Printed in the United States of America
on acid-free paper

I should like to thank Tom Ban, Barney Carroll, Max Fink, David Healy, and Gordon Parker for a close intellectual companionship over the years that has made this book not only possible but inevitable.

Contents

Preface

BARNEY CARROLL IS a large, ruddy Australian psychiatrist who does not suffer fools gladly. In 1968 he figured out that there is a biological marker—a chemical indicator—for the form of serious depression called melancholia. The article in the *British Medical Journal* in which he announced this finding aroused a certain passing interest. But then several official commissions, staffed by people who had little curiosity about the endocrine system (where Carroll's test was active), decided that his test, called the dexamethasone suppression test, was not really all that revealing. Carroll, it must be said, did not handle this situation as well as he might have. He became irascible, further alienating people. Psychiatry lost interest in Carroll's test and went on to decide that there was actually no difference between serious and minor depression, that they were all the same thing. Carroll's finding passed into oblivion, and the idea that serious depression has a biology of its own became substantially forgotten. Instead, people with emotional issues ended up with the diagnosis of major depression, for which, of course, there was no biological marker. That is the situation in the new millennium: Almost everybody is depressed. This is a scientific travesty. How did it happen?

Take the women that you know. About half of them are depressed. Or at least that is the diagnosis they got when they were put on antidepressants. But depression is a mood disorder. It means the mood is sad, the opposite of euphoria (which would be mania). These women are not necessarily sad, sobbing at home. They go to work, but they are unhappy and uncomfortable; they are somewhat anxious; they are tired; they have various physical pains—and they tend to obsess about the whole business.

What's Up with That?

There is a term for what they have, and it is a good old-fashioned term that has gone out of use. They have nerves, or a nervous illness. It is an illness not just of mind or brain, but a disorder of the entire body. That is what this book is about.

How about men? Do they get nervous too? Yes they do, although not in the same proportion as women. Also, men tend to express their dysphoria more by getting into bar fights, in sociopathy, rather than with nervous symptoms. Still, nervousness is a disorder of both sexes, one that is present in all cultures—although the predominant symptom may differ. We have a package here of five symptoms—mild depression, some anxiety, fatigue, somatic pains, and obsessive thinking—and the symptom that is most salient may vary from culture to culture. The depressive component, for example, is played down in Chinese culture.

We have had nervous illness for centuries; it may be a constant in the human condition, and seems to have a significant hereditary component. If your mother was nervous, you may be nervous too. When you are too nervous to function, things ratchet up by a peg and you have a different illness: it is a nervous breakdown. But that term has vanished from medicine, although not from the way we speak.

In medical parlance nervousness has turned into depression and anxiety, although so slowly over so many years that physicians themselves have tended to lose sight of this subtle—but hugely important—linguistic drift. The nervous patients of yesteryear are the depressives of today. That is the bad news, because their basic problem is not really sadness. The good news is that nervousness is treatable,although maybe not with Prozac-style drugs.

By this point I know that some readers, especially psychiatrists and neuroscientists, will themselves have become nervous: Is Shorter proposing to revise this antique term nerves for use in disciplines that pride themselves of being scientifically advanced and future-oriented? I should say at the very beginning that I am not insisting that depression be rebaptized nervousness. There is indeed such a thing as serious depression as an independent entity (melancholia). Rather, I want to show that history offers a template for a much needed rebaptizing of some kind. There is a deeper illness that drives depression and the symptoms of mood. We can call this deeper illness something else, or invent a neologism, but we need to get the discussion off depression and onto this deeper disorder in the brain and body. That is the point.

Edward Shorter
Toronto
May 2012

How Everyone Became Depressed

1

Introduction

FOR THE PAST 40 years, the diagnosis of depression has been steadily increasing. The prevalence of serious depression in the middle third of the twentieth century was less than one in a thousand; today, it is measured in the double digits *per hundred*. In an outpatient medical practice in New York, 18.9% of the patients had a diagnosis of major depression.[1] On a lifetime basis, one American in five will receive a diagnosis of depression.[2] This is a real puzzle.

Given that these millions of patients with purported depression are not necessarily sad and have scads of other symptoms, it is not clear what the basis is for calling them depressed. Maybe they have some other diagnosis?

The extreme form of being very ill was historically the nervous breakdown, involving melancholia, panic, overwhelming fatigue, and bodies that felt and moved like lead. Lesser forms of nervous illness were simply called "nerves." Were these nervous patients simply depressed? Or is it we who are the nervous?

This is a subject that we as a society have not lost interest in. "Government on the Verge of a Nervous Breakdown" was a page one story on the cable channel MSNBC in 2011, as Congress teetered on the point of passing the controversial deficit reduction plan.[3] So the nervous breakdown has not gone away after all! Just when psychiatry, with all its talk about depression, thought diseases of the nerves were dead, the concept turns out to be alive and well among the public. Take the HBO comedy-drama "Enlightened": When Laura Dern, as troubled corporate executive Amy Jellicoe, has a nervous breakdown, every system of her body screams stop! This is way beyond depressed. Then when she returns from a New Age spiritual healing colony in Hawaii "after swimming with the turtles," everything has been buffed. She's a "new person."

People can relate to nerves as a disease of the entire body, whereas depression, in the sense of a sad mood, is a bit of a stretch. Many patients who are called depressed are not sad. And you can have a nervous syndrome without necessarily crying all the time. In fact, in serious depression, mental pain and bodily anguish are the disturbing symptoms, not tristesse in the style of a French romantic movie. Patients complain about the "inability to feel," not about sad feelings.

The difference between depression and nerves is that depression is considered a mood disorder whereas nerves is a disease of the whole body. Melancholia, for example, the quintessence of the nervous breakdown, reaches deep into the endocrine system, which governs the thyroid and adrenal glands among other organs.

The Japanese have retained this concept of mood disorders as an illness of the entire body far more than we. Junko Kitanaka, in a history of depression in Japan, writes in 2012, "Japanese psychiatrists have continued to combine the technical, neurochemical imageries of depression with familiar cultural idioms that present depression as a *generalized* illness of both mind and body." In 2006 one Japanese investigator described depression as a "temporary decline of vital energy" and a "generalized illness of the whole body … and the whole person." The Japanese tend to see what we call depression as "a cold of the heart." This thinking arose from Japanese notions of neurasthenia earlier in the century.[4] We Atlantic types are therefore not the first civilization to conceptualize mood disorders as nerves and to surveil the entire body for its symptoms.

Nerves are a kind of package. It includes such common symptoms as mildly depressed mood, anxiety, fatigue, somatic symptoms such as insomnia, and a tendency to obsess about the whole business. These might be considered a nervous syndrome, though physicians in the past did not use that exact term; instead they spoke rather vaguely of nervousness, nervous illness, and the like. Since the 1940s this useful nerve category has been discarded in favor of a disease, considered to be mainly of *mood*, called "depression." Today, "depression" has become the disease most commonly diagnosed in medicine. Worldwide, literally hundreds of millions of people are now thought to suffer from depression, or to have a history of it in their past, or the likelihood of another episode in the future, unless they are treated with drugs called "antidepressants." In the United States, in 2005–2008, according to data from the National Center for Health Statistics, almost a quarter of all women (22.8%) were on antidepressants.[5] This is an appalling story of scientific error that has resulted in a public that believes itself to be, more or less, depressed.

How could we have been led into this blind alley? In psychiatry, cutting nature at the joints, or coming up with true disease entities, is devilishly difficult. Barney Carroll says, "On ward rounds we direct the attention of medical students to the woman pacing the corridors, wailing, shredding her clothes, appearing unkempt, importuning staff. We tell the students the diagnosis is melancholia. Then we enter another room where a patient is lying mute, inert, with bedsores from immobility and wasting from lack of nutrition. We tell the students again that the diagnosis is melancholia. Not surprisingly, the students are perplexed. So we invent qualifiers. We call these cases agitated depression and retarded depression, respectively. By means of the nominalist fallacy (I name therefore I know) the students are then satisfied."[6]

What do these patients really have? Patients do not turn up with diagnoses stamped on their foreheads but with collections of symptoms, a story that they relate orally. With a few exceptions, there are no blood tests or biological markers in psychiatry that let us bypass the story and announce "diabetes"! Trying to align these symptoms and signs into diseases is the purpose of "nosology," or classifying diseases on the basis of cause. And from the beginning, clinicians have been mindful of what they are up against. James Sims, president of the London Medical Society, wrote in 1799 of the "various kinds of alienation of the mind": "… In distinguishing disorders which have an affinity to each other, there will, in particular cases, be great difficulty; the shades of difference, as they approach, being so very minute, as almost to escape the most experienced mind. Every thing in Nature is a continued chain, without those breaks and intervals which even the accurate describer is obliged to make, in order to keep up due discrimination, and to render himself intelligible."[7]

Thus, Sims said, we do need to discriminate among distinctive diseases, because, though clinically very close in appearance, they have different responses to treatment and different outcomes. Thus to render ourselves "intelligible"—I love the concept! for otherwise we would be unintelligible—we need to consider the differences among the diseases.

Today, in the study of the different diseases of mood, we have become close to unintelligible. The current classification is a jumble of nondisease entities, created by political infighting within psychiatry, by competitive struggles in the pharmaceutical industry, and by the whimsy of the regulators. Yet this book is not a diatribe. Rather, we want to consider how the majority of illnesses of body, mood, and mind were once understood and how the story has come out today. How everybody has become depressed in other words.

In emphasizing nerves and the whole body rather than just mood, we join a worthy tradition of biological thinking in psychiatry, seeing so-called mental illness as brain disease, not the kind of frank pathological brain lesions studied by neurologists, but disorders of neural biology. Yet impulses from the brain are modified by thought, culture, and society before they turn into behavior. These things have to be kept in balance: the body's chemistry driving the deep story, the psychoanalysts of the 1930s and 1940s turning the story's course in certain directions, and the pharmaceutical industry today turning it in others. At a meeting in 1988, Joseph Zubin, a neuroscientist from the University of Pittsburgh, said with the wisdom of his 88 years, "The biological variables we talk about have primarily been wired in through evolution. The psychosocial variables came much later, when culture took over. Cultural transmission is not as efficacious, not as direct, and not as built-in as the biological, yet it presents a very basic underpinning of total behavior, including biological behavior."[8] So the churnings of the American Psychiatric Association, the group that produced the radical new reordering of psychiatric diagnosis in 1980 called *DSM-III*, meaning the third edition of the official *Diagnostic and Statistical Manual* of psychiatry, will receive equal billing with the disorders of the body's endocrine axis that seem to twin with melancholia.

The story is driven by the shift from nerves to depression. And the major players are the big-dome German psychiatrists of the late nineteenth century who rather arbitrarily hit on "depression" as preferable to older labels. Then the psychoanalysts, the adherents of Freud's doctrines, burst on stage in the 1920s; they ditch biological thinking completely, putting neurosis arising in the mind in the center spotlight. Then the analysts, too, fall from grace. After the 1970s, psychiatry, with artful new depression diagnoses at the bowsprit, acquires a kind of mass audience attuned to every fresh diagnostic quiver. And the pharmaceutical industry deftly markets these new diagnoses to the tune of billions of dollars in drug sales. Yet this is a story in which not just vast social tides but ideas make a difference.

In the area of mood disorders, which is to say the gamut of affective styles that runs from euphoria to anxiety and sadness, medical ideas do matter. In the past, the notion of nerves suggested that patients had an illness of the entire body, that spa treatments, for example, could correct. The caress of the healing waters restored equilibrium; the walk at eleven in the spa park before lunch while the band played was calmative. The body was calmed. There were medications such as opium that effectively treated nervous illness and melancholic breakdown as well. Today, with the ubiquity of the diagnosis of depression, we have the idea that low mood and an inability to experience pleasure are our main problems; we see ourselves as having a mood disorder situated solely in the brain and mind that antidepressants can correct. But this is not science; it is pharmaceutical advertising. Meanwhile, the serious, melancholic depressions are missed. The consequence is many suicides that otherwise might have been prevented, and a population taking antidepressants as though they were Tums—and getting all of the side effects and few of the imagined benefits of these medications.

But what if what we have is really nerves, and when things go awry what we experience is not major depression but a nervous breakdown? What then?

2

Nerves as a Problem

Motto: "Once upon a time I was falling in love
Now I'm only falling apart."
BONNIE TYLER, "Total Eclipse of the Heart"

IN 1996 THE *Wall Street Journal* noted, "The nervous breakdown, the affliction that has been a staple of American life and literature for more than a
century, has been wiped out by the combined forces of psychiatry, pharmacology and managed care. But people keep breaking down anyway." Indeed they
do keep breaking down. Kitty Dukakis, wife of former presidential candidate
Michael Dukakis, remembered lying in bed doing nothing. "I couldn't get up
and get dressed, but I couldn't sleep either."[1]

What was the matter with Kitty Dukakis and millions of sufferers like
her? Depressed?

What does psychiatry think? In psychiatry there are a few distinct, sharply
defined diseases that would be difficult to miss, such as melancholia and catatonia.
These tend to be psychotic illnesses, involving loss of contact with reality in the
form of delusions and hallucinations, though not always. Then there is the great
mass of nonpsychotic ill-defined illnesses whose labels are constantly changing
and that are very common. Today these are called depression, often anxiety,
and panic as well. These are all behavioral diagnoses, suggesting that the main
problem is in the mind rather than the brain and body.

Yet there is a tradition, now almost lost, of viewing psychiatric symptoms
as a result of body processes, and it has always been convenient to speak of
these as "nervous" diseases, even though much more of the body than the
physical nerves may be involved. Writing in 1972, English psychiatrist Richard
Hunter directed attention toward the body as a whole. "Many diseases are
ushered in by a lowering of vitality which patients appreciate as irritability
and depression. The mind is the most sensitive indicator of the state of the
body. An abnormal mental state is equivalent to a physical sign of something
going wrong in the brain."[2]

The Nervous

The term symptom cluster is popular today,[3] but that is jargonish, so let us call these patients "nervous." Their distinguishing characteristic is that they do not have the "C" word, as Eli Robins at Washington University in St. Louis used to call it, meaning that they are not "crazy." This distinction between insane and noninsane illness has existed for many years. Parisian psychiatrist Jules Falret said of the diagnosis hysteria—meaning excessive emotional lability—in 1866, "It's a nervous disorder not a form of insanity."[4] Nerves and psychosis are separate concepts. Historically, the label nerves has not always been used, although it has a sturdy pedigree reaching back into the eighteenth century. Symptoms of nerves include tiredness, anxiety, mild depression, compulsive thoughts and actions, and a rash of physical complaints without an obvious organic cause. Some of these are frankly psychiatric, such as mild anxiety and depression (the severe forms of both seem to be different illnesses entirely). Some relate to the physicality of the body, such as somatic symptoms of fatigue, pain, ill-functioning bowels, and the like. Not all patients will have all five domains, given the enormous variability from person to person that exists in subjectivity. Indeed, it is quite possible to feel just uncomfortable in nervous illness, without being anxious or depressed. Yet the presence of this five-pack of symptoms across the ages is quite constant, although the attention of physicians and patients at any point in time may be focused on one or the other.

It was thus a bit like assembling an Easter basket. A nervous patient would have a symptom from each of several domains. Here is Maurice de Fleury, a 44-year-old Parisian psychiatrist, describing in 1904 the "neuropaths" in his extensive private practice:

They come through the door and announce themselves: "Docteur, je suis neurasthénique." Doctor, I'm neurasthenic. The patient might take from his pocket the papers on which he has written down all his symptoms. This was the kind of patient that Jean-Martin Charcot, the great Parisian neurologist, had called "l'homme aux petits papiers," or "the patient with the little slips of paper."

What's the matter with the patient?

The first symptom, said Fleury, is "profound lassitude." "His legs scarcely hold him up." Fleury said there was a kind of "chronic sadness of those with nervous exhaustion, which is only the vague and confused awareness of their state of physiological misery and functional lassitude."

Then the neuropath suffers sleeplessness: "The nights are deplorable." He has trouble falling asleep, is "torpid" with the digestion of the evening meal, and then awakens toward midnight.

On the somatic side, "The pains that plague the neurasthenic are infinitely variable," said Fleury. And the digestive tube: "Frequently those with nervous exhaustion are subject to stubborn constipation and, following, to muco-membranous enteritis," a popular diagnosis in which patients believed they could identify "membranes" from the gut in their stools.

In terms of frank psychiatric symptoms, said Fleury, "things are in disarray. Their memories have lost in precision. Some patients have lost almost completely their memory of numbers, and proper names, and are subject to obsessive thoughts. I know some who go back up their five sets of stairs two or three times to reassure themselves that they have locked their door."

Fleury likened neurasthenia to what he called its "baby sister" melancholia. Melancholia, like neurasthenia, had depressive and anxious forms. He described a borderland between the two diagnoses as "serious anxious neurasthenia, with progressive wasting, obsessive thoughts, self-accusations, and quite close to melancholia" (for which Fleury used the older French term "lypemania"). "Melancholia can supervene, and push the patient to suicide."[5] Thus we are not just dealing with self-centered middle-class people who eat too much and are tired all the time despite spending their days sitting down. These are serious though nonpsychotic disorders and it is important to bear in mind that these patients have real illnesses and are not just victims of "medicalization," or the conversion of normal sensations into medical diagnoses. Fleury was typical of many writers on neurasthenia: It was an illness that drew upon the entire body in different domains, not at all just a mental illness.

What did the concept of nerves mean to Marion D, 49, a patient of Frederick Parkes Weber, a fashionable consultant on Harley Street in London's West End? On July 27, 1906, she saw Parkes Weber because of headaches "for the last five years." As well, "A great trouble is 'nervousness,' worst between 4 and 5 pm … Very often she has feelings of depression, but commonest—she gets neurasthenic 'irritable weakness'—Sometimes she goes 3 days without these feelings—such attacks last hours." "Patient used to have nervous feelings at night—for instance, that if she went to sleep she would never wake up again. (This was owing to feeling so weak and wretched—no real delusion.)" Parkes Weber's diagnosis at this point was "climacteric neurasthenia, with vascular excitability." (Climacteric means menopause.)

Six months later, in January 1907, he saw Marion D again. "She feels giddy and muddled in her head and dreadfully 'tired.' … She says the urine has been rather thick. Bowels regular." Parkes Weber changed her medications from bromides and valerian to Ichthyol pills (ammonium bituminosulfonate, now used as a skin cream).

Alas, the change in medication was for the worse. When she returned again in April 1907 Parkes Weber noted that "[She] mentally feels wretchedly, depressed and weak and has no energy." Later that year, she moved on to a private sanatorium in Buxton, and Parkes Weber lost her from view.[6]

Marion D was a splendidly ordinary example of the nervous patient. She experienced crushing fatigue, was mildly depressed, terribly anxious about waking up in the morning and in her late-afternoon episodes of "nervousness," and reported somatic symptoms of various kinds such as headaches. Parkes Weber does not mention obsessive thoughts but the entire story has an element of obsessiveness as she fretted about her nervousness and her medications. She was neither psychotically depressed nor anxious, and suffered, as far as she herself was concerned, from "neurasthenia." Almost all his patients also obsessed about which continental watering places they should visit, and Parkes Weber, a specialist in balneology, seconded these ruminations with claims about the supposed virtues of Plombières versus Bad Homburg.

By the 1920s, terms such as "neurasthenia" had gone out of style ("tired nerves," oh dear); rocketed by psychoanalysis, "neurosis" was coming into style. Yet plenty of nonanalysts found the term neurosis useful for patients who were troubled but did not have a major mental illness. Angelo Hesnard, professor of nervous diseases at the French naval medical college, distinguished between—the French here is so delicious that I'm going to use it—"les petits névropathes" and "les grands névropathes." "Les petits," the patients with lesser neurotic illnesses, would never consult a psychiatrist but were treated in family medicine, or self-treated, and had a variety of nonorganic complaints. Hesnard furnished a list of all the illnesses they thought they had but did not: heart, gut, kidney, liver, and so forth. "Les grands névropathes," by contrast, had serious obsessional ideas about health and would likely be treated in private nervous clinics—which then abounded in Europe. But they were not "insane" in the classical sense, and would not be found in psychiatry textbooks.[7]

What did these neuropaths, or neurotics, really have? Hesnard said they could be broken down into several main groups, and it is these groups that guide us in much of our analysis: First came the fatigued, formerly known as the neurasthenic, a term that by the 1920s by going out of style but was a mixture of tiredness and dysphoria; then there were the anxious, with their "neuropathic anguish" (a term for somatic anxiety); Hesnard included the obsessives and the phobics; finally, those with "hysteria," a term that I do not find useful but that in the 1920s meant more or less physical symptoms caused not by lesions but by the action of the mind. This schema could be simplified even more for the general practitioner; as Joseph Collins, a neurologist at the New York Post-Graduate Medical School, put it in 1909: "Finding the patient lachrymose and emotional, he calls the disorder hysteria; if depressed and inert, he calls it neurasthenia."[8]

These are the five domains that add up to the concept of nerves and nervousness: (1) pathological fatigue, not just tiredness at the end of the day but nervous exhaustion; (2) mild depression, by which is meant nonmelancholic depression; melancholia is another kind of depressive illness entirely and is considered in Chapter 6; (3) mild anxiety, by which is meant, nonpsychotic anxiety; psychotic anxiety, again, is a different illness; (4) somatic symptoms, such as chronic pain, insomnia, and disordered bowel function; and (5) some variation of obsessive thinking, the mind dwelling on certain themes even with the realization that this behavior is irrational. In 1913, the great German psychopathologist Karl Jaspers said that obsessive thoughts (Zwang) were present in all pathological psychic processes,[9] and indeed this domain of obsessiveness is part of the larger package of nervousness. These five domains represented an illness entity that exists in Nature and cuts Nature more closely at the joints than do notions such as major depression and general anxiety disorder today, which are considered to be independent illnesses. It is important to mention that these five domains cannot be boiled down to the concept of a mood disorder.

It is in the context of these domains that we are better able to situate depression, which is on the face of it a mood disorder not a disorder of the whole body. Depression means low mood, and the term has been in use for at least two centuries. Here is Clara Bloodgood, an actress who in 1908, playing the leading role at the Academy Theater in New York in Clyde Fitch's comedy "The Truth," committed suicide in her hotel room. "She was always extremely nervous," said her manager. The newspaper account ascribed her death to a "nervous breakdown." But it was William Courtenay, her leading man, who invoked the "d" word: "Of course, I know that Mrs. Bloodgood was subject to spells of nervous depression," he said. Today, the headline would read depression (although newspapers have stopped putting supposed mental states in the headlines of suicide stories). But Mrs. Bloodgood was laughing and gay hours before her suicide, and was not clinically depressed in any meaningful sense.[10] She was nervous.

None of these various domains of the nerve syndrome include psychosis, meaning loss of contact with reality in the form of delusions and hallucinations. The presence of psychosis automatically changes the frame and we are no longer dealing with nerves. One English psychiatrist in 1854 was describing a female patient, formerly very ill with "insanity," who now had recovered and was working usefully around the asylum but from time to time experienced the odd auditory hallucination. "The patient knows that she has a nervous disease and consequently is no longer insane."[11]

Among experienced clinicians, the view predominated that the neuroses (when used in a nonpsychoanalytic sense meaning nervous illnesses) were a completely different breed of animal from the psychoses. Lothar Kalinowsky, trained in the German tradition, with years of experience in the university psychiatric clinic in Rome behind him (as a Jew, he had fled Germany to Italy), ended up by 1944 as a staff psychiatrist at the New York State Psychiatric Institute. With this vast wealth of experience, his view of the complete difference between neuroses and psychoses is interesting. In a discussion in 1944 he noted that patients with "anxiety neurosis" responded poorly to electroshock treatment, but those with "agitated depression," meaning melancholia, responded splendidly. "[This] is another argument in support of the opinion that the neuroses and the psychoses have a different basis. I do not think a typical anxiety neurosis ever passes over into the psychotic picture of an agitated depression."[12] The distinction between nerves and insanity is therefore an important one.

Nervous illness was like a bucket of water: It is pointless to draw lines in it or make sharp demarcations. All the domains flooded together. Hesnard was leery of too much classifying because deep down there was a kind of "unity of the neuroses," rooted in our "affective," or emotional, life.[13]

Many asylum psychiatrists had a similar unitarian perspective. They discussed "the unity of the psychoses," the idea that there was really only one underlying form of psychotic illness, but that it went through different stages. This was known in German as "Einheitspsychose," or unitary psychosis. Hesnard did not coin the term "Einheitsneurose," but he might well have. (Of course, it was the last thing he would have done because in these years French and German physicians were at daggers drawn.)

For some writers, the concept of nervousness implied a kind of psychic precursor, or stem cell, from which specific diagnoses arose. Oswald Bumke, professor of psychiatry in Munich, said in 1924 that neurasthenia, or constitutional nervosity, an inborn state of nervousness, "represents the primeval muck from which all functional psychoses [severe illnesses] are differentiated."[14] According to this concept, nervous illness was not a specific diagnosis but rather a constitutional substrate from which specific symptom patterns evolved. The idea is appealing and over the years has had great resonance among those who believe in genetically determined constitutions.

Yet nervousness is not just a predisposition, as Bumke believed, but a specific syndrome. Historically, it seems clear that fatigue, anxiety, mild depression, somatic symptoms, and obsessive thoughts held together in a continually recurring pattern, and that the term nerves or nervousness refers to this package, or syndrome. I just want to introduce this concept here; it will be elaborated on later. A big point now is that we cannot be overly precise in this domain because the different symptoms and syndromes blend together, now one, now the other catching the light. As Columbia psychologist Joseph Zubin once said, "Only in mathematics can definitions be foolproof and rigid. In biology rigidity of definition falls by the wayside, and the power of the defined concept to integrate observations becomes the criterion of a good definition."[15] So in nerves we are integrating observations about various behavioral domains into a larger concept, however uncrisp at the edges the image may be.

A Peek Forward in Time

Now let us put on our seven-league boots and vault ahead to the late 1970s. "Nerves" have now vanished, but the specific components of the package of nervous disease remain with us. Anxiety, for example, was still considered by many as part of a larger package. Katherine Halmi, a psychiatrist at the University of Iowa, told an advisory committee of the United States Food and Drug Administration in 1977, on the subject of using antipsychotic drugs in the treatment of anxiety, that "anxiety" could not be narrowly defined in the list of indications for a drug. "The thing that bothers me about this is that the patients that come for anxiety are not just anxiety patients … In some cases, they do have in fact discrete psychiatric diagnoses. In many cases, they do not." The bottom line is that "Any patient who comes to a physician's office does not have just anxiety."[16]

So the understanding had continued that apparently specific terms such as anxiety were in fact markers for larger disorders. This is never spelled out in any official handbook of diagnostics, yet is clearly part of the profession's operating rules. In the late 1980s, when the Eli Lilly Company in Indianapolis was developing Prozac, they constructed a "dictionary" of the exact meaning of symptoms that might be reported in the scattered trials. Charles Beasley, the Lilly scientist in charge of the Prozac program, later said, "The dictionary that was being used at the time contained distinct entities of 'nervousness' and 'anxiety.' And guess what? Getting any degree of agreement from amongst 10 psychiatrists on how you slice and dice these two terms or what the distinctions between them are … would be, I think, virtually impossible."[17] Thus, when many clinicians wrote "anxiety," they thought "nervousness."

Anxiety remained part of a larger package going into the 1980s. Authors David Goldberg and Peter Huxley, psychiatric epidemiologists, wrote in 1980, "Minor affective disorders—that is to say, anxiety states, minor depressive illnesses—account for the vast majority of [psychiatric] illnesses seen in a primary care setting." Goldberg had done a survey of the symptoms of 88 patients "diagnosed as psychiatrically disordered" in several family practices in Philadelphia: 82% of them had "anxiety and worry"; 71% had despondency and sadness together with fatigue; 52% reported somatic symptoms; and 19% had "obsessions and compulsions." There was indeed in Philadelphia a coherent syndrome of what we might call nervousness, although the authors preferred the label "conspicuous psychiatric morbidity of general medical practice."[18]

Physicians of every epoch focus on the symptoms of nervousness that make most sense to them in terms of their larger theories. Fleury concentrated on fatigue and "nervous exhaustion." Today, a medical community drenched in talk of "affective disorders" would see the sadness, insomnia, and phantom pain that Fleury mentions as evidence of major depression. The point is that the terms nerves and depression both tell us the same thing: The problem is not a disorder of mood; the problem is a disturbance of the entire body. But clinicians today are more conditioned to see the affective side than, let us say, the tar-ball stomachs, the early-morning vomiting and diarrhea, and the leaden fatigue of the somatic side.

By the 1970s, the term nervousness, grievously assaulted by psychoanalysis in previous decades, was almost extinct in medical diagnostics, although not in the minds of patients. We catch a last gasp in 1972 with a new set of diagnostic criteria put forward by the department of psychiatry of Washington University in St. Louis, a group of important clinicians known as the "St. Louis school." Among the diagnostic criteria for "anxiety neurosis," they specified "chronic nervousness with recurrent anxiety attacks … "[19] But the St. Louis group soon abandoned "nervousness" as they moved into the language of mood disorders centering about "depression."

Now, in switching from nerves to mood diagnoses such as depression, the idea was that depressed people are basically sad, rather than having whole-body diagnoses. The essential concept of a mood disorder is that your mood is either euphoric, as in mania, or sad, as in depression. Yet depressed mood is often not present in depression as the term is used today (see also Chapter 11). As Philadelphia psychiatrist Aaron Beck discovered in the 1960s: Of patients with mild depression, only 50% had a dejected mood; of those with moderate depression, 75% had it.[20] These are the great majority of depressions. So moving the spotlight from nerves to depression has illuminated a large number of people who are not sad at all, but are discouraged, or unhappy, or uncomfortable. All these people, however, are encouraged to think that they have a mood diagnosis called depression and that their moods are down. As Max Hamilton, the great English student of mood disorders, said in 1989 of patients with depression and anxiety, "Not all of these have a depression of mood. In a sense, we have the paradox of depression without depression."[21]

The Ranks of the Nervous

The frequency of nervous illness gave its stamp to an era. Robert Musil, the great Viennese novelist who in 1930 composed *The Man Without Qualities*, spoke of "a nervous age" (ein nervöses Zeitalter).[22] And the ranks of the nervous were indeed numerous.

There are formal epidemiological data. One German epidemiological survey conducted in 1935–1938 found the "nervous" to number about 9% of the population of a rural area. Of the 284 nervous individuals identified in a door-to-door count, 74 also had organic illnesses; 59 had a "neurasthenia" that was "not immediately conspicuous"; and 13 had "nervous disorders of a clearly psychogenic nature." Of the nervous, a further 50 individuals had thyroid problems (thyroid difficulties can have psychic ramifications). The nervous were thus almost one in ten.[23] In rural Sweden in 1947, the lifetime incidence of the population suffering from "neurosis" was put at 7.0%.[24] A survey of morbidity in general practice in England in the mid-1950s estimated the prevalence of "psychoneurotic conditions" as about 7.4 per 100 population.[25] These studies are not readily comparable but they do indicate that those suffering from nerves in one form or another represented a not inconsiderable share of the population.

There was a reason that German psychiatrists were called "nerve doctors" (Nervenärzte), and when they left the asylum for community practices, it was nerves and not insanity that they saw. In 1882, Conrad Rieger, a psychiatrist in Würzburg, tried to advise his colleague Emil Kraepelin, then in Leipzig (who was shortly to become world famous for devising the diagnoses "dementia praecox" and "manic-depressive disorder"), about how to plan Kraepelin's future career. "As near as I know the situation in Leipzig, you would have, as an assistant at the university psychiatric outpatient clinic, a good opportunity to found a private psychiatry practice on the side. Erb [Wilhelm Erb, director of the outpatient clinic] would probably try to give you a boost rather than make things difficult, and the whole business would be just terrific for you. You've actually seen enough 'mentally ill patients' in Munich [where Kraepelin earlier worked at the Munich asylum]. And I'm finding increasingly that it's precisely the middle classes, that one never sees in an asylum, who are very common in a private nervous practice."[26]

In Britain, the ranks of the nervous were legion. In 1968, at a conference at McGill University celebrating the 25th anniversary of the founding of the Department of Psychiatry, London psychiatrist Stephen Taylor (later Lord Taylor) described community nervousness. In 1959, he and Sidney Chave had done a survey: "We found, among people who were not necessarily attending their doctors, a sub-clinical neurosis syndrome. The symptoms, which tend to cluster, are: mild depression; undue irritability; 'nerves' or excessive nervousness, and insomnia. This group constitutes about 30 per cent of the population."[27]

Nervousness also seemed quite well represented in the United States. When Herbert Berger began practicing family medicine in the early 1930s in "a semi-rural community," he said that he had "the certainty that I lived in a belt of inbred neurotics ... It felt fairly certain that the residents of my community had intermarried (with some poor stock to begin with) and that this explained the large number of functionally incompetent individuals whom I met." But now on Staten Island in 1956 as an internist, Berger said, "I see even more neurotic personalities." "Gradually I have come to recognize that these individuals never wish to be told that they are *just* nervous. The word 'imagination' is anathema to them for they are certain that they are seriously ill, and they expect and demand that the physician treat their disease with considerable respect. It is often necessary to medicate these people." The remark lets us understand why the flood of psychoactive drugs—Miltown (meprobamate) being the first blockbuster in 1955—was received with such gratitude by community physicians. In rural New York, and on Staten Island, nervousness was as common as in rural Germany. Berger had to explain to his patients time and again that "This is not insanity and that nervous individuals never become insane."[28]

Today in the United States, epidemiological surveys conducted on a door-to-door basis by the federal government at the national level show that about one American in seven is "nervous," whereby respondents were left to define nervous themselves: In 2010 19.4% of the population told interviewers they had "nervousness either all of the time or some of the time" (18.0% of the men and 20.6% of the women): one woman in five![29] For people in general, the concept of nervousness remains very much a reality.

3

The Rise of Nervous Illness

IT IS MUCH better, people think, for the nerves than the mind to be ill. The nerves are physical structures, and heal in the way that all organs of the body heal naturally. Disorders of the mind are frightening because they are so intangible, and, we think, may well lead to insanity rather than recovery. From time out of mind, people have privileged nervous illness over mental illness.

From time out of mind, societies have had expressions for the varieties of frets, anxieties, and dyspepsias to which the flesh is heir. In France and England in the seventeenth and eighteenth centuries, one term was "vapours," a reference from humoral medicine to supposed exhalations of the viscera that would rise in the body to affect the brain. A major apostle was London physician John Purcell, writing in 1702, of "those who have laboured long under this distemper, [who] are oppressed with a dreadful anguish of mind and a deep melancholy, always reflecting on what can perplex, terrify, and disorder them most, so that at last they think their recovery impossible, and are very angry with those who pretend there is any hopes of it."[1] He emphasized melancholia and anguish, and for him the "vapours" were something more than a mild attack of the frets.

But this was not for everyone. Lady Mary Wortley Montagu, now 60 and living in exile in Italy, described to her estranged husband in 1749 Italian health care arrangements, and how physicians visited rich and poor alike. "This last article would be very hard if we had as many vapourish ladies as in England, but those imaginary ills are entirely unknown here. When I recollect the vast fortunes raised by doctors amongst us [in England], and the eager pursuit after every new piece of quackery that is introduced, I cannot help thinking there is a fund of credulity in mankind ... and the money formerly given to monks for the health of the soul is now thrown to doctors for the health of the body, and generally with as little real prospect of success."[2] In a similar tone, Louis Sébastien Mercier, a late-eighteenth-century French littérateur, mocked the "vapours" of the society women: "Our doctors, accustomed to taking the pulse of our pretty ladies, now see only the vapours and nervous illnesses … A pretty woman with the vapours does nothing other than drag herself from her bath to her toilette, and from her toilette to her couch."[3] Vapours released their grip only slowly. In 1821, French psychiatrist Étienne-Jean Georget deplored that medical writers were still using the term "vapeurs," rather than the modern expressions hysteria and hypochondria that Georget favored.[4]

But then vapours went out of style. The great term for neurological and psychiatric illness of a nonpsychotic nature that dominated public and medical profession alike from the mid-eighteenth to early twentieth century was "nervous illness," implicitly assuming that mental symptoms were reducible to the nerves of brain and body as explicitly neurological symptoms.

The term "nervous diseases" reaches way back in medicine, without any particular author taking priority for first describing them. In 1602 Felix Platter, the official physician of the city of Basel, described a patient who had a lip pain so intense that it felt as though a "red-hot iron" was burning him. Platter noted "that such conditions come from the nerves, and that some nervous disorders [Nervenleiden] are capable of inflicting chronic distress without there being otherwise the slightest hint of disease, is amply illustrated in my practice."[5]

But it was unquestionably Oxford physician Thomas Willis who in his 1667 work *Pathologiae Cerebri*, translated into English in 1684 as *An Essay of the Pathology of the Brain and Nervous Stock*, introduced the concept of the nerves to academic medicine in a rigorous scientific way as a cause of disease: through autopsies. On the causes of epilepsy, he wrote, "As to the places affected, for the seat of the irritative matter, although this brings hurt in any part of the nervous system, yet for the most part, it is wont to become most infestous [troublesome], when it is fixed near the beginnings or the ends of the nervous system, or about the middle processes of the nerves … " How wrong other observers had been! "I know that very many ascribe these convulsive passions … to the vapours rising from the spleen: but it seems much more reasonable to deduce them from the convulsive matters laid up within the brain, and rushing upon the beginning of the nerves." Thus, the "passions commonly called hysterical" originated in the head, not the uterus.[6]

Willis's easy use of the adjective "nervous" gave rise to the term "nervous disease." As early as 1739 we find London society doctor George Cheyne trying to convince the novelist Samuel Richardson that his various nervous flutterings were not evidence of a grave disease. This is before Richardson lapsed into frank melancholia. Cheyne: "Your noise in your ears is a common symptom of nervous Hyp and of no possible consequence." ("Hyp" was another term for nervous ailments.) Later that year: "All your complaints are vapourish and nervous, of no manner of danger, but extremely frightful and lowering." Richardson's friend Mrs. Leake had sent to Cheyne a portion of a letter by Richardson that reflected, Cheyne told Richardson later, "the pain, anxiety, and discouragement your symptoms give you." But take heart: Such symptoms, "I must sacredly assure you, are merely nervous and hysterical." Later in 1742 Richardson's "dejection and lowness" had reached such a state that Cheyne cautioned him, "Nothing hurts weak nerves so much as melancholy stories and despondency." "If you would honestly have my opinion about the cause and origin of your disorder I take it you were born originally of weak nerves." Cheyne's wise advice might have echoed down the ages: "You will be sometimes better and sometimes worse. You will be a constant weather machine, and this last plunge has been entirely owing to this boisterous, moist, and rainy season. Every single individual of my nervous patients have suffered, some more, some less, and I myself to a very considerable degree, but all without danger [of death]."[7] The concept of nervous disease—to mean the aggregation of mild depression, anxiety, fatigue, somatic complaints (such as Richardson's tinnitus, or the ringing in his ears), and obsessive preoccupations—was thus well established within London society by the early 1740s.

In 1765 Robert Whytt, professor of medicine in Edinburgh, then the most distinguished medical center in the world, shifted the academic discussion from vapours to nerves. In a work that, for its comments on the "sympathy of the nerves," continued his efforts to lay the basis for modern neurophysiology, Whytt offered observations on "those disorders which have been commonly called nervous, hypochondriac, or hysteric." He said that the term "nervous" had previously been applied to "almost all the complaints to which the human body is liable." Whytt had a different, much more limited conception: " ... It is only proposed to treat of those disorders, which in a peculiar sense deserve the name of nervous, in so far as they are, in a great measure, owing to an uncommon delicacy or unnatural sensibility of the nerves."[8] This was the true intellectual founding of the concept of nervous disease.

Several years later another Edinburgh professor, William Cullen, placed the concept of nervous in the context of diseases in general. In his general classification of all diseases, or nosology, entitled *First Lines of the Practice of Physic*, published initially in Latin in 1769, 4 years after Whyte's work, he described "neuroses or nervous diseases," including neurological afflictions such as apoplexy and palsy, but also "hypochondriasis, or the hypochondriac affection commonly called vapours or low spirits." Describing a mixture of depression, anxiety, and apprehension of illness, he wrote in the English edition that appeared some years later, "In certain persons there is a state of mind distinguished by a concurrence of the following circumstances: A languour, listlessness, or want of resolution and activity with respect to all undertakings; a disposition to seriousness, sadness, and timidity; as to all future events, an apprehension of the worst or most unhappy state of them; and therefore, often upon slight grounds, an apprehension of great evil."[9] Hypochondriasis is one of those old-fashioned terms for low mood, in addition to its modern meaning of unreasonable fear of illness, and what Cullen had done here was to draw together the various skeins of what would later simply be called nervous illness.

The Spreading of Nerves

Nerves began very much as an Edinburgh concept. In 1769 Edinburgh physician William Buchan, together with William Smellie, then a medical student and later a famous obstetrician, helped bring the diagnosis of nervous disease to the great public in one of the most successful medical advice manuals of all time, *Domestic Medicine, or, a Treatise on the Prevention and Cure of Diseases*. He told his breathless readers that "nervous diseases … generally begin with windy inflations or distentions of the stomach and intestine; the appetite and digestion are usually bad … Excruciating pains are often felt about the navel, attended with a rumbling or murmuring noise in the bowels." What else? Pains all over: "flying pains in the arms and limbs; pains in the back and belly … " Then came the mental part: "Alternate fits of crying and convulsive laughing; the sleep is unsound and seldom refreshing … As the disease increases … the mind is disturbed on the most trivial occasions, and is hurried into the most perverse commotions, inquietudes, terror, sadness, anger, diffidence, etc. The patient is apt to entertain wild imaginations, and extravagant fancies; the memory becomes weak, and the judgment fails. Nothing is more characteristic of this disease than a constant dread of death." So nerves were a serious business, and nothing to trifle with.[10]

Patients in their turn embraced the diagnosis of nerves because it sounded modern and up to date, unlike those hoary old humoral terms such as hypo and spleen. Nerves seemed medical—the nerves are organic structures—and it is probably close to a general rule that patients prefer organic-sounding diagnoses to mental-sounding ones. (In the United Kingdom today, individuals who cluster together in support groups to complain of fatigue refer to their condition as "myalgic encephalomyelitis," or "ME"—inflammation of the brain and spinal cord causing muscle pain—rather than as chronic weariness.) In 1786 Mary Wollstonecraft, then 27 and not yet embarked upon the literary career that would make her famous as an early champion of the rights of women, wrote to her sister, "A whole train of nervous disorders have taken possession of me—and they appear to arise so much from the mind—I have little hopes of being better." A bit later that year she wrote that "My nerves are so impaired I suffer much more than I supposed I should do, I want the tender soothings of friendship." In 1788, now in London and actively writing, she complained to a friend of "the return of some of my old nervous complaints … A nervous head-ache torments me, and I am ready to throw down my pen." By this point, she had evidently abandoned a mental theory of her sufferings in favor of a somatic one: "Nature will sometimes prevail, 'spite of reason, and the thick blood lagging in the veins, give melancholy power to harass the mind; or produce a listlessness which destroys every active purpose of the soul." Again, Mary Wollstonecraft showed every evidence of a typical nervous illness: She was downcast, anxious, fatigued, and had a somatic "headache."[11]

Thus did the illness attribution nerves spread among the British upper class. In 1811, George Gordon Byron, Lord Byron, then 23 years old, wrote a pal from Cambridge, "I am growing *nervous* (how you will laugh!)—but it is true,—really, wretchedly, ridiculously, fine-ladically *nervous*. Your climate kills me [writing from Newstead Abbey]; I can neither read, write, or amuse myself, or any one else. My days are listless, and my nights restless; I have very seldom any society, and when I have, I run out of it.... I don't know that I sha'n't end with insanity, for I find a want of method in arranging my thoughts that perplexes me strangely; but this looks more like silliness than madness."[12] Thus Byron exhibited a bit of dysphoria, some anxiety about madness despite a bluff front to a college buddy, and insomnia with his restless nights. Byron was quite correct about his nervousness: Today we would call it depression, but nerves is a better diagnosis.

Elsewhere, nerves had an equally brilliant course, though it was only the name that was new, not the symptoms. In Germany, the young Franz Baader, later to become a famous Roman Catholic philosopher, confided to his diary the morning of April 13, 1786, "On awakening I felt myself rather leaden and apathetic, but calm. I blame the increased sensitivity and weakness of my nervous system, which these days I so notably feel. [He also blamed his dietary fasting]. I read some of the [poet] Klopstock's odes, but became totally out of sorts since my spirit was, rather unusually, not able to soar along."[13] In some of these passages we detect the romantic spirit of the day, and the moods of the young romantics were highly changeable. Yet it is interesting that, unlike earlier times, they now indicted their nerves.

The Marquis de Sade put a positive spin on nerves. In 1801 we encounter his great fictional heroine, the dominatrix Juliette, who unlike the poor martyred Justine, triumphed over all her male and female sex partners before, following her usual wont, killing all the participants in the scene. Juliette is talking with an equally fearsome female companion named Clairwil. They are discussing poisoning all the participants in an episode of group sex.

JUSTINE: "Most assuredly I will follow your lead, Clairwil. I have always loved the idea of poisons."
CLAIRWIL: "Ah, my angel. It is delicious to dominate over the lives of others."
JUSTINE: "For sure I'm going to come all over the place when this happens [une grande jouissance], because at the very moment when you first spoke to me of this plan, I felt my nerves vibrate. An incredible fire seized their mass, and I am sure that if you touch me, you will see that I'm totally wet."[14]

So, nerves were not all negative.

Neurosis Is Introduced

The eighteenth century was the era of the great classifiers of natural phenomena, whether the Swedish botanist Carl Linnaeus's taxonomy of plants in 1735 or French physician François Boissier de Sauvages' classification of human diseases in 1763. Above, we saw the Scotsman William Cullen trying his hand at classification in 1769.

In Europe the term "neurosis" received a major boost when French psychiatrist Philippe Pinel included the term in his own nosology of illness in 1798. Paris was then seen as the epicenter of the learned world, and Pinel's *Nosographie philosophique* proposed "névroses" as the "fourth class" of diseases. Neuroses for Pinel more or less mirrored Cullen's scheme, which he had translated into French, including vesaniae [major mental illnesses], spasms, convulsions, pains, "comatose affections," and paralyses. "The brain, the cerebellum, the spinal cord and the nerves are without doubt the prime organs for the origin of these varied disease pictures."[15]

The writing of Cullen and Pinel combined to insert "neurosis" into the medical vocabulary by the early nineteenth century. The term did not take the medical world by storm, in the later way of "neurasthenia," because it embraced such a vast range of psychiatric and neurological phenomena. (Neurasthenia, as we shall see, was much more specific, and materially rewarding as well. It became the intellectual basis of an entire world of expensive private psychiatric clinics.) Yet early on, neurosis did enjoy a certain amplitude. In 1823, for example, C.-H. Machard, chief of hospital services in the little French town of Dôle on the Doubs River in the Jura Department—a complete nobody in other words—said in his "medical topography" that "Hypochondria, hysteria and in general the various *névroses* are the lot of those people here with temperaments fatigued by excess and psychological afflictions." Happily, such conditions were not common in Dôle, he said.[16]

How did neurosis differ from psychosis? In the beginning, the meaning was the exact opposite of that we assign today. In 1845 in his textbook of psychiatry, Ernst von Feuchtersleben, 39 years old and secretary of the Medical Society of Vienna, took a new run at defining the difference between psychiatric and neurological illness, because until then the term "neurosis" embraced both. Neurosis, said Feuchtersleben, was as Cullen and Pinel had described, the entire range of illness having a physical basis in the brain. Yet some disorders had primarily mental symptoms, although situated in the brain, and Feuchtersleben proposed calling them "psychoses." (Later usage reversed this completely, making "neuroses" the minor mental illnesses and "psychoses" the major.) Feuchtersleben wrote that "Every psychosis is simultaneously a neurosis, because without the agency of the nervous system no change in psychic expression could emerge; but not every neurosis is at the same time a psychosis, as the examples of convulsions and pain very well demonstrate."[17] It is actually hard to think of a neurological illness that does not have some kind of psychiatric symptoms, but Feuchtersleben's idea was that apparently organic illnesses such as epilepsy (which he called "neuroses") had no mental symptoms, whereas all behavioral symptoms, such as mania ("psychoses"), must have a basis in the brain. In the next half century there would be a dramatic upturn in the use of the term "neurosis," but in the modern sense, not in Feuchtersleben's.

Nerves and the Abdomen

From the very beginning, interest in the symptoms of nervous illness had a somatic side, and for a century and a half this interest was centered on the stomach and intestines. This is not to hold these early writers up to ridicule for the falseness of their ideas, but to reinforce the point that "nerves" had an irreducible bodily dimension: The condition has never been just a "mental illness."

In his *First Lines* in 1769 Cullen said, as we have seen, that "vapours or low spirits" were the same thing as "hypochondriasis," a kind of minor depression dependent on "a certain state of the body." Yet the curious thing about Cullen's hypochondriasis was that it was localized not in the mind but in the stomach. What was the cause of hypochondriasis? In many cases it was "dyspepsia ... a symptom of the affection of the stomach."[18]

This is interesting. Here we have a major medical writer telling us that the seat of an important mental malady is in the stomach. It is actually not far fetched that nervous illness of the mind and brain might have a connection to the digestive tract. The stomach and colon have quite a refined nervous system of their own, and several hormones that serve as nerve transmitters in the gut, such as cholecystokinin (CCK), are also neurotransmitters in the brain. One observer said, "Gastroenterologists are just psychiatrists that look like doctors."[19]

As the nerve story gets going in the eighteenth century, not only are the bowels closely associated with the brain, they are thought to be among the primary causes of nervous illness. The humoral doctrines of the day easily associated mental symptoms with gastrointestinal events. Among the earliest writers was Richard Blackmore, London society physician and poetaster (whose "heroick poem in ten books" was attacked by a contemporary scribe whom Dr. Samuel Johnson pronounced "more tedious and disgusting than the work which he condemns."[20]) In 1725 Blackmore composed *A Treatise of the Spleen and Vapours* in which he presented hypochondriasis, "vulgarly called the Spleen," as attended with a long suite of abdominal complaints: "First, a depraved disposition of the stomach, and an impaired digestive faculty," the organ "filled and distended with storms of hypochondriacal winds ... This receptacle, and the inferior neighbouring parts, seem a dark and troubled region for animal meteors and exhalations, where opposite steams and rarified juices contending for domination, maintain continual war." And mentally, what were these patients like? They were not psychotic or demented. "Yet a considerable inequality is observed in the operation of their intellectual faculties; for some seasons they discover great impertinence and incoherence in their thoughts, and much obscurity and confusion in their ideas, which happens more often, and lasts longer in those who are far gone in this whimsical distemper. These patients are likewise very various and changeable in their judgment, and unsteady in their conceptions of persons and things." Blackmore described an almost manic-depressive temperament in these hypochondriacal patients: "Sometimes they are gay, cheerful, and in good humour; and when raised and animated with wine, they acquire an extraordinary degree of mirth ... But though these delightful scenes exhilarate the hypochondriacal man, yet when they are past, his spirits are exhausted and sunk; and suddenly relapsing into his dull and lifeless melancholy, he pays dear for his transient, voluptuous satisfactions."[21]

Let us say you are a man with a "gouty humor" and a temperament disposed to melancholy: This unhappy combination of humor and temperament might lead you, said Edinburgh's Robert Whyte in 1765, to develop "a great depression of spirits and sometimes very uneasy distracting thoughts," a reference to suicide. But in a patient with a different constitution, the same humor might produce gastrointestinal upset rather than thoughts of suicide. Or "low spirits in hypochondriac and hysteric cases may be frequently owing to some morbid matter in the blood, flatulent and improper ailments, or other causes affecting the stomach and bowels with a particular sensation, which, though not painful, nevertheless is attended with great dejection of mind." Thus did low spirits, melancholy, and flatus all come together. There was, however, good news for sufferers: "When low spirits or melancholy have been owing to long continued grief, anxious thoughts, or other distress of the mind, nothing has done more service than agreeable company, daily exercise, especially travelling, and a variety of amusements."[22] As we wrestle with these issues today, we do well to keep this cheery advice in mind.

Whyte, like most of his contemporaries, moved within the hypochondriasis frame: troubles supposedly associated with the intestines, meaning below the hypochondrium (under the diaphragm), that produced mental changes. In the world of nerves, hypochondriasis was often the diagnosis par excellence for men. The preferred diagnosis for women was "hysteria." Only later did hypochondriasis take on the exclusive meaning of preoccupation with the risk of falling ill.

In *Domestic Medicine* in 1769, Buchan assigned hypochondriasis to "men of a melancholy temperament ... in the advanced periods of life." Among the causes, "the suppression of customary evacuations ... obstructions in some of the viscera, as the liver, spleen, etc." The remedy? "The general intentions of cure, in this disease, are to strengthen the alimentary canal, and to promote the secretions."[23]

Thus, for the public, it was self-understood in the eighteenth and nineteenth centuries that brain and bowels were linked. In 1814 Lord Byron wrote to an undoubtedly riveted Lady Melbourne of his taste for pleasure: "I began very early and very violently—and alternate extremes of excess and abstinence have utterly destroyed—oh! unsentimental word! my *stomach*—and as Lady Oxford used *seriously* to say a *broken heart* means nothing but *bad digestion*. I am one day in high health—and the next on fire or ice—in short I shall turn hypochon*driacal*—or drops*ical*—whim*sical* I am already."[24]

The nineteenth century accented strengthening the constitution through spa and seaside treatments. In 1845, Edward Bulwer Lytton, seeking succor at the spa at Malvern for his weakened nerves, said, "I was thoroughly shattered. The least attempt at exercise exhausted me. The nerves gave way at the most ordinary excitement—a chronic irritation of that vast [gastrointestinal] surface we call the mucous membrane, which had defied for years all medical skill, rendered me continually liable to acute attacks … "[25] As with many patients at the hydros, the healing waters calmed the irritated membranes and restored nervous strength.

And sea bathing! Louis Verhaeghe, a spa doctor in Ostende, Belgium, explained in 1850 how beneficial it would be for hypochondriasis, a disease seen mainly in men with digestive problems such as his patient, "le docteur M," 43 years old, from a large German city: "He fell ill as a result of excessive fatigue accompanied by some reversals of fortune. His digestive process was at first painful and gave rise to a great malaise. Thousands of belches emitted from his mouth during the passage of the food through his stomach; then his head became heavy; he had palpitations sometimes in the region of the heart, sometimes in the epigastrium. Constantly pursued by fear of being stricken with a grave disease of the abdominal organs, possibly incurable, the patient became gloomy, oneiric [rêveur], and nothing could distract him. During the day, chimerical terrors assailed him; at night, his sleep was troubled by terrifying dreams." After 9 months of this "painful existence," Doctor M finally sought help at Ostende, a seaport and watering place in West Flanders, where under the guidance of Dr. Verhaeghe a course of sea-bathing soon restored him. Dr. M was, according to his medical advisor, a typical "nervous" patient, with hypochondriacal symptoms attributable to the digestive tract.[26]

These beliefs in bowel function as a cause of nervous and mental disease lingered long in medicine, perhaps with some justification, although there were excesses: Toward the turn of the century at Ticehurst Asylum, a private psychiatric hospital for the better classes in England, it was standard practice to administer laxatives therapeutically. "We have had many strikingly rapid recoveries by unloading the intestines in cases of subacute, sometimes almost amounting to typical acute mania." The administration of a large dose of olive oil, per mouth or per rectum, worked wonders said superintendent Herbert Newington in 1901.[27]

Today, there is considerable evidence that patients with depression have more than their share of gastrointestinal upset. In 1990 a team of psychiatrists at the University of Iowa led by Michael Garvey found that among 170 patients with a diagnosis of major depression, 27% had constipation associated with their depression.[28] There is a substantial literature on the role of psychological factors in the irritable bowel syndrome,[29] and the historical evidence as well gives every reason to think that this combination of constipation, diarrhea, and abdominal pain has been a regular companion of nervous conditions.

At a symposium in 1959, Willi Mayer-Gross, a refugee from the Holocaust who became director of a mental hospital in Scotland and at 71 years old was one of the grand old men of British psychiatry, said, as the discussion wandered toward somatic symptoms, "The fact that the digestion, or more broadly the intestinal tract, is so closely linked up with depression has been known for a long time … Such symptoms can be thought of as the shields or disguises of a depressive illness. I find an astonishingly large number of patients who have come to me finally with depression who have been investigated extensively for gastro-intestinal disorder."[30]

Whether the depression was masked by the gastrointestinal symptoms, or whether all these symptoms, mental and somatic alike, were part of a larger parcel of nervous illness, was not debated at the symposium. But the generation of psychiatrists and physicians who preceded the participants believed it, and maybe they were right.

The Heyday of Nervous Illness

To launch nerves center stage, something more was needed than anatomy. A physiological basis for the concept that weak and irritated nerves caused nerve disease was supplied in 1844 by a young German psychiatrist named Wilhelm Griesinger, then 27 years old and a resident in the Department of Medicine of the University of Tübingen; Griesinger had just finished a 2-year stint as an assistant physician at a nearby mental hospital and was full of theories about mind and brain. "It is much less pathological anatomy than physiology that causes brain disease in insanity." To be sure, he continued, psychiatry had labored for years under physiological theories that implicated the spine, in "spinal irritation," but the real problem lay in the "irritable weakness" (reizbare Schwäche) of the brain itself. " … Early exhaustion gives rise to conditions of weakness and pain."[31] We could not imagine that the ratiocinations of such a young and unheralded scholar would have such an impact. Yet Griesinger, alternating between internal medicine and psychiatry, went on to have a brilliant career, becoming professor of psychiatry in Zurich in 1861 and in Berlin in 1864. The first edition of his textbook, published in 1845, had moderate success; the second edition in 1861 became the leading international textbook of psychiatry and firmly established the biological doctrine that "mental disease is brain disease."[32] Nerves sailed forward in history under the banner of irritable weakness.

The spas, especially those offering the hot springs and mineral-water-by-the-cup of hydrotherapy, unfurled their banners for nerves in anticipation of their later reception of neurasthenia (see below). Here, for example, is Ewald Hecker, who together with his teacher Karl Kahlbaum, coined the diagnosis hebephrenia in 1871, a precursor of schizophrenia.[33] In 1882 he had just founded the Clinic for Nervous Illness at Geisenheim near Wiesbaden, in the Rhine valley, on the site of a former hydrotherapy station. What kind of nervous diseases did they treat? All kinds: peripheral nervous diseases such as paralyses; chronic brain and spinal diseases; general neuroses, such as "hysteria, chorea, hypochondria and spinal irritation; general nervosity, such as chronic headache, insomnia, general nerve irritation, psychic dysphoria, mood changes." In addition, they also treated "Patients recovering from psychoses."[34] These are, for the most part, all real illnesses, but to group them tidily in the same facility and pour water on all the patients shows the firmness of the conviction that much illness was reducible to nerves. Within this vast panoply of nervous problems, however, the core was the nervous syndrome, and in treatment, Hecker over the years drifted ever more in the direction of psychotherapy.

The golden years of nerves were from about 1860 to World War I. In 1872 the little section for the electrical treatment of nervous diseases that James J. Putnam had just founded at the Massachusetts General Hospital served just over 70 patients. By 1903 this unit, now the Out-Patient Department for Diseases of the Nervous System and still under Putnam's direction, had, as historian Eugene Taylor tells us, "moved into successively larger quarters three times … and in that year handled between 6,000 and 9,000 patient visits." Most frequent of these "nervous conditions" were "epilepsy, chorea, neurasthenia, and hysteria."[35]

Patients were no less full of talk about nerves than physicians. Young Russian Maria Bashkirtseff, a teenager living in Paris and aspiring to be a painter, was dying of tuberculosis; she wrote in her diary in 1874, "I want to live faster, faster, faster!" She knew that her time was growing short. Later in 1875 she wrote that "I am so nervous that every piece of music that is not a gallop makes me shed tears…. Such a condition of things would do honor to a woman of thirty. But to have such nerves at fifteen, to cry like a fool at every stupid, sentimental phrase I meet, is pitiable."[36] For this heart-rending young woman, nerves was more reduced to sadness, an affective disorder, yet she interpreted her mood as nervous in nature, not depressive.

By 1900 nervous disease had divided into two distinct populations: first, a nervous basin for those suffering every neurological and psychological ailment imaginable, a broad band of diseases that indicates that the term had no specificity at all; and second, the highly focused population of those with the nervous syndrome, or nervous package, that included depression, anxiety, fatigue, somatic symptoms, and obsessive thoughts.

This latter meaning of nervous syndrome was in its twilight toward 1900, although it was still powerful. In 1908 a "private select home," meaning psychiatric unit, in Dundrum near Dublin offered "rapid and perfect cures" to "nervous ladies and voluntary boarders," the latter meaning patients who voluntarily agreed to admission and could sign out again (almost) any time.[37] Family physicians recognized at once the significance of a term such as "chronic nervous patients": They might find your office after a long surgical history, as W. Gray Schauffler, with a 9-year practice in Lakewood, New Jersey, told the medical society of that state in 1906: "If a woman, she has already been the rounds of the gynecologists with varying degrees of relief and has realized that they can do nothing more for her; and if a man, the chances are that surgery has long since done its utmost by removing a doubtful appendix. And so the poor creature comes into our hands in a truly pitiable condition of suffering and despair."[38] There clearly was an army of the nervous out there, who together with their physicians had initially defined their problems as organic and correctible with surgery, only later to come to the end of the road.

Thus all orders of society knew nervous disease, from the small towns of New Jersey to the top of the London social heap. Alfred Schofield had a fashionable nervous practice in Harley Street in the west end of London, the street where elite medical specialists with brass plaques at their front gates tended to cluster. And Schofield was quite sympathetic to the many women and men—many more of the former than the latter—who came to see him for nervous irritability, neurasthenia, and the like. "The battlefield of life is increasingly on a psychic rather than a physical plane," he wrote in 1906, at age 60 years. What if the patient had "nervous irritability," the Griesinger diagnosis, rather than "nervous debility," or fatigue (which will be treated in the next chapter)? In that case she cannot be "put to bed," meaning given the rest cure. Send her away to a spa with "an experienced nurse-companion," until her "nerves are stronger and quieter; and then may come travel or a restful voyage."[39] It is impossible to read these lines today without thinking that they must have been written on a planet other than the one we inhabit. But Schofield's patients had the same illnesses that we do today.

Shortly, the nervous syndrome would disappear and be replaced by depression. Nervous disease as a long spectrum of quasiphysical illness would be replaced by psychological disease.

Let us look now at the specific components of the nervous syndrome one by one. What did it consist of?

4

Fatigue

LET US TRY to unpack nervous disease. What does it consist of? For one thing, most of the patients are tired, even exhausted, and one of the main components of the nervous picture is fatigue.

Today, psychiatrists do not think of fatigue as a terribly important symptom. After such obvious sources as iron deficiency have been eliminated—and it has been determined that the patient is not suffering from one of those quasidelusional disorders such as "chronic fatigue syndrome"—most clinicians would be inclined to ascribe fatigue to depression. For patients, however, fatigue remains a hugely important matter. A study of Stirling County in Canada's Atlantic provinces in 1970 found that only 6% of psychiatrists considered fatigue to be serious; by contrast, people in the community reported "feeling weak all over" as one of the most serious symptoms among a list of 46.[1] In hospital charts today it is not uncommon to see the acronym "TATT," Tired All The Time.

The complaints of the fatigued and weary echo across the ages. In 1712 Lady Mary Wortley Montagu, en route in a journey, complained to a correspondent, "This is what writing tackle the Inn affords, and my head and hand are both disorder'd with fatigue, both of mind and body."[2] Lest psychological fatigue be thought mainly a women's complaint, one of the "grand asthenics" of all time was Parisian novelist Marcel Proust, who, around the turn of the century, was so droopy with fatigue—his medical father had written a book on the subject![3]—that he barely made it from his bedchamber. His correspondence from 1909, for example, mentions fatigue throughout. On Friday, November 26, after his guests had departed, "I set about demolishing what I had written. And over my heart, fatigued from this absence of repose, voilà the fog that rolls in again. It's about three in the afternoon and [another nervous] crisis seems to be starting up."⁴

Whatever period or social class is under discussion, fatigue simply tumbles from the page. A keen young female scholar studying working-class housewives in a German industrial city just before World War I described a wearying struggle just to make ends meet: "A tired indifference speaks from the eyes of these women, who only seldom muster the strength to express a wish or a hope." When asked where and how they might like to spend old age, they respond, "Where we get enough to eat our fill."⁵ The fatigue of grinding poverty is well known, and had they been prosperous enough to see a doctor, which of course they weren't, their fatigue would doubtlessly have been medicalized with a diagnosis such as "neurasthenia." The point is that the grinding conditions of life can produce disorders that seem to pivot about exhaustion.

This fatigue of the miserable bears a superficial resemblance to the fatigue of bored, upper-middle-class London women in the 1920s. Archibald J. Cronin, a young Scottish doctor just trying to build a practice in London, discovered how many of his well-heeled female clients were "rich, idle, spoiled, and neurotic." "I even invented a new disease for them—asthenia." This magical word opened many a salon. His patients might say to each other, "Do you know, my dear, this young Scottish doctor—rather uncivilized, but amazingly clever—has discovered that I'm suffering from asthenia. Yes ... asthenia. And for months old Dr. Brown-Blodgett kept telling me it was nothing but nerves." Cronin began giving his patients strengthening injections. "Again and yet again my sharp and shining needle sank into fashionable buttocks, bared upon the finest linen sheets.... Asthenia gave these bored and idle women an interest in life."⁶ This is not the same fatigue, of course, that these worn-down German women endured—yet the denizens of these London salons believed themselves to be tired and not just suffering from "nerves."

Thus fatigue occupied center stage in the nervous illnesses. George Waterman, a neurologist at the Massachusetts General Hospital, said in 1909, "Taking the various forms of the psycho-neuroses as a group there is no one symptom so frequently encountered as that of fatigue."⁷ Asked about "fatigue, weariness and downheartedness," a third of the women in a rural area of Sweden polled in 1947 responded yes (a much smaller percent of the men).⁸

Psychiatry has always tried to bind fatigue into larger concepts. In the past fatigue was central to the nervous package. As German psychiatrist and philosopher Karl Jaspers worked during World War II on the last edition of his great textbook of psychopathology that he would personally edit, he noted that "tiredness" was "one of the basic concepts of neurophysiology." Any theory of how brain and mind worked, he said, would have to come to grips with tiredness and exhaustion (Ermüdung and Erschöpfung). Indeed, said Jaspers, the main theorists of the twentieth century, such as Pierre Janet and Sigmund Freud, had postulated "energetic" theories of mental phenomena: "Energetic theories regard the subconscious mind as a force that has quantitative properties. This force can ebb away, is subject to change, can pile up at obstacles and thereby increase in pressure; it can bind itself to particular objects, and transfer itself from one object to another."[9] Thus tiredness sits at the middle of the whole diagnostic basin of nerves.

A Brief History of Fatigue

Let us attempt first a brief history of fatigue before looking at the psychiatry of it. The exercise is somewhat academic because today, of course, fatigue has vanished from psychiatry.

The first point is separating the history of subjective sensations of fatigue and weariness from the history of medical interest in the subject. Before 1900, real levels of fatigue would be expected to be very high, for several reasons.

One is the exhaustingly long work day in farm and craft shop, where most people labored before the great expansion of urban life began around mid-nineteenth century. For most urban dwellers at the beginning of the twenty-first century, it is simply unimaginable how long and hard people used to work—and how exhausted they were from their labor. Just before World War I, a young German doctoral student named Maria Bidlingmaier, who died during the war, did a work–time study of women's days in a rural community in Württemberg. This was an era when women were fully engaged in farm work in addition to running the household and raising the children. Bidlingmaier interviewed 77 married women obligated to work in the family fields: Their average work day lasted 14 hours, leaving home for the fields around 6 am and returning evenings around 8 or 8:30 pm. The women's entire work day, household chores included, was 17–18 hours. Bidlingmaier commented: "In these numbers lies much secret grief for the peasant women, much courageous determination to get it done, much weary dragging home on dusty country roads, torrents of sweat in the heat of the summer, much staunch persistence in the work that is their duty, much resentment against the harshness of fate, and much exhaustion ... "[10] The work of these Württemberg farm wives was unusually well documented. Yet their world was typical of an entire way of life that once prevailed in Europe and the United States when, in a premechanized era, work was done by hand, hour after endless hard hour, in the fields and the carpentry shops. This is now all vanished in the West, and our conception of hard work, though hard for us, has nothing in common with this former reality for millions of people.

Yet few of the physicians of the day saw "fatigue" as a medical complaint. In the older medical literature, there are almost no references to fatigue or any of its synonyms as medical complaints. At the end of the eighteenth century, a literary genre called the "medical topography" arose, in which local physicians described the hygienic and medical conditions of their district. There are hundreds of these. In almost none of them is fatigue ever mentioned, despite the local population having conditions of work as exhausting, or even more so, than those described by Bidlingmaier.[11] Medical historian Peter Voswinckel notes the appearance of "fatigue" in German medical writing only toward the end of the nineteenth century.[12]

After the last third of the nineteenth century, these brutal working conditions started to come to an end. Objectively, we would expect real levels of fatigue in the population to decline. Time becomes available for recreation. Field and shop become mechanized with the advent of the electric motor. Work times in establishments become regulated. Unions demand the 10-hour day, then the 8-hour day. People begin to eat more protein and fat as they can afford to add meat to diets that previously consisted heavily of starchy porridge.[13] Iron-deficiency anemia was once a major cause of women's fatigue in particular, owing to chronic blood loss from the menses and repeated childbearing. Low iron in your hemoglobin means fatigue, and it is interesting that in Britain the percentage of women admitted to hospital with "chlorosis," the old-fashioned term for iron-deficiency anemia, dropped from 23.2% in 1901–1903 to 8.4% in 1913–1915, evidence of a meatier diet. (Hemoglobin rates rose correspondingly.)[14]

As well, postinfectious fatigue was once very common, meaning the exhaustion that patients experience after a severe infection. But with the urban hygiene movement of the nineteenth century, infectious illness began to decline. The last major pandemic western society experienced occurred in the years 1917–1923 with influenza, together with an associated epidemic of encephalitis lethargica (the two are not the same disease). And encephalitis lethargica, also called "Von Economo's disease," carried with it a crushing postinfectious feeling of fatigue, hence the term "lethargica."[15] As these terrible epidemics died away, the total fatigue burden of the population would have lessened.

Yet paradoxically, at the same time medical interest in fatigue quick-ened. Physicians who previously could not have cared a hoot about their patients' tiredness now came alive to it. Scottish psychiatrist James Crichton-Browne, who in his 80s produced several charming volumes of puckish medical observations, gently mocked his colleagues in 1926 for their fatigue alarmism: "Fatigue, over-fatigue, is one of the great dangers of our day, and the ease with which it is [medically] induced is perhaps one of the signs of our degeneracy." He contrasted a tough-minded Scottish dowa-ger, "vigorous and sarcastic at the age of ninety-six," portrayed in a contem-porary novel, with her greatgrandniece, Miss Douglas, who constantly was running off to the South "on account of her health." It was not the dowager who was fatigued.[16] Still, there is a serious point here. The medical discov-ery of fatigue, as Anson Rabinbach notes, marks "the association of fatigue with pain," in contrast to the older perception "of fatigue as the necessary accompaniment of work."[17] Rabinbach might have extended the point to include not just pain, but depression, anxiety, and somatic symptoms other than fatigue as well, plus a kind of obsessive fretfulness in general—that were all the companions of nerves.

Several new phenomena in the patients' world might have elicited this new interest among physicians. Exactly what happened here is still quite obscure, and key events antedate the popularizing of the term "neurasthenia" in 1869, so it is not simply that a medical term for fatigue arose and the patients oblig-ingly followed by reporting tiredness.

One development is situated not in the world of peasants and laborers but among the upper middle classes, quite particularly among society women. It concerns women wealthy enough to have servants, who "take to their beds," and stay there for months, years, and decades. Medically, they were known as the "bed cases," or the "sofa cases," les femmes à chaise longue, and they were common among the upper-middle-classes of the big cities. What exactly was wrong with these women was never really clear, but they did complain of fatigue despite endless bed rest.

It was around the age of 37, in 1839, that Harriet Martineau, later to become a popular English author, took to her bed. Offspring of a well-off English provincial family, she had been sickly as a child and complained often of fatigue, but finally as an adult she had become "exhausted" by it and sought the sick room. Her self-pitying account "Life in the Sick Room," published anonymously by "An Invalid" in 1844, struck a nerve and became widely read. In addition to "long hours of weary pain," she suffered from "beset-ting thoughts," insomnia, and, as she put it, "nature's feebleness and apparent decay."[18] Looking back on these years in her autobiography, she mentions "a depressing malady."[19]

Harriet Martineau's autobiography, written in 1855 but not published until 1877, emphasizes fatigue more strongly. " ... Considerate persons will at once see what large allowance must in fairness be made for faults of temper, irritability or weakness of nerves ... in sufferers so worn with toil of body and mind as I, for one, have been. I have sustained, from this cause [her deafness], fatigue which might spread over double my length of life." This is not to belittle the sufferings of the deaf, of course, but to show that she experienced them as fatigue. Soon, her writing had put her in a state of "nervous exhaustion." She numbered herself among the "brain-worn workers" and was at pains "to save my nerves from being overwhelmed." By her early 30s she was, she reveals, "exhausted with fatigue," her nerves "overstrained." After the end of her "sick room" reclusion, around 1845, she continued to suffer subjective debility while maintaining an active and successful literary career. At age 52 she apprehended the approach of death (in fact she lived another 20 years) and experienced "a *creaking* sensation at the heart" and "sinking fits." The litany of woe and fatigue then comes to an end because, believing that death was nigh, she hastily concluded her autobiography.[20]

Harriet Martineau was singular in her literary talent but typical of an entire social class of invalids and shut-ins whose nerves were exhausted and were now taking to their sofas and beds. In 1881 Silas Weir Mitchell, a leading scientific figure in neurology who also had an upscale private practice in Philadelphia, referred to "hysterical motor ataxia," the inability or unwillingness to walk based on psychological grounds. The disease, he said, "adds many recruits to that large class which some one has called 'bed cases,' and which are above all things distinguished by their desire to remain at rest."[21]

The second half of the century saw the foundation of many high-end private nervous clinics and sanatoriums, catering to the fatigue crowd (on the owners' fondness for neurasthenia as a diagnosis, see below). It was a whole art, judging where to send patients who suffered from "general weakness," and in 1882 a German spa guide cautioned, above all, not to refer them to places with a high-altitude "strengthening" climate. Much more advisable were watering places in the front ranges and in valleys, "depending on the degree of weakness and especially on the amount of energy that is present in the nervous system."[22]

Thus was the spa world crafted for the weary. The Sanatorium Val-Mont in Montreux-Territet, a pricey Swiss spa-resort, featured in 1908 as an indication for admission "fatigue resulting from overwork."[23] Perfect. Whom should we find there in 1913 but Marcel Proust.[24]

Fatigue thus slumbered on, in a sense, for decades and centuries as plain old weariness, or as part of a larger nervous picture, until it suddenly became a disease of its own. This is usually bad news for patients, when a symptom turns into a disease. Maurice Craig, a psychiatrist at Guy's Hospital in London, deplored in 1917 "the mistake of naming a disease according to its most prominent symptom." He was talking about "depression," because low mood is found in many different disorders.[25] But the stricture applies to fatigue as well. This kind of medicalization fixes attention on a given symptom so that it becomes the elephant in the room rather than just a found-in. Today, this has happened with vague bodily pains as they turn into "fibromyalgia," ensuring that the bearers of the fearful diagnosis will become disabled.[26] In the past this happened with fatigue in the form of "neurasthenia." Boston neurologist James J. Putnam, who established the first nerve clinic in the United States at the Massachusetts General Hospital, said in 1899, "To feel 'tired' may be bad enough at the best, but it makes a world of difference whether one accustoms himself to take the term as meaning the fatigue of a person who expects in due time to be rested, or as a bottomless pit of exhaustion, demanding sighs and groans."[27] It was this that "neurasthenia" accomplished.

Neurasthenia

What fixed the attention of everybody—doctor and patient alike—upon the phenomenon of tiredness, to the exclusion of everything else in the nerves package, was the coining of the diagnosis "neurasthenia" by New York electrotherapist George M. Beard in 1869. To be sure, the term neurasthenia had been used before and Beard did not literally coin it. But his 1869 article in a prominent American medical journal, and following book in 1880, gave the diagnosis a kind of viral spread.

Beard's neurasthenia bombshell burst into the medical world with an article in 1869 in *The Boston Medical and Surgical Journal*, which was the forerunner of the *New England Journal of Medicine*. In a talk in 1868 to the New York Medical Journal Association, Beard said, "I am to speak to-night of a condition of the system that is, perhaps, more frequently than any other, in our time at least, the cause and effect of disease. I refer to neurasthenia, or exhaustion of the nervous system." Thus at the beginning, Beard appeared to be referring not to a whole syndrome but to the specific symptom of tiredness, the result of the central nervous system becoming "dephosphorized ... and as a consequence becomes more or less impoverished in the quantity of its nervous force." But attentive listeners on that evening would have learned that Beard was in fact speaking more of a nervous syndrome than an isolated symptom: "If a patient complains of general malaise, debility of all the functions, poor appetite, abiding weakness in the back and spine, fugitive neuralgic pains, hysteria, insomnia, hypochondriasis, disinclination for consecutive mental labor, severe and weakening attacks of sick headache, and other analogous symptoms ... we have reason to suspect that ... we are dealing with a typical case of neurasthenia."[28] So, from the outset, neurasthenia was really just a synonym for nerves, but one that focused in particular upon the component of fatigue.

Beard's 1880 book, *A Practical Treatise of Nervous Exhaustion (Neurasthenia),* reached a wide medical audience and was at once translated into the most important medical language of the day: German. Indeed, it was dedicated to the Heidelberg neurologist Wilhelm ("William") Erb, one of the major international authorities, with whom Beard was by now bosom buddies. Here Beard made it clear that he included in neurasthenia a variety of anxiety disorders, including phobias and obsessive-compulsive traits (one of his patients was unable to "go more than half a mile in a straight line"); others displayed what would later be hived off as "social anxiety disorder": "This aversion of the eyes is so constant a symptom in neurasthenic patients that I often make the diagnosis as soon as they enter the office, before a word has been spoken by either party, and even before the patient has had time to be seated."

And insomnia! "One man finds no difficulty in getting to sleep on retiring, but soon wakes, and must remain awake for the rest of the night." Beard's patients had disorderly intestinal tracts. "Flatulence with annoying rumbling in the bowels these patients complain of very frequently; also nausea and diarrhoea."

Some of the symptoms of neurasthenia were almost certainly the result of medical suggestion, such as "crawling, creeping, and burning sensations" along the spine, a holdover from the days of "spinal irritation" (which Beard considered part of neurasthenia).

Beard believed "nervous exhaustion" to be synonymous with neurasthenia, and in the 1880 book he dilated upon, "This feeling of exhaustion, though not exactly pain in the usual sense of the word, is yet, in many cases, far worse than pain." Exhaustion might come on in what would later be called "panic attacks": a kind of "going-to-die feeling," Beard said. Beard avoided describing symptoms of depressed mood, probably because he did not want to risk having his precious diagnosis conflated with melancholia or even with what people were already referring to as "depression." Yet he could not avoid the subject. On variations in muscular strength, he said, "One may have great mental depression at times, or at all times may have neurasthenic asthenopia, the various forms of morbid fear, general debility in its various phases, and yet be capable of great muscular endurance." One of his patients, a physician, "gave a perfect history of the disease [neurasthenia]; but when I asked him if he was subject to mental depression, he replied: 'I passed through all that;' and this I observe oftentimes of neurasthenics in middle life, that symptoms of the early stages of the disease, such as mental depression and dyspepsia, have ceased their annoyances."[29] So mild depression was definitely part of the picture.

The many advocates of neurasthenia in the decades ahead increasingly avoided the expression "nerves," which now seemed too old-fashioned, and shunned as well phrases conveying mood disorders, because they wished to cling to the organicity of neurasthenia, rather than turfing their booty to the psychiatrist.

But booty there was aplenty. Medical empires became founded on neurasthenia. Physicians set up profitable consulting practices as neurasthenia specialists, not psychiatrists to be sure, but not your ordinary run-of-the-mill doctor either. Paul Hartenberg in Paris saw mainly patients with hysteria and neurasthenia and profiled his high-end practice along those lines. Yet, trained by internist and hypnotherapist Hippolyte Bernheim at Nancy, he was not a psychiatrist. He was 41 years old when in 1912 he published his widely read *Treatise on Neurasthenia*, featuring patients such as "the forty-ish man who entered my office and said to me, 'Docteur, I've come to consult you because I am always fatigued and incapable of working. When I get up in the morning, I am tireder than the night before. During the whole day, I feel my body, my limbs all stiff. The slightest effort exhausts me, and I can no longer go for walks or take any physical exercise. Even standing upright is painful.'"

Thus far, a clear-cut fatigue case, right? But there is more. "But I'm tired, not just in the body but in the head. There is constantly a tension band about my skull. I feel that my head is empty. My mind refuses to work. My thoughts are confused and I can no longer fix my attention. My memory is shot. When I read, I no longer know by the bottom of the page what I've read at the top. I forget my appointments, my business affairs." This certainly sounds like depression.

And it is: "With all that, I'm sad. I am bored to death everywhere and always. Everything that other people find amusing leaves me flat. I take no pleasure at anything." These are classic symptoms of depression. But Hartenberg's patient was also anxious: "I am worried about everything. The slightest problem alarms me. The least upset exasperates me." Moreover, this forty-ish man had "lost his appetite, slept poorly and had no sexual desire."[30] Doctor, your diagnosis? Today we would say unhesitatingly "major depression," with comorbid anxiety. But there is nothing that differentiates Hartenberg's patient from the many other nervous patients of history, merely that both the patient and Hartenberg chose to focus on the man's fatigue, rather than on his anxiety or dysphoric mood. Fatigue is not a medical emergency. The complete absence of pleasure in life is, because these patients are inclined to suicide.

Every big city had its Doctor Hartenberg, the neurasthenia specialists who sometimes were genuine scientific figures as well, such as Hermann Oppenheim in Berlin, or sometimes they were just medical businessmen. Oppenheim, a leading neurologist of the day, also received nervous patients from all over the world in his private clinic. He wrote in his *Textbook of Nerve Diseases*, a leading neurology textbook, "Neurasthenia has become a widespread illness in our society. One encounters it with special frequency among the residents of the big cities. Even though it might have been present in all epochs, and has long been familiar under the term nervousness, nonetheless in recent decades it has doubtlessly increased phenomenally, with the constantly growing haste and unrest of existence, with the extreme increase in challenges that life, work, livelihood, and pleasure-seeking that all demand."[31]

What gave impetus to the business side of neurasthenia was the discovery in 1875 of a "cure" for it: Weir Mitchell's rest cure. Rest cures had a long history in medicine, putting patients to bed in the hopes that they would more or less recover. But in a world awash with neurasthenia, Mitchell's particular rest cure was a brilliant innovation as it involved isolating the patient in a private room, subject completely to the authority of an authoritarian physician (and enforced by Amazonian nurses); a milk diet to fatten up these emaciated women—and they were almost all women—many of whom had been eating poorly; small peripheral doses of electricity to get those exhausted muscles contracting again; and vigorous massage: some claim that by introducing massage into medicine, Mitchell was the founder of physiotherapy.[32] Because the rest cure demanded private rooms, special nurses, electrical apparatus, and other equipment, it could be most easily performed on in-patients, and the number of physicians willing to raise the capital for exclusive private clinics catering to wealthy female neurasthenics was very large. Of course these private clinics treated nervous and mental diseases other than neurasthenia, but it was a flagship diagnosis, and in their advertising to the medical profession, the owners featured it prominently, along with the availability of the "milk diet," as the Mitchell cure was often called in Europe, among other physical and dietetic treatments.

The private clinics that conducted rest cures were legion, but to give a concrete sense let's look at Anton Frey's "Sanatorium Frey-Gilbert" in Baden-Baden, Germany, an exclusive watering-place noted for its casino—one that exists even today, along with the famous Brenner's Park Hotel—and for Baden-Baden's numerous private clinics located near the warm springs. (It was to these springs that the town owed its rise to fame, in contrast to the cold springs that previously had ridden the hydrotherapy crest elsewhere; Baden-Baden physicians claimed to treat nervous disease in particular.) At the Frey-Gilbert sanatorium, nervous diseases were the first order of clinical indications for admission, and included "neuralgia, neurasthenia, hysteria, hypochondria, and insomnia." Therapeutically, the clinic specialized in dietary cures, especially the "milk cure—Mitchell, Playfair."[33] (Named after William S. Playfair, the London gynecologist who introduced the Mitchell rest cure to England in 1881.)

In the United States, neurasthenic patients had an array of choices, including Weir Mitchell's own private clinic in Philadelphia. Yet there were private nervous clinics in many places; in Des Moines, Iowa, neurasthenics were received at "The Retreat: A Private Hospital for Nervous and Mental Cases." Led by Gershom Hill, then 67 years old and a graduate in 1886 of Rush Medical College in Chicago, the Retreat billed itself as "a large, quiet home, for neurasthenic and mild mental cases." Its treatments included "rest."[34] The "Oconomowoc Health Resort for Nervous and Mental Diseases" in a town by the same name in Wisconsin, "three hours from Chicago" by rail, possessed an imposing building, newly built in 1913, and equipped "to supply the demand of the neurasthenic, borderline [psychotic] and undisturbed mental cases."[35] These private clinics were substantial affairs, and neurasthenia was a diagnosis one could take to the bank.

In these private sanatoriums for "nervous and mental disease," neurasthenia was definitely a nervous condition, not a form of madness. It was psychiatrists who treated "mental disease," meaning patients who were psychotic, melancholic, or demented. Psychiatry entailed insanity; nervous disease represented a physical condition of the nerves of the body, those exhausted nerve centers, as Beard put it, that just needed some phosphorus.

As neurasthenia sat on the cusp between internal medicine and psychiatry, who should march into the office of one of the London west end's neurasthenia specialists, Frederick Parkes Weber on fashionable Harley Street, on June 29, 1907, but the Reverend X, age 50. Parkes Weber was the son of Sir

Hermann Weber, who had emigrated earlier from Germany to England and specialized in spa referrals. Frederick was similarly a spa consultant, and his wealthy patients often spent the summer season traipsing from one continental hot spring to another. For the Reverend's "neurasthenic condition (irritable weakness)" Parkes Weber thought it right to send him initially to the English watering-places Buxton and Harrowgate.

But fate took a different turn. There was news from Parkes Weber's father, Sir Hermann: In January 1908, while stopping at the Grand Hotel in the French spa of Grasse, Reverend X had a "nervous breakdown" and in a private clinic on the French Mediterranean coast was administered the Weir Mitchell "cure"; in his notes, a skeptical Parkes Weber put "cure" in quotation marks.

Sufficiently restored to travel to America, Reverend X returned from his travels in October 1908 and came to see Parkes Weber. Apparently America had not gone well, and the Reverend "spent part of the time in bed." He was now gripped with somatic complaints. Noted Parkes Weber in the Reverend's chart: "Mr X is an example of the 'neurasthenic' or 'asthenic' constitution (probably with a certain amount of gastroptosis etc [a supposed sinking of the stomach in the abdomen] and some 'American neurasthenia' superadded."

Reverend X drifted from spa to spa, taking a "quack remedy" called "Antineurasthin," and experiencing at the German watering-place Bad Nauheim a "nerve storm." Things went decidedly better after Reverend X tried what Parkes Weber referred to as "some new sedative," but that was, in fact, one of the powerful new barbiturates, Medinal (barbital), that had recently been introduced in England. Yet sedation is not a cure, and the Reverend X, over an illness trajectory that lasted yet a decade, continued to suffer "feelings of nervous exhaustion" and other flutterings.[36] Parkes Weber, a kind man and generous with his patients, did not see medicine as a business but as a science, and several eponyms are associated with his name (for example, Rendu Weber Osler disease, or hereditary hemorrhagic telangiectasia). He certainly did not regard himself as a psychiatrist, nor did he use psychiatric lingo in his chart notes.

Yet contributing to the ultimate decline of the diagnosis of neurasthenia was its increasing association with psychiatry. As London psychiatrist and medical historian Simon Wessely points out in his overview of the history of neurasthenia, the disorder went out of style as a diagnosis because it lost its organicity, and became transferred from "central nervous" models to psychological models.[37] Neurasthenia occupied an increasingly prominent place in psychiatry textbooks. This was a literature written by psychiatrists, not neurologists or electrotherapists. Maurice Dide and Paul Guiraud were both clinicians at the Braqueville mental hospital in Toulouse. Their guide to psychiatry for the family doctor, published in 1922, makes neurasthenia sound very close to depression, with its psychomotor slowing and its sensations of "ennui." "This volitional distaste for acting and reacting is well translated by the English word *spleen*," they noted. "Although the neurasthenic is often dismissed as a 'malade imaginaire,' it would not be accurate to reduce this syndrome to the exaggeration of a thousand small psychological miseries which, normally, pass unperceived. His suffering is real and involves a state of nosophobic preoccupation [fear of disease] that is continually reactivated."[38] This does not sound like "exhausted nervous centers."

Simultaneously with its englobement by psychiatry, neurasthenia began to leach out of family medicine. In 1921, Tom Williams, a District of Columbia neurologist, writing for an audience of family doctors, found neurasthenia a useless term; the patient's symptoms could almost always be attributed to some physiological or psychic cause.[39] The typical family doctor who is dealing with nonorganic illnesses, said German psychiatrist Kurt Schneider in 1933, "calls the male cases neurasthenics, the female cases hysterics; or the doctor calls the patients whom he finds unsympathetic on a human level hysterics, and the people he finds sympathetic and wants to treat as ill, neurasthenics."[40] The term had become effectively deorganicized.

Neurasthenia came to divorce itself from the notion of nervous disease as something encompassing the entire body and started to refer solely to a disturbance of affect, hovering in a disembodied manner in the space of the mind without physical attachment to the rest of the body. Among academic English neurologists at the National Hospital for the Relief and Cure of the Paralysed and Epileptic at Queen Square in London, neurasthenia was assimilated to the "psychoneuroses" by 1932; the term disappeared after 1941.[41]

Outside of psychiatry, progressive figures such as English neurologist Farquhar Buzzard had started to decompose neurasthenia into depression and anxiety. In 1930 Buzzard, who had just become Regius professor of medicine at Oxford (and who as all neurologists in those days saw many psychiatric patients in his private practice), said that " ... out of any 100 patients sent or brought to me suffering from depression, insomnia, loss of concentration, and fatigability, 99 are labeled neurasthenia or neurosis, and perhaps one a possible manic-depressive psychosis. After investigation the proportion is probably fifty-fifty." (The other fifty being not neurasthenia but anxiety neurosis.) He proposed the term "autonomous depression" to describe those patients "in the dump of neurasthenia." The two alternative diagnoses to weigh, said Buzzard, were anxiety neurosis and autonomous depression.[42]

Yet despite the doubting neurologists, in psychiatry, neurasthenia sol-
diered on, possibly because of the sanctity Freud had lent the term in 1898
by calling it one of the "actual neuroses," unlike the "psychoneuroses," actual
meaning caused by current events rather than anomalies in early childhood
development; Freud considered neurasthenia the result of masturbation and
coitus interruptus.[43] (Yet Freud himself took little interest in the diagnosis and
many of his followers pooh-poohed it entirely.[44]) Neurasthenia survives even
today in the international classification of diseases (ICD) of the World Health
Organization, where it is ranked among the "neurotic, stress-related and somatoform disorders" (the WHO distinguishes among a variety caused by mental
effort and another associated with physical weakness, and insists that it be differentiated from asthenia, burn-out, malaise, and psychasthenia, among other
diagnoses.[45] None of these possibly quite valid diagnoses exists in American
psychiatry! It will be interesting to see if these diagnoses escape alignment with
the *DSM* in future editions of the ICD series.). Neurasthenia appeared in the
second edition of the *Diagnostic and Statistical Manual of Mental Disorders*
("DSM") of the American Psychiatric Association, published in 1968, as "neurasthenic neurosis (neurasthenia)"; this *DSM* edition also featured an "asthenic
personality"; neurasthenia vanished from American psychiatry thereafter.[46]

Neurasthenia ebbed in the public discussion as well. It never amounted
to much in the press. The first reference to it in the headlines of the *New
York Times* occurred only in 1898: "Boy Ate a 'Whisky Biscuit': Young Samuel
Guttman Suffers from Neurasthenia for His Experience."[47] The decade before
World War I saw a few more mentions, likewise a few after the war, the last
being in 1935 ("Sir John Collie Dead; Neurasthenia Expert").[48] *The Times* got
much more excited about nervous breakdowns (see Chapter 7).

In international psychiatry, however, neurasthenia has led a robust existence almost to the present as a synonym for minor affective disorder, or minor
depression, in contrast to melancholia, which is very serious depression. We in
the United States do not have the *concept* of minor depression, because all acute
depressions are "major depression." Nor do we have the *term* minor depression—
because the insurance companies will not pay for anything minor. So American
nervous disorders have always tended to be Texas-sized, bigger than what they
are. But at an international level, as stated, neurasthenia cuts still quite a figure.

Nervous Exhaustion

The most severe form of neurasthenia was nervous exhaustion, a synonym
for nervous breakdown; it was several orders of magnitude more severe than

garden-variety neurasthenia, or nervous illness. To qualify for admission to the Homewood Retreat, a private psychiatric hospital in Guelph, Ontario, led by psychiatrists, someone would have to be fairly ill. Cheryl Warsh has tabulated the symptoms of the patients admitted with neurasthenia between 1883 and 1920; of their 687 symptoms, 12.6% of the total were melancholic in nature, the most frequent kind of symptom. Almost 7% displayed delusions. Many others hallucinated. Only 2.9% of the symptoms were "fatigue or weakness."[49] Although the Retreat apparently did not use the term nervous exhaustion, these are the patients who would qualify for it: psychotic, melancholic, and incapable of dealing with the stresses of normal life, in other words, the kind of nervous breakdown called nervous exhaustion.

In understanding the relationship between simple nervous disease and nervous exhaustion, there are two traditions. One was established by Beard himself, who considered nervous exhaustion to be synonymous with neurasthenia. This tradition viewed exhaustion as a familiar physiological state arising from stress and overwork, really the equivalent of neurasthenia. Weir Mitchell deplored the "sexual excess" of the young and saw it as a cause of "nervousness." "I presume that the term nervous exhaustion is as good a label as any," he sniffed in 1877.[50] Investigators such as Angelo Mosso, professor of medical physiology at the University of Turin and author of an influential book on fatigue, fed into this tradition by regarding the subjective sensation of exhaustion ("épuisement," which he also called "la fatigue intellectuelle") as characteristic of any chronic nervous disease: It was omnipresent.[51]

For Emil Kraepelin, the German psychiatrist who initiated the modern system of classifying psychiatric disorders, "nervous exhaustion" (nervöse Erschöpfung) was just a synonym for Beard's neurasthenia. Kraepelin put it among the "psychogenic illnesses," while he assigned manic-depressive illness and dementia praecox—the major diseases—to weightier categories entirely. "The prognosis of simple nervous exhaustion is seen as thoroughly favorable," he wrote in 1915, "in so far as the causative agent is removed," which he mainly considered to be overwork.[52] (By this final edition of his textbook in 1915, Kraepelin viewed nervous exhaustion more benignly than he had earlier, when he classed "chronic nervous exhaustion" among the "exhaustion conditions," alongside "acute dementia" and other nontrivial disorders.[53] Why his own thinking evolved along these lines is unclear, possibly because so many private nervous clinics had sprung up, with good treatment results, that exhaustion symptoms no longer seemed so alarming, or maybe it was that Germany was now in a terrible war, where gravely damaged men were continuously invalided back from the trenches and the problems of the "weary" appeared comparable to those of patients with unruly stomachs.)

But another tradition believed there was really no such thing as simple neurasthenia and that nervous exhaustion was a serious disease of its own, entailing melancholy and psychotic symptoms together with admission to a hospital. These were true nervous breakdowns, although the term was not yet in use. "Clinically," said German psychiatrist Heinrich Averbeck in 1886, the chief physician at a private nervous clinic in Bad Laubbach on the Rhine River, "acute neurasthenia is the collapse of nervous energy, the bankruptcy of the nervous system." This sudden exhaustion might affect the brain, or the spinal cord, the sympathetic nervous system, or the entire central nervous system, but it could be abrupt in onset and overwhelming in impact. He described high officers who felt their minds had become deadened. The stuffing seemed to come out of them: "Acute neurasthenia is seldom fatal, but it imprints upon the patient the stamp of being 'finished,' used up; the patient has become 'old before his time'; not just physically but also morally; these patients become 'broken existences,' 'ruins' of earlier greatness."[54]

This picture of ruin and collapse in acute neurasthenia is quite different from the tense businessmen Beard described. Averbeck's account captures perfectly the image of people's lives coming apart without their being formally "crazy": For this is the essence of the nervous breakdown: Your life, as you knew it, has come to an end because you can no longer cope. Yet you are not "nuts," which is what psychosis means. And today we have only the concept of psychosis to convey this sense of breakdown.

American observers saw in "exhaustion" this sense of things coming apart. Charles Dana, who at 50 years old had just become professor of neurology at Cornell Medical College in New York, thought the essential form of neurasthenia, if one were even to retain the term, was psychotic, not benign. He preferred the term "exhaustion neuroses" for the lesser forms of neurasthenia and did not believe in any form of neurasthenia not caused by the psyche. Then there were "neurasthenic psychoses," such as "the melancholic neurasthenia of later life." If all these major illnesses are cut out, "one has cut out about 50% of neurasthenia. What is left is usually not a general neurasthenic state, but a local disorder. So ... we may yet end in finding that there is no such thing as neurasthenia at all." In this talk to the Boston Society of Psychiatry and Neurology, which in January 1904 he had come up from New York to give, he told his audience that if neurasthenia turns out not to exist, "America has been deleted of one of its most distinctive and precious pathological possessions. If no longer able to claim any disease as specially our own [neurasthenia was often described as "the American disease"], or point with pride to a national and neurasthenical syndrome, there is removed ... an important stimulus to patriotism and racial solidarity!" But he was kidding (or at least I hope he was). The point is that if neurasthenia existed at all, then it was as a psychosis. (He proposed the term "phrenasthenia," that didn't catch on.)[55]

The most influential advocate of neurasthenia as a form of madness, not of nerves, was the Austrian psychiatrist Richard von Krafft-Ebing, who would win international notoriety with his *Psychopathia Sexualis*, published in 1886, an explicit catalogue of every sexual practice that diverged from the missionary position. Yet it was in his psychiatry textbook that Krafft-Ebing influenced the field of psychiatry. The first edition, written in 1872 when Krafft-Ebing was 32 years old, did not even mention neurasthenia. But in the third edition in 1888, he embraced neurasthenia as mainly a form of madness. He conceded the existence of a benign neurasthenic neurosis that usually ended favorably in those blessed with healthy constitutions. But in those born predisposed to illness, neurasthenic "psychoneurosis" was a terrible disorder, leading often to terminal decline and madness. "On August 14, 1882, Herr H, railway station employee, 41, was brought to the Graz University Psychiatric Clinic because on August 12 he had suddenly become insane, considering himself the stationmaster and behaving accordingly." Krafft-Ebing had not yet assumed the professorship of psychiatry in Vienna and was still professor in the provincial city of Graz. "The patient behaves in a confused and irritated manner, and demands to be taken to his office, because he is the chief of the station. He does not belong here. He doesn't know that he is in a hospital, feels perfectly well, and is justifiedly irritated only because the previous station master is unwilling to submit to his authority." We will not follow the further progress of the case, which ends well for the railway employee, except that he loses his post, becomes destitute, alcoholic, and is readmitted. Krafft-Ebing does not use the diagnosis "nervous exhaustion," because for him the term "psychoneurosis," or what was later called simply "psychosis," tells the whole story.[56] Krafft-Ebing's psychiatry textbook had a large international impact, and the last edition, published in 1903 a year after his death, was even more adamant about neurasthenia as a form of madness. So, with Krafft-Ebing the nervous exhaustion approach—or its functional equivalent—was gathering steam.

In the 1920s and after, as nerves and neurasthenia were ground to bits by the diagnoses of anxiety and depression, nervous exhaustion maintained itself, and even increased in prominence. This shows a growing need for a kind of time-out diagnosis that did not indicate madness. In a sense, it sounds much more sympathetic to say, "How could you expect the poor thing to carry on! Her nerves were exhausted," than to say, "How could you expect the poor thing to carry on! She was psychotic." Eduard Hirt, consulting physician for a health insurance fund in Munich, who had a good overview of diagnoses in private practice, said in 1926, "The word neurasthenia has certainly become seldom in medical outpatient practice, but 'chronic nervous exhaustion' has unfortunately become expanded today to mean not just the now abolished neurasthenia but a host of other psychogenic conditions and other syndromes of degeneration."[57] Exhaustion was becoming a fig-leaf, in other words, for other diagnoses that people did not readily wish to admit having and Hirt deplored the consequences for insurance reimbursement. What might some of those conditions be? In Germany in the 1920s, just after the World War I (according to Maximilian Laehr, a veteran asylum psychiatrist in Berlin-Zehlendorf), the conditions being diagnosed as "acute and chronic exhaustion" included posttraumatic neuroses (which would include psychologically disabled veterans), chronic occupational intoxications (lead poisoning and the like), and various addictions—none of which would be gladly discussed in company. The limits of the concept, said Laehr, were psychically abnormal behavior that disturbed others, and disorders that required constant supervision.[58]

The Great Depression seems to have dramatically increased the number of people with nervous exhaustion. So grim were conditions that Adolf Hoppe, a sanatorium doctor in north Germany, said, in language that reminds us of the Great Recession of our own time, that we are no longer talking of the "exhausted" but the "ground down." "Sanatorium treatment used to help the exhausted relax and rebuild. But for those who are ground down, the therapeutic goal can only be to help the convalescent solely to increase his powers of resistance, to hold out and to endure."[59]

Yes indeed: the victims of economic disaster were not crazy, just exhausted, a point made at a meeting of the Clinical Society in London, in April 1931, when Philip Seymour-Price, who had run a high-end practice for almost 30 years at exclusive Sloane Gardens in London, "asked whether it was not possible for nervous exhaustion to be a pure and simple exhaustion of nerve energy, a case of a really tired-out nervous system, which with rest and treatment might get perfectly well. Was it any wonder that the business man of to-day, with things as they were on the Stock Exchange or in the City, or the woman of to-day, with things as they were in domestic service [not being able to hire domestics] became utterly exhausted? These people should be not labeled psychotic or anxiety-neurotic; they were just ordinary people very short of nervous energy."[60]

Nor did the flatness and fatigue of emotional exhaustion spare Americans during the Great Depression. On May 1, 1934 Patrolman Alfred Herbstsomer in Millburn, New Jersey, answered the phone, to hear a man's voice say "casually and unemotionally," "This is Percy Layman. I just shot my wife, Herby, and now I'm going to shoot myself. You'd better come over right away." Within minutes police arrived to find Layman's body on the kitchen floor, his wife scarcely breathing beside him with a fatal wound in her right temple. The cause of such distress? Said the *New York Times*, he had recently been discharged from a sanatorium as cured, Yet "his business ventures since were reported to have met little success."[61] This is so sad. As I write these lines in the summer of 2012, and look about at the massive unemployment in our own society, the anxious home owners whose mortgages are underwater and dread the sheriff's knock, there is a good deal to be said for these sentiments about breakdown and exhaustion, even though they have nothing to do with neurotransmitters.

In any event, long though nervous exhaustion lingered as a synonym for nervous breakdown, it did cede to the advancing tide of depression diagnoses and vanished beneath the waves. By the advent of *DSM-III* in 1980, fatigue had gone out of psychiatry.[62]

5

Anxiety

*Motto: At a meeting of the Psychopharmacologic Drugs Advisory
Committee of the U.S. Food and Drug Administration, November
1980, on what drugs should be prescribed for insomnia:*
JOHN KANE (LONG ISLAND JEWISH HILLSIDE MEDICAL CENTER):
*"Prior to the prescription of sedative hypnotics other conditions
which might be responsible for insomnia, for example, anxiety,
depression, psychosis, should be ruled out."*
DONALD M. GALLANT (TULANE MEDICAL SCHOOL):
*"Well, by ruling out anxiety I think you would rule out the entire
population of this country."*[1]

IN 1970 AUBREY Lewis, the past master of the Maudsley Hospital, England's premier psychiatric facility, was 70 years old. In his long decades of experience, he was puzzled by the rise of anxiety as a popular stand-alone diagnosis. The evolution of the term, he said, had gone through two phases. The first was using anxiety "as a qualifying term for the agitated depression of melancholia." Anxious melancholia meant melancholia out of control. In the second phase, anxiety became "a qualifying term for a neurosis in which subjective feelings of alarm are associated with visceral disturbances." This would be Freud's anxiety neurosis. He noted that the number of articles on anxiety in the scientific literature had increased from three in 1927 to 222 in 1960—and was still rising.[2] As Lewis wrote in 1970, anxiety was about to undergo a third phase in its evolution: Anxiety, or panic, attacks would shortly occupy center stage.

Anxiety, another part of the nervous syndrome, has a distinctive story line: For most of the history of psychiatry, it was considered part of some other disorder, or not really attended to at all. Clinicians paid no particular heed to whether their patients were worried or fearful: These emotions were part of the human condition. Augustin Jacob Landré-Beauvais, professor of clinical medicine at the Salpêtrière Hospice in Paris, in his great catalogue of signs and symptoms written in 1809, takes it for granted that anxiety will be present in infectious illnesses. "Anxiety accompanies the better part of acute illnesses and some chronic illnesses, and is produced by various causes," he said, and considered it an advance warning of an attack among "hypochondriacs, hysterics, and epileptics."[3]

Then throughout the nineteenth century anxiety became part of the nervous package. As the nervous syndrome disaggregated in the early twentieth century, anxiety was spun off to become a free-standing disorder, "anxiety neurosis" in psychoanalytic parlance. More recently, anxiety *tout court* has morphed into panic disorder, and we shall shortly watch panic stride to the center of the stage.

Yet anxiety is rarely found alone. William Sargant, an influential biological psychiatrist at St. Thomas's Hospital in London, said in 1962, "Pure anxiety states are rarely seen in clinical practice because secondary symptoms of hysteria, depression or obsessional thinking generally complicate the picture."[4] (Today, in drug trials, the rule is, as George Beaumont, a clinician with Geigy Pharmaceuticals, said in 1996, that a virgin anxiety patient is "worth his or her weight in gold."[5]) Yet there is such a thing as psychotic anxiety, a quite different disorder, and it is often found alone and not part of a larger syndrome. On the fringes of anxiety are phobias, panic reactions, and even obsessive-compulsive disorder. Trying to draw sharp boundaries among these neighboring conditions is like trying to draw lines in a bucket of water.

But our purpose here is not clinical. It is to see how common illnesses such as nerves lose their credibility and dissolve into other syndromes that are, at the end of the day, less credible. Anxiety disappears from the nervous package by taking on an independent existence.

Anxiety

Anxiety means various things. Anxiety can be a clinical *syndrome*, a combination of symptoms that anxious patients often display, such as mental worry, plus a sinking in "the pit of the stomach," plus diarrhea. It is a ubiquitous *emotion*, synonymous with apprehension, and familiar in normal behavioral states. In post-World War II American psychiatry anxiety was considered a "*neurosis*," a vague term for any behavioral disorder that was not psychotic. And in the world of psychoanalysis, anxiety was deemed "the chief characteristic of the neuroses,"[6] meaning that it was a supposed intrapsychic *mechanism* for dealing with conflict. Otto Fenichel, one of the main interpreters of Freud's doctrines for the American public, wrote in 1945 of "anxiety hysteria": "A part of the dammed-up energy [in neurotic conflict] is discharged, but in such a way as to intensify the defense against the rest. The typical neurotic symptom expresses drive and defense simultaneously."[7] Thus in the United States in the middle of the twentieth century, anxiety was absolutely center stage.

Yet not all believed the psychoanalytic version. One day, in a discussion of anxiety with Robert Spitzer (the architect of "*DSM-III*"), New York psychiatrist Max Fink said, "It's complicated for me, because I don't define anxiety very easily. Anxiety is a poorly-described term. There is the overt anxiety where a person is tremulous, sweating, tachycardia, fearful, etc. There is the precipitated anxiety by lactate, where you get an acute syndrome [lactate can precipitate a panic attack]. There is the stage fright which you call anxiety. In many depressed people, they are frightened and they're nervous, and we say they're anxious and depressed."[8] Clearly, for biologically oriented psychiatrists such as Fink, anxiety was not so central.

Indeed, anxiety was so vague as often to be useless as a drug target. Pioneering psychopharmacologist Fritz Freyhan of the University of Pennsylvania told the First International Congress of Neuropharmacology in Rome in 1958, "I have come to suspect that anxiety, whatever its manifestations, is now treated with tranquilizing drugs just as fever, regardless of cause, has been treated with antibiotics. Anxiety is as vague a therapeutic target as is body temperature."[9] So anxiety is in some ways like a handful of smoke; in other ways it is a very solid and overpowering disorder.

Anxiety may either be considered a disease in its own right, which is this book's take on psychotic anxiety (see the section below on Juan Lopez-Ibor), or as one symptom among many in larger disease entities; in the psychiatric illnesses, anxiety is quite common, and we see garden-variety anxiety as part of the larger package of nervous illness that includes depressed mood, fatigue, obsessive thinking, and various somatic symptoms of a nonorganic nature.

Others too see anxiety as just one symptom among many, rather than as a separate disease. In 1985 a team from Yale University called efforts to "distinguish anxiety disorders as separate diagnostic entities" problematic, "because the subjective features of anxiety are often difficult to describe uniformly, anxiety is a ubiquitous emotion in normal behavioral states, and symptoms of anxiety are common in most psychiatric syndromes."[10] So a few clinicians still adhere to the former view that anxiety is not a distinctive disease such as mumps. Yet there are not many such observers because the pharmaceutical industry has marketed anxiety so relentlessly as a separate disease. The official view in the diagnostic manual of the American Psychiatric Association, currently in its fourth edition (*DSM-IV*, 1994), is that anxiety is a stand-alone disease, quite separate from depression. (And as I write now, it looks as though this state of affairs will persist in *DSM-5*.)

One more thing. Anxiety may or may not include tension. There are anxious patients who are not tense, but few tense ones who are not anxious. Veteran psychopharmacologist Tom Ban remembered from his days of training in Budapest in the early 1950s, before he decamped for Canada in the Hungarian Revolution of 1956, "The Hungarians qualified anxiety by saying whether it's tense or not. It was a subclass of anxiety."[11] Said New York family doctor Harry Friedlander in 1953, reporting on clinical trials of a new drug, mephenesin, the first of the anxiolytics, in combination with a barbiturate: Something was needed other than the plain barbiturates to "cope with the tremendous increase in recent years of what we have come to call anxiety tension."[12] And the combo did seem to release patients from the grips of tension. (Or at least it was the barbiturate that did so[13]; mephenesin soon vanished, replaced by its more powerful cousin meprobamate—Miltown.)

Tension thus rings down over the years in the patients' charts and the pharmaceutical ads. In 1953, Ciba Pharmaceutical Products (now Novartis) launched the drug reserpine (Serpasil) for "anxiety, tension, nervousness and mild to severe neuroses" as well as for hypertension.[14] By 1958 Merck Sharp & Dohme was marketing the drug benactyzine (Suavitil) for "tension, mild depression, anxiety, fears."[15] Tension made sense to many patients and their physicians for decades as part of a larger group of troubles, before vanishing from the language of psychiatry. *DSM-IV* makes no use of tension as a diagnostic concept, save for glancing references to "muscle tension."[16] (In the draft *DSM-5* "tension" appears occasionally in the disorder descriptions alongside "anxiety," yet is not an independent diagnosis.)

So official diagnostic concepts are of little help. Worry, tension, somatic anxiety, psychic anxiety: all are jumbled together. Rather than insisting on precise definitions let us see if we can figure out what ordinary people usually had in past times, and today.

Among the nervous patients in Frederick Parkes Weber's west end London practice was Frau X, 38 years old when he saw her in 1922; she had a long history of divorce and personal disruption behind her as, for family reasons, she navigated between Germany and England. Parkes Weber suspects hyperthyroidism to be the cause of her nervous problems, including paroxystic accelerations of her heart rate. Also, she has trouble swallowing. We pick her up again in April 1927, when "during her last (short) Easter holiday she had again her troublesome vegetative nervous system attacks—in these attacks she becomes altogether a prey to cramps of the stomach or oesophagus, cardiac palpitation, paroxysmal, angiospastic conditions [contraction of blood vessels], with pallor of the upper and lower limbs." She is relieved by "high frequency electrical current."

At mid-life Frau X resolves to undertake a new career in one of the professions, and the studying and examinations are hugely stressful for her. She continues to have "nervous attacks" with cardiac and circulatory symptoms "necessitating day and night nurses." (Almost all Parkes Weber's patients were from a social stratum that could afford such attention.) She begins taking the barbiturate Luminal (phenobarbital).

In December 1927 she was admitted to a German nervous clinic in Degerloch near Stuttgart in "a complete nervous collapse with a continuation of her obsessive and anxious states," as her German doctor told Parkes Weber. "She is fearful of every terrible event imaginable, that she could become mentally ill or have a stroke or a heart attack and become completely incapable of working. She has continuous attacks of convulsive swallowing and she struggles for air." Parkes Weber added in his note next to the letter of this German physician, "I think this is a kind of nervous visceral (spastic) tic." The German doctor's letter resumes: "She also suffers from complete insomnia and loss of appetite and the general consequential weakness. Recently, she has been unable to arise from bed, the more so because she suffers from highly copious menstrual bleeding, and she is not able to write you yourself." The German physician predicted, however, a complete recovery, which in fact took place.

By October 1928 she is back in the large German city where she lived, "depressed." Parkes Weber reflects about her case in his notes: "She was certainly born with an excitable and easily upset vegetative [autonomic] nervous system ... easily influenced by excitement and emotions of all kinds. (Even after her marriage she could hardly sleep in a room by herself without a light; she was, I believe, fearsome in other respects, and her daughter [name omitted] has an abnormal dread of dogs; abnormal fear of cows is present in the female members of the family.)" Parkes Weber has now abandoned the idea that Frau X ever had hyperthyroidism, save perhaps symptoms from taking too many thyroid tablets. She was depressed, anxious, spent long periods in bed, had a riot of somatic symptoms, and obsessed about fate and death. In Parkes Weber's eyes, the emphasis was on her anxiety, but in fact she seems to have been a typical nervous patient. The case shows well how "mental" symptoms such as anxiety and depression in fact represent illnesses of the whole body.[17]

The History of Anxiety in the Nervous Syndrome

Anxiety and anguish, sturdy terms, have always been part of patients' everyday language. Gerolamo Cardano, a Renaissance mathematician and physician with a long history of physical woes, said in his autobiography in 1575 that "I have discovered by experience, that I cannot be long without bodily pain, for if once that circumstance arises, a certain mental anguish overcomes me, so grievous that nothing could be more distressing."[18] Anxiety and anguish are among the most basic of emotions, and of course people have always had words for expressing them.

Similarly, the term anxiety has been part of the descriptive vocabulary of medicine since time out of mind. In 1602 Basel's municipal physician, Felix Platter, whose *Observations* contained numerous psychiatric cases, described a melancholic patient "who complained about ever more severe mental anxiety [Seelenangst] and became so agitated that she ... ran back and forth from room to room."[19]

To be sure, anxious behavior has not always been called anxiety. Vincenzo Chiarugi of Florence, whose concept of the therapeutic asylum was spelled out in his three-volume textbook in 1793–1794, counts as one of the early pioneers of psychiatric diagnosis and treatment. In this work he lays out the various stages through which melancholia progresses: "We shall call true melancholia all that which is accompanied by sadness and fear [timore]."[20] Strictly speaking, fear is not exactly anxiety, because the latter is often said to lack a specific object. Yet the word anxiety was not yet current in the Italian medical vocabulary, and from the case reports in Chiarugi's study, anxiety is meant as well as concrete fears of given things. Philippe Pinel, another founding figure in psychiatry, chief of the Salpêtrière hospice in Paris, described in his large classification of diseases in general, published in 1798, melancholic illness as figuring among the "neuroses." He wrote of the "causes" of melancholia: "sadness, bitter disappointments, fear, office work, tiredness of life ... an imagination that infinitely multiplies and exaggerates the misfortunes of life ... " As for the symptoms of melancholia, Pinel wrote, "The sleep is agitated and troubled by terrifying objects and lugubrious images; the patient is constantly tormented by singular ideas."[21] Again, this is anxiety in so many words.

During the nineteenth century psychiatrists made great progress in describing individual symptoms, which is the science of psychopathology, and in sorting symptoms into various diseases, which is the science of nosology. Both of these sciences of exact description focus ever more on anxiety as a symptom, not as a disease of its own. John Haslam, the apothecary of Bethlem Hospital, a famous asylum in London, was not a great innovator in describing symptoms, but in an account of his cases in 1809, he does attribute "anxiety" to several of them, such as the 36-year-old woman who in a postpartum depression killed her baby, then "became more thoughtful and frequently spoke about the child; great anxiety and restlessness succeeded."[22] By contrast, a major innovator in the exact description of disease was the Leipzig asylum psychiatrist Christian August Heinroth, who in his 1818 textbook uses the term anxiety (die Angst) as a symptom, not just a state of mind. In an account of "mixed forms of mood disorders," he said of the march of symptoms, "Anxiety and melancholy [Angst und Schwermuth] increase from hour to hour; no consolation, no kindly words help; the patient is mute and deaf to all intervention, to all urging ... "[23] This is, to my knowledge, the first time that anxiety was used in a clinical sense in German psychiatry.

By mid-nineteenth century, anxiety had become well-established as a symptom of psychiatric diseases of various kinds. One footnote: In retrospect it is tempting to see the 1844 book of Danish philosopher Soeren Kirkegaard, *The Concept of Anxiety*, as an important milestone in this forward progression. It is not. Kirkegaard was writing of the existential anxiety that many Christians felt when confronted with the prospect of choosing their own eternal salvation. His book was entitled in Danish *Begrebet Angest*, translated in the German edition as *Der Begriff Angst*, or *The Concept of Anxiety*. Yet Kirkegaard's book appeared in German only in 1923, in French in 1935, and in English in 1944 as *The Concept of Dread*. Only the Princeton translation in 1981 used the term anxiety in the title.[24] Although of great importance to subsequent philosophical discussion, Kirkegaard's book had almost no impact on medicine during the nineteenth century.

In the second half of the nineteenth century, as psychiatric historian German Berrios points out, French writers began a distinguished tradition of refined symptom description.[25] Joseph Guislain, professor of psychiatry in Ghent, Belgium, and 55 years old at the time of publication of his important psychiatry textbook in 1852, for which he chose the unfortunately idiosyncratic title *Phrenopathies*, linked anxiety firmly to depression. "There is a whole series of melancholias in which the patient is dominated by vague worries. He feels ominous premonitions. He doesn't feel well in any sense; terrible misfortune seems to threaten him; he's fearful of everything, afraid of everything." This clearly detached anxiety from specific worries and gave it an unanchored, inchoately menacing sense.

Guislain also distinguished between anxiety and anguish. "In the melancholia that is characterized by fears, the patients experience feelings of anguish. They are either profoundly dejected or else unable to remain still for a minute." So that was anguish: fearfulness in the context of what is called psychomotor change, speeding up or slowing down. By contrast, "anxiety" for Guislain meant strange somatic feelings: "It is the melancholy that I call anxious, or pneumomelancholy, with respect to trouble that reigns in the organs of the chest ... Anxious melancholy is sometimes preceded by a painful feeling that the patient experiences in the region of the heart."[26] (Later, these meanings would be reversed, anguish meaning somatic sensations and anxiety being the mental perception.)

But it is the Germans who, in the second half of the century, come to dominate the understanding of anxiety, and this German supremacy begins with Wilhelm Griesinger, professor of psychiatry in Berlin when in 1861 he published the influential revised edition of his textbook, *Die Pathologie und Therapie der psychischen Krankheiten* (*The Pathology and Treatment of the Psychiatric Diseases*).[27] He described the "unsettling" feelings (Beängstigung) "which often emanate from the epigastrium and region of the heart, and appear to rise upwards. 'Here,' say many of these patients, and point to the pit of the stomach, 'Here something is sitting like a stone. If I could only get rid of it!' These feelings of anxiety increase then to an intolerable condition, a desperation that often passes over into mania."[28] There were not a lot of new concepts in Griesinger's text, but it did become the leading German language reference book, and therewith the premier psychiatric textbook of the world.

Emil Kraepelin, the great German clinician and nosologist, wrote the final chapter in the German anxiety story just before World War I. For Kraepelin, there was no question of anxiety being an independent disease, or even an important symptom that required its own extensive description. He said it was omnipresent in psychiatric illness, especially in "the depressive conditions of circular insanity." (By circular insanity he meant manic-depressive illness.) Anxiety, he said, often lacked a specific object, and represented a "union of dysphoria with inner tension." This was quite an authoritative statement. Yet in Germany, Freud's psychoanalysis was already shaking the ground under Kraepelin, and after World War I these thoughts about anxiety as one symptom among many, "the commonest of the pathological changes of mood," would be forgotten.[29]

The English in these years rather limped along behind the German heavyweights. To be sure, the concept of anxiety as part of some larger nervous disease gained ground in England, as elsewhere, and in 1866 William Murray, who lectured on physiology at the College of Medicine in Newcastle-on-Tyne, offered one of the speculative theories about neurophysiology that abounded in the late nineteenth century: The seat of "emotional diseases" must lie in the "defective nutrition of the nervous centres, irregular distribution of the blood inducing paresis through the capillaries of the brain," and so forth, all highly reminiscent of Beard's theory of neurasthenia. Yet Murray focused not on fatigue but anxiety: "Foolish fears are no longer dismissed by sober sense, the risings of morbid feelings are no longer controlled by the will ... and thus the way is open for the rushing in of vain imaginations, groundless fears, or absurd suspicions ... The man is not insane ... but he is the victim of emotional disease, which, while not causing him to be haunted by positive delusions [madness], leads him irresistibly to view the dark side of everything, to entertain the most distressing fears where none ought to exist, till life is made gloomy, morbid, miserable."[30]

Murray and his ratiocinations about "the cerebrospinal system" passed unheralded from the scene. Yet neither his nor anyone else's writings about anxiety made any difference in clinical practice in England. Even though anxiety was accepted as part of some larger package—call it "emotional disease" if one will—these academic musings made little difference in the actual practice of psychiatry. And this is known because the patient records of a semicharitable private psychiatric hospital, the Holloway Sanatorium in Virginia Water, just to the west of London, have survived for the late 1880s and early 1890s. We can see what the clinicians are thinking in their daily practice. At the Holloway Sanatorium, the physicians were astute clinical observers, but on the open service at least (for voluntary boarders), they were often reluctant to make diagnoses. They simply described what they saw. In August 1895 Arthur W, a middle-aged man, was admitted. He "has a restless, anxious, careworn expression." Mentally, the patient "cannot settle down to anything, is inclined to worry in an undue way over trifles and is in a vague state of dissatisfaction with himself. Does not know what to do, keeps asking for advice, and then wandering away in the course of conversation from the subject matter in hand. Sleeps badly." Clearly, there was some larger problem with Arthur W. His physicians noted his anxiety together with other symptoms that sounded like a larger nervous syndrome. And indeed there was some larger problem: 8 months after admission he was certified and sent to the closed service for patients with major illnesses.[31]

On the women's service on the closed side, Rosetta X, 19 years old, came in on April 16, 1889. The admission medical certificates—two were required—claimed that she was psychotic and heard God telling her to do various things, but at admission this "healthy looking, well-developed girl, with freckled face, moist skin, auburn hair and blue eyes ... appears to be of an extremely nervous disposition. She will not look in your face when shaking hands or answering questions. She is incessantly moving her hands, fingers or head ... Mentally she appears to be suffering from the 'impulsive insanity of adolescence,' intermingled with 'hysteria.'" On the unit she kept to herself, "answers only in monosyllables when questioned without raising her head, and silently does the needlework put into her hands." She was discharged "recovered" almost a year after admission.[32] Here again, her anxiety leaps to the eyes. Yet for her clinicians it had no particular significance. She had a "nervous" disposition.

This was the picture of the nerve syndrome on the ground: anxiety blended in with the other components of depression, fatigue, compulsive thoughts (Rosetta, as she told her mother in letters, obsessed about the food on the unit), and somatic symptoms to form a pattern that was easily recognizable without any particular component standing out. Once we encounter the rise of the affective disorders, this will change.

The Beginnings of Panic

Panic would rank high in a list of disorders composing the nervous breakdown. Panic patients may be immobilized with fright, and may become withdrawn recluses in their efforts to avoid further panics. It is a true breakdown.

The concept of panic disorder is not new. Eighteenth-century English novelist Fanny Burney (Frances D'Arblay) had panic attacks, and she uses that term . In August 1778, at 25 years old, she was a guest at the Thrales, a noted literary couple, and heard one of the company, not knowing she was the author, make an unflattering remark about the novel *Evelina* that she had just published anonymously. "My heart beat so quick against my stays, that I almost panted with extreme agitation at the dread either of hearing some cruel criticism or of being betrayed, and I munched my biscuit as if I had not eaten for a fortnight." Indeed, her mouth was so dry that she was unable to swallow, and had to ask Mrs. Thrale for water, imploring her in private not to identify her, Fanny, as the author. That night at the Thrales passed in disquiet. "When Mrs Thrale came to me the next morning, she was quite concerned to find I had really suffered from my panics. 'O Miss Burney, cried she, what shall we do with you? This must be conquered ... '"[33] Fanny Burney was a nervous creature, and in May 1792 she confided to her diary about her unease in the company of strangers: " ... The panics I have felt upon entering to any strange company, or large party even of intimates, has, at times, been a suffering unspeakably, almost incredibly severe to me."[34] For this Englishwoman panic was a real entity.

Psychiatry was somewhat slower to discover panic. We are about to watch anxiety states sailing off on their own in the form of panic disorder, phobias, and even obsessive thoughts and compulsive actions. It is a bit of a perilous voyage, and where one cuts Nature at the joints not always clear.

A core symptom of the nervous breakdown, as people generally conceived it, was becoming panicky in public. Panic in open places has long been recognized in medicine. The old spa doctors realized that many of their patients were highly anxious and that the warm spa waters could calm them. In 1844 Anton Theobald Brück, the spa doctor in tiny Bad Driburg, in a memoire praising the waters, said there were all kinds of dizziness (Schwindel), and that dizziness in open spaces represented an ideal indication for the waters of Bad Driburg: One of their patients, a priest, "perceived the most profound anxious dizziness (Schwindelangst), just as soon as he was no longer safe at home. He needed a solid floor underneath him, just as others require this kind of solidity, in order to avoid dizziness. If he had to cross a field, where the wide heavens stood open above his head, he would be gripped by unspeakable anxiety, and creep about on detours, under hedges and trees, and even, if all else failed, open up his umbrella." This would later be seen as a panic attack, but Brück did not assign the syndrome, associated with pounding hearts and other forms of somatic anxiety, a particular name.[35]

A very preliminary step toward panic as an independent diagnosis was the concept of "precordial anxiety," proposed in 1848 by Carl Friedrich Flemming, director of the Sachsenberg asylum in North Germany. "Often when we examine a person with insanity," said Flemming, "he complains of a feeling of anxiety that has its seat in the breast and upper abdomen, and is connected with the sensation of internal heat and the feeling that a rock is pressing in on him or an iron band is tightening about his body." The anxiety struck paroxystically. "In more severe cases, the patient feels the need for frequent deep breaths, so that it seems like a real gasping for air." There were spasmodic changes in the pulse and slowing of the heart rate alternating with acceleration. The feelings of anxiety often followed the somatic sensations. An obsessive-compulsive element was strong: "The patients say they are anxious because they cannot fend off terrible thoughts, and because sad things, ugly words and immoral acts occur to them of which they cannot free themselves and they feel compelled to tell others." Flemming described a woman plagued by anxiety who believed herself guilty of the death of her child from measles. She recovered, then 4 years later "had to endure bravely the unexpected death of her husband and the deterioration of her material circumstances ... Two years after the death of her husband she was obliged by her employer [she was working as a live-in servant] to sell the clothes, previously kept under lock and key, of her late husband. She got to work cleaning them. The sight of these clothes made such a strong impression on her, that a nameless anxiety befell her, which in the course of several hours had so intensified that people were obliged to protect her from herself."[36] This is nervous-breakdown-level panic, on the basis of chronic anxiety and melancholia.

Here is Frau M, 23 years old, in a Viennese private nervous clinic around 1890: At age 16, just married, she had a spontaneous abortion, with significant blood loss. As her clinician Hanns Kaan, tells her history, "From then on she became insomniac and anxious; for example she had to arise at night and check whether she had truly extinguished a match she had lit earlier. When she fought against this impulse, she was overcome by a nervous crisis, with heart palpitations [Herzbeklemmung], shortness of breath, and anxious sweating (precordial anxiety)."[37] Frau M, young and nervous, was clearly having panic attacks.

Using the term "mood-depression" (Gemüths-Depression), in 1859 Flemming described somatic anxiety as a traveling companion of melancholia. As the illness advances, "The feeling of oppression and anxiousness, which had accompanied the entire symptom train, now mounts to a powerful, nameless anxiety, the seat of which the patient localizes in the cardiac area, the upper abdomen, the lower chest, or under the sternum." The patient describes the feeling "as though he had a stone lying upon his heart, an iron wheel compressing his chest, a rope that is squeezing his body together." Patients consistently used these images, said Flemming.[38]

Free-Standing Anxiety

A key development in the story is removing anxiety from the nervous syndrome and seeing it, at least in its spasmodic forms, as a free-standing illness. Severe forms of anxiety were regarded as part of the nervous breakdown by the laity. It is therefore interesting to watch anxiety emerge from the soup of melancholia, at an epoch when melancholia meant severe illness of various kinds.

The first big step in liberating anxiety from melancholia was taken in 1866 by Jules Falret, son of Jean-Pierre Falret (who in 1851 had been the first to offer a careful description of bipolar disorder). Jules Falret said there was a form of rational insanity that he, with a clunky touch, proposed to call "partial insanity with predominance of the fear of contacting external objects." Noting that his father had proposed the term "fearfulness disorder" (maladie du doute) for it, Falret junior offered a close clinical account: "The true core of this disorder consists above all in a general disposition of the mind to ceaselessly return to the same ideas or the same acts, feeling the continuous need to repeat the same words to accomplish the same actions, without ever succeeding in satisfying the need or being convinced, even by evidence." This was a partial insanity: "These patients are perfectly aware of their state [of illness]; they recognized the absurdity of their fears and seek to extract themselves, but they don't succeed in this and are, despite themselves, obliged to return to the same ideas and to accomplish the same acts." "It takes them quite a while to put on their makeup, to decide to come to the table, and they even fear bringing the food to their mouths. They are afraid to take walks, in the fear of sullying their feet with the ground; they shun the company of other people to avoid shaking hands ... " Although previous authors, such as Falret senior, had alluded to the existence of obsessive thinking and compulsive actions, Falret junior assembled the entire package (and has received from historians almost no credit for this because he chose such an opaque designation). Falret junior said that the disorder erupted in paroxysms: "It is remarkable, in fact, that this mental state, which may extend itself for one's entire life with the irregular alternation of paroxysms and sometimes very pronounced remissions, never ends in true dementia."[39]

Another classical account stems in 1866 from the pen of Bénédict-Augustin Morel, chief of the mental hospital at Saint-Yon near Rouen. He described what he called "emotional psychosis" (délire émotif), a picture of excess emotivity in combination with chronic somatic symptoms of anxiety, and obsessive-compulsive symptoms such as fear of touching things; Morel, who introduced with great certitude the concept of "degeneration" into psychiatry in 1857, was just as confident about the causes of this new "délire": it emerged from the autonomic nervous plexuses of the abdomen; the diagnosis did not catch on.[40]

Wilhelm Griesinger, professor of psychiatry in Berlin, read Falret's piece and reflected about some of his own patients. In March 1868 Griesinger described to the local Society for Medical Psychology in Berlin a remarkable syndrome that he had never previously encountered, certainly not in the asylum patients that were the meat and drink of Berlin psychiatry, but not often in outpatients either: They were unable to keep themselves from asking silly questions in an obsessive and uncontrollable manner, even though they knew the questions—such as "why are there not two suns and two moons"?—were ridiculous. The behavior was definitely not part, he said, of "the customary depressive sensations of anxiety." Two of the patients Griesinger had seen only briefly; a third, a young man of 21, he had gotten to know better. Griesinger also mentioned the latter patient's susceptibility to paroxystic symptoms of somatic anxiety: "His sleep is troubled; the patient often has a 'headache in his nerves,' as he puts it, 'from the continuous thinking and rumination.' Now and then he feels his heart pounding.... Frequently a slight tremor of his facial muscles is apparent, more evident in his hands; not infrequently he has the sensation that his entire body is vibrating." Griesinger believed the patient was making his symptoms worse with continuous masturbation, and adopted the patient's own term, "Grübeln," or obsessive rumination, as a name for the new syndrome.[41] After Falret, this constitutes one of the earliest mentions of paroxystic anxiety as a symptom independent of melancholia or depression with somatic as well as mental symptoms.

There now emerged a series of reports on what was probably somatic anxiety. In 1871 Jacob DaCosta, a Philadelphia internist who had served as an army doctor during the Civil War, described "irritable heart," a condition he had seen in many soldiers accompanied by "dizziness and palpitation, with pain in the chest." The symptoms oppress the sufferers, who perceived cardiac "palpitations," and fear they are about to die. The troops develop other symptoms as well, such as aphonia, "inordinate sweating," and "dimness of vision and giddiness." "Pain was an almost constant symptom, I cannot recall a single well-marked instance of the complaint in which it was wholly absent ... It was generally described as occurring in paroxysms, and as sharp and lancinating." The pulse was accelerated and the patients were short of breath. DaCosta believed that the action of the heart in these otherwise healthy young men was actually disordered, the organ enlarged. (He had no x-rays to verify his physical examination, and could only percuss the heart to determine its size.) DaCosta, bent upon demonstrating organicity and not hysteria in the troops, does not comment upon their mental states, but some sound anxious: Some had "smothering sensations."[42] (English cardiologist Thomas Lewis, who served as an army doctor in World War I, revisited in 1918 the subject of what he was now calling "soldier's heart" and "the effort syndrome"; he implicated "neurasthenia," and said, "A large proportion of the men are of highly-strung nervous temperament, an unusual number are sensitive or querulous, others are apathetic or depressed."[43] Therewith, irritable heart was on its way out.)

As we saw above, it was actually Brück who was among the first to describe a panicky fear of open spaces. But he did not name it, and he who names a phenomenon owns it. In 1872 Carl Westphal, 39 years old, associate professor of psychiatry in Berlin, described panicky responses to open spaces under the term "agoraphobia," linking anxiety specifically to the sudden onset of physical symptoms. Westphal's first patient, a traveling salesman of 32, was incapable of "traversing public squares. A feeling of anxiety overcomes him immediately as he tries it." Westphal said the seat of the anxiety was more "in the head than in the cardiac region." It was easier for him to navigate open spaces in company with someone else, so in the evening, to find his way home, he might chat up a prostitute for part of the way, then strike up a conversation with another to continue on, "gradually reaching his home." He also reported a strong tremor in his hands during these "anxiety attacks" (Angstzufälle).

Westphal's next patient, a young man of 24, also had "powerful feelings of anxiety" when attempting to cross public squares that caused "an ascending feeling of warmth beginning in his lower abdomen accompanied by cardiac palpitations." The patient also reported "generalized tremor." Neither patient had a mood disorder. Westphal discounted earlier reports that fear of open spaces was linked to dizziness, and called it a phenomenon of anxiety. He concluded that "In the preceding observations, I have called attention to a psychic symptom that is, in essence, a previously unknown general neurosis."[44] Westphal's patients were otherwise not nervous. This was a big milestone in detaching anxiety—or at least the episodic form—from nervous illness and assigning it to the nervous breakdown.

Five years later, in 1877, Westphal, by now a professor of psychiatry in Berlin, made it clear that he was separating the new disease of "fear of public places" from traditional "nervous illness."[45] Animated by the criticisms of nationalistic colleagues that "agoraphobia" was too Latinate and that a solid teutonic expression was preferred, he now called the disorder Platzfurcht, fear of public squares; there was some back and forth between defenders of Brück, who thought *fear* of fainting in open places and other settings the essential, and Westphal, who found fear of *open spaces* themselves the essential.[46]

In 1877 Westphal also established as a general disease category, "obsessive-compulsive disorder," in which he no longer considered anxiety the primary disturbance but a consequence of the illness. Westphal's change of heart led to later views that "obsessive-compulsive disorder" (OCD) was not really an anxiety disorder at all, a view quite incompatible with the historical record.[47] (In a rare reversion to tradition among the disease-designers, in *DSM-IV*, OCD ranks among the anxiety disorders.)

There is such a thing as anxiety without panic, and it, too, can occur in a paroxysmal rather than a continuous chronic form. English psychiatrist Henry Maudsley at the West London Hospital, who would shortly introduce the term "panic" into psychiatry (see below), in 1867 called this "paroxysmal anguish," and associated it with melancholia.[48]

Yet it was the French who undertook systematically the parsing of anxiety into subtypes divorced from melancholia. This began a process that has reached its ultimate form today in dividing anxiety into microfragments that themselves have little credibility as independent entities but have turned out to be highly profitable for the pharmaceutical industry.

In 1875 Henri Legrand du Saulle, 45 years old and at the time an assistant physician at the famous training ground, the psychiatric clinic of the Paris Prefecture of Police, took the first step in this literature of exact description of anxiety by carving out obsessive thoughts together with a compulsive fear of touching things (La folie du doute avec délire du toucher). Legrand was quite immersed in the growing culture of interest in obsessive-compulsive symptoms in France in these years: He was a former student of Morel's and a close friend of Jules Falret's. Given the great tension that prevailed between France and Germany in these years—France had just lost a war to Prussia in 1870—he acknowledged a number of French forbears in the study of such disorders but did not mention Westphal. Legrand portrayed a malady that by stages went relentlessly downhill, ending in the social isolation of the victim who became afraid of contact with everything imaginable. At the Prefecture of Police he saw a lot of psychopathology, and some of that experience made its way into the pages of his 1875 book. But the relentless progression of the illness by clearly demarcated stages that he described came more from an obsession of the late nineteenth century with finding the iron laws of everything, whether economics (Marx) or evolution (Darwin). Legrand called it a "neurosis" (une névrose), but otherwise it had little in common with the nervous syndrome. Legrand's patients were plagued with anxiety, and he refers a number of times to their "anguish." Of interest, however, is Legrand's account of what sound very much like panic attacks in the second phase of the illness: the sudden onset of headaches, sweating, spasms, feelings of fainting, "and the turbulent excitation that ends in constituting a real morbid picture ... that lasts from two to twenty-four hours, but more commonly five or six hours." Legrand used the adjective "paroxystic" to describe the temporal course of the disorder.

Typically, Legrand's patients realized that their obsessive thoughts and compulsive refusals were irrational: the girl of twelve, who believed that "all the objects at home were more or less impregnated and covered with cancerous matter [a person with a facial cancer had visited the home] recognized perfectly that her terrors had no basis, but she could not banish them from her mind." (She recovered, in turn married and became a mother, and then was again visited by the same kinds of fears, this time of a "rabies powder" that supposedly enveloped her home.[49])

What separates anxiety definitively from the nervous syndrome is not really obsessive-compulsive thinking and actions, because nervous patients were subject to plenty of obsessing about their condition. It is rather the condition of panic, which occurs in discrete bursts and is overwhelmingly somatic, with pounding heart, sweating, and so forth. In 1890 Édouard Brissaud, trained more as a neurologist than a psychiatrist (and at the time, at age 37, occupying the history of medicine chair of the Faculty), gave a formal description of panic attacks, which he termed "paroxystic anxiety." (Anxiety for him was "intellectual anguish," which is the modern distinction between somatic anguish and mental anxiety.) He reported a patient suffering from "l'anxiété paroxystique" who would arise in the night fearful that "he is going to die suddenly." He has no chest pain or shortness of breath, "but he cannot stave off the presentiment of immediate death." He also has daytime crises "of the same apprehension of dying." His legs almost give way. "The thought that this crisis might occur at the moment when he is crossing a big street has caused him to adopt the practice of taking narrow streets." But it is not agoraphobia because these crises recur in the middle of crossing even the little streets and passers-by have to assist him. For the past 5 years he has had "very violent cardiac palpitations with sharp intercostal [at the ribs] neuralgia accompanied by anguish and a tendency to faint." "Since then, his palpitations have occurred in the paroxystic form and always accompanied by great anguish."[50] This is sometimes seen as the first formal description of panic attacks, but as we have seen, numerous observers preceded him *avant la lettre*. It is important that the transition from phobias such as agoraphobia to panic was seamless; at the beginning these shrewd observers discerned little difference between agoraphobia and panic. Later, these were to be sundered as separate conditions.

This French thread of refining anxiety reached a final way station in 1901 with Paul Hartenberg's creation of the diagnosis of timidity, today called social phobia, the last of the anxiety syndromes to spin off before Janet closed the discussion with psychasthenia—and Freud's "anxiety neurosis" then reunified the anxieties. Hartenberg, who specialized in the walking wounded with their various anxieties and phobias, believed timidity to be a distinctive disorder: "The emotion of timidity seems to be a combination, in varying proportions, of fear and shame." To emphasize its distinctive nature, Hartenberg did not use the term anxiety. To be sure, "The patient's emotions ... are revealed in palpitations, anguish, a cold sweat." "And when does this emotion surface? In a unique circumstance, in the presence of a human being."[51] The "crises" of timidity sounded very much like panic, and the background emotional symptoms seemed very much like garden-variety anxiety, but once the carving up of anxiety has begun there is really no stopping it, as we know today, because it is so difficult to prove that a given combination of symptoms is not a disease of its own.

Then the carving up of anxiety stopped. Pierre Janet, a student of Jean-Martin Charcot's with his own psychological laboratory at the Salpêtrière Hospital, put a cap on the whole anxiety discussion in 1903 when he announced that there was only one underlying nonpsychotic disorder, and it was psychasthenia. Obsessions, compulsions, and phobias were all psychasthenic in nature, the result of a weakened will, or aboulia, that permitted such disordered behavior to break through. Janet had been trained as a psychologist, but then Charcot encouraged him to study medicine and Janet became a psychiatrist. In his laboratory Janet, 44 years old in 1903, saw a long series of obsessional patients, including a man of 52 whom Legrand had treated 20 years previously. (Legrand had apparently been quite forceful with him and had shoved him around and shaken him up.) The patient had not, however, recovered from his agoraphobia and here he was at the beginning of the new century unable to cross squares and fearing instant death. "When he approaches a square, he shakes himself, he breathes laboriously, he displays his tics, and he repeats this absurd phrase, 'Maman, ratan, bibi, bitaquo, je vais mourir [I'm going to die].'"[52] Summing up, Janet said that although neurasthenia represented physiological insufficiency, in psychasthenia, the insufficiency was psychological, including "phenomena of abulia [lack of will], aprosexia [inability to sustain attention], indifference, and the apathy that we have frequently studied, all as diminutions of the sense of reality. We understand by this term psychasthenia, the totality of psychological functions that play the principal role in the precise adaptation of the individual to a given reality." And what were those positive qualities that psychasthenia negated? "The will, attentiveness, the belief in that which exists in the present, pleasurable or painful sensations—all in rapport with this reality."[53] We sometimes have the feeling that Janet has been deprived of his fair place in history, marginalized by Freud's much grander but much more fanciful ideas. In understanding nervous disease, this might have been a point of departure, but the opportunity passed and the world moved on.

The bottom line is that there are forms of anxiety that occur together with other symptoms, such as depression and fatigue, historically recognized as the nervous syndrome. There are forms of anxiety that occur in the guise of panic, in obsessions, compulsions, and phobias. In their severe form, the public would consider them part of the nervous breakdown. Freud, like Janet, asserted that there was but a single anxiety. Yet like the horse galloping out of control, he took this bit in his teeth and ran away with it.

Anxiety in the Age of Psychoanalysis

It was under psychoanalysis that anxiety became an independent disease entity. How did this happen?

In the 1890s several Central-European clinicians argued that anxiety and anxiety attacks were among the commonest symptoms of neurasthenia.[54] This literature has now been forgotten because the attention of historians has been fixed upon one of these investigators (whose main contribution was in quite a different area, hebephrenia), simply because Freud rather ruefully identified him as having been the first to describe anxiety neurosis. This was Ewald Hecker, whom we met doing the spa treatment of nerves and who by 1893 had moved his water-cure institute from a small village on the Rhine River to Wiesbaden. At a meeting of the Southwest German Psychiatric Association in Wiesbaden in November 1893, Hecker argued for the existence of "atypical anxiety conditions" in neurasthenia. In neurasthenia, "anxiety attacks" (Angstanfälle) could occur either sporadically or chronically. Hecker said that for a number of years he had been calling attention in neurasthenia to anxiety equivalents (larvierte Angstzustände), such as asthma or dizziness, that are "present in well defined attacks without being accompanied by mental feelings of anxiety."[55] This observation would probably have perished in oblivion—for it was obvious that nervous patients had all kinds of somatic symptoms without necessarily feeling anxious—had Freud not picked it up.

In 1895 Sigmund Freud, a young Viennese neurologist of 39 years, truly did describe an independent anxiety syndrome, which he called "anxiety neurosis," arguing that it was separate from neurasthenia. Among the characteristics of this new neurosis were general irritability, anxious anticipation of dreaded future events, somatic anxiety attacks such as pounding heart, and the kinds of anxiety-equivalents that Hecker had suggested, among other symptoms. Freud's account of anxiety neuroses was clinically shrewd, psychologically astute, and kicked neurasthenia over the side. Freud did write, "I am calling this symptom complex [syndrome] 'anxiety neurosis' because all of its components may be grouped around the chief symptom of anxiety. I had imagined that my conception of the symptoms of anxiety neurosis was quite original until an interesting lecture by E. Hecker crossed my desk, in which I found my particular interpretation laid out with clarity and completeness."[56] (It is unimportant that Hecker had not done this at all. Yet Freud was showing himself to be a generous colleague in giving Hecker, a water-cure-institute doctor, so much credit.)

Three years later, in an 1898 essay on "Sexuality in the Etiology of the Neuroses," Freud explained that anxiety and neurasthenic neuroses alike were "actual neuroses," caused by current sexual events in the patient's life, while obsessive-compulsive phenomena and hysteria were "psychoneuroses," caused by sexual events in development. Neurasthenia was caused by excessive mas-turbation and anxiety neurosis by coitus interruptus, abstinence, or frustrated arousal.[57]

These were concepts that had an enormous impact, not just on psychiatry but on western society. It took a while for them to be picked up, in these and Freud's subsequent writings. But by the decade before World War I, anxiety neurosis had become a common diagnosis. In the United States, some of the great names in neurology—it was then the neurologists who did private-practice psychotherapy—seized upon anxiety neurosis. In 1912 Smith Ely Jelliffe, a professor of neurology in the New York Post-Graduate Medical School, reviewing patients recently seen in their outpatient clinic, said, "Some of our cases of menopause psychoneuroses are probably anxiety neuroses. The increase of the libido ... accounts in large part for many of these cases. The histories are too direct and to the point to permit dodging the Freudian conceptions of these states notwithstanding one's reluctance to accept an idea which at first sight seems far fetched."[58]

In Zurich, Ludwig Frank, who had a psychiatric private practice and at age 50 was no inexperienced shave-tail, wrote at length in 1913 about "anxi-ety neuroses and the suppression of the libido."[59] After the war he developed a whole scheme of "thymopathies," meaning anxiety, inhibition, feelings of inferiority, and other "dysphorias."[60]

In Paris, society nerve doctor Paul Hartenberg gave anxiety neurosis (la névrose d'angoisse) huge play in 1901, bringing anxiety from the wings onto center stage.[61]

The English have always been cool to psychoanalysis, yet Aubrey Lewis, an Australian who came over from a U.S. post to join the Maudsley Hospital in 1928, held the opinion that whatever interest his colleagues had been able to muster in anxiety was largely due to the influence of Freud. He said in 1971 that "There can be little doubt that the attention paid to anxiety in the last ten years or more has been largely due to the adoption of Freudian concepts and ... of Freudian metapsychology."[62]

In other words, the impact of Freud's anxiety neurosis on international psychiatry was immediate and profound. As Freud's acolyte Wilhelm Stekel said in 1936, just 2 years before he was forced to emigrate from Vienna to London, where he died by suicide in a lonely hotel room, "The picture of neurosis has changed extraordinarily in the course of recent decades. Hysteria has almost disappeared, obsessive-compulsive neuroses and organ neuroses, anxiety conditions, schizophrenia and disturbances of affect have stepped into the foreground."[63] Indeed, the revival of anxiety was part of a larger pivot of diagnosis from hysteria and neurasthenia to disturbances of mood and affect. In doing so, nervous illness too was left behind. Freud himself had almost no interest in fatigue.[64] And he considered neurasthenia too uninteresting for words.[65]

The tradition of identifying anxiety with unconscious Freudian processes lasted long in American psychiatry. In 1971, in an effort to grab the attention of a psychiatric audience still more fixed upon Freud than psychopharmacology, the Hoffmann La Roche company flogged its drug Librium as good for anxiety using the psychoanalytic formulation, "The most characteristic and common feature of neurotic habits is anxiety."[66] The Freudian triumph of anxiety was almost complete.

Anxiety Neurosis Part of a Continuum, or Not?

Were all these new diagnoses pretty much of a muchness, or not? Were serious anxiety and melancholia diseases of their own, or did they merge imperceptibly into all the other diseases? Were illnesses such as melancholia a different order of magnitude from less severe diagnoses of the nervous syndrome, or does it all blend together? The English poet Thomas Gray, then 26 years old, took the two-level approach, though he would not have formulated it in those terms, when contemplating his own symptoms. The two levels existed within him. As he wrote to classmate Richard West in 1742, "Mine, you are to know is a white melancholy ... which though it seldom laughs or dances, nor ever amounts to what one calls joy or pleasure, yet is a good easy sort of a state, and ça ne laisse que de s'amuser [stops me just short of enjoying myself]. The only fault of it is insipidity [lifeless, dull, flat]; which is apt now and then to give a sort of ennui, which makes one form certain little wishes that signify nothing." So here Gray is telling West that he feels mildly dysphoric from time to time and even toys with suicide; from other letters it is clear that he is a bit anxious on occasion, but nothing more really; he might have accepted that at moments he was nervous.

Gray continues: "But there is another sort, black indeed, which I have now and then felt ... for it believes, nay, is sure of every thing that is unlikely, so it be but frightful [meaning he is delusional]; and, on the other hand, excludes and shuts its eyes to the most possible hopes, and every thing that is pleasurable; from this the Lord deliver us!"[67] This black melancholy, in other words, brings paranoia, anhedonia, and hopelessness with it, all symptoms of melancholia. Gray did not experience these different illnesses as a continuum; he did not have them both at the same time; but both dwelt within his breast.

At a meeting of the British Medical Association in 1926, swords clashed less poetically over the same issue. Edward Mapother, the superintendent of the recently opened Maudsley Hospital, England's premier center for the study of psychiatric illness, expressed dubiety about the wisdom of drawing sharp lines. He said it could happen that Freud's new diagnosis of anxiety neurosis might easily "merge in the same patient, and by a perfectly continuous gradation in a series of patients, into agitated melancholia."

Robert Dick Gillespie, a brilliant young clinician and scientist at the Cassell Hospital at Penshurst and known as "R.D.," was in the audience. Gillespie said that melancholia and anxiety neurosis had little overlap. "Who had heard of a melancholic of the manic-depressive type who was well and at ease while he sat in the garden, but was plunged into misery when he returned to the drawing-room? [in other words, manic-depression was a chronic illness not relieved by an afternoon of sun in the garden but anxiety could be dependent on the situation] Dr Gillespie had at the present time a patient with such an anxiety state."[68] Clearly, there were forms of depression, such as Kraepelin's manic-depressive illness, the depression of which was melancholic, that differed not just in degree but in kind from the anxiety and depression of nervousness. As we watch anxiety liberating itself from melancholia, we keep in mind that some of this new freedom was justified and some was an arbitrary shattering of a real nervous syndrome: Agitated, anxious melancholia was, and is, a real disease.

Psychotic Anxiety as a Distinctive Breakdown

There are different kinds of paroxystic anxiety, of anxiety attacks, and of panic disorder that sweep over the individual with hurricane-like force. The classic authors tended more to sense this rather than characterizing it neatly, and terms such as "anxious melancholia" and "anxiety psychosis" abound in the literature. Some of this extreme anxiety may be psychotic, involving delusions and hallucinations, and other forms may not. My purpose here is to acquaint readers with a clear historical strain that we have forgotten today and that comes as close to a complete nervous breakdown as anything we encounter in these pages. Readers may judge for themselves whether this is a separate diagnostic entity or not.

In 1852, Joseph Guislain in Ghent was among the first to introduce the notion of "anxious melancholy, sometimes preceded by a painful feeling that the patient localizes in the region of the heart." Suddenly the disorder erupts: "the patient is sleepless, assailed by sad ideas, his personality comes apart. A feeling of anguish accompanied by vague terror announces the beginning of the disorder." Guislain demonstrated to the medical students a patient "who is terrified of her present situation. She says, 'I don't know what I'm doing. I'm capable of wreaking a tragedy. I'm good for nothing. It seems to me that I am suffocating.'"

Guislain continues the presentation: "Sometimes her feelings of anguish erupt suddenly. They compel her to be agitated in every possible way. She walks about her apartment and courtyard fifty times in a row. Frequently she repeats the name of someone or some thing. She's filled with lamentations; her thinking grows cloudy and she acts impulsively. Each attack may last only a few hours, or days and weeks." Guislain thought this was the same condition as Flemming's precordial anxiety.[69] But it is dramatically different from any form of anxiety previously considered in this chapter. Heinrich Schüle, director of the Ilenau asylum in Germany, said in 1878 of anxiety-melancholia (die Angst-Melancholie) that "restlessness of the muscles results in an illusory rerouting of all the senses in the direction of fear of destruction ... There is an anxious agitation that lasts day and night with a pathological feeling of having sinned."[70]

Anxious melancholia thus embedded itself in psychiatry for the next half century, the extreme form being a panicky, psychotic eruption that had little in common with the anxiety of nervous illness or that of phobias and obsessions. It borders on the delirious mania of catatonia. In 1896, Emil Kraepelin wrote in his psychiatry textbook, which became in his day what the "*DSM*" of the American Psychiatric Association is in our own, that "There are pronounced anxiety conditions, which take on an extraordinary force and degree. It is such cases that used to receive the name anxious melancholy [Angstmelancholie]. I have recently become convinced, that between them and simple sad mood disorders there are no sharp lines of division. Either anxiety accompanied the entire illness course with many fluctuations, or it occurs in single attacks, that suddenly erupt and are accompanied with severe, even psychotic, disturbances of conscience (Raptus melancholicus)."[71] Anxiety and anxious melancholy vanished from the 8th edition in 1913, as Kraepelin got rid of them altogether as distinctive illness entities.

It was Carl Wernicke, professor of psychiatry in the East German city of Breslau (and who in 1874 identified a brain region named after him), who in 1900 liberated extreme panic and anxiety from melancholia and made them, in the form of psychotic anxiety (Angstpsychose), a separate condition. Wernicke presents to the medical students a 55-year-old man who is anxious, groans lightly, answers questions slowly (there in front of the students), and has difficulty collecting himself. In addition to his anxiety, he seems to understand little of what is going on around him. His chief complaint is "incessant anxiety at the region of the heart." He feels that it will "crush" him. Also, he cannot catch his breath. Why is he so anxious? He fears decapitation. He also believes that his family has suffered a catastrophe (untrue), that he hears the voice of his young son, who has had "nothing to eat for three weeks." (In fact, he hallucinates the presence of the son in front of him.) And he believes that everything is his fault, above all, because he masturbated as a youth. He is "a great sinner and is persecuted by Satan." Not panicky but severely anxious, the patient spontaneously recovers and is well again. In Wernicke's view, such patients have "the primary symptom of anxiety as the exclusive basis of the illness." It sits first of all in the epigastrium, next most commonly in the head, and third commonest "in the entire body." The somatic symptoms are mainly motor agitation, crying, hand-wringing, and sweating. Almost all the patients with this disorder are suicidal. It is the anxious ideation, said Wernicke, that means the patients do not have an "affective melancholia." He said this psychotic anxiety was very different from the neurotic sort.[72] In retrospect, this is a kind of anxiety that certainly has a different feeling from the other anxieties in this chapter, and justifies weighing the possibility that there might be several different kinds of anxiety, though not the kinds featured in the *DSM* manual today. (It does not appear to be a subtype of melancholia.[73])

Wernicke's "psychotic anxiety" never took off, probably because, as one researcher explained in 1905, "the disease cannot be accommodated in the Kraepelinian School's forms of diagnosis."[74] Then the psychoanalysts gained the ascendancy in psychiatry and the field lost interest in these refined forms of diagnosis, particularly in the field of psychosis, with which the analysts never felt comfortable because psychotic patients could not enter into a transference relationship—essential in psychoanalysis for recovery from illness.

Panic Becomes Familiar

Once Freud had put "anxiety neurosis" on the table, many non-Freudians began to interest themselves in the study of anxiety as well. Inevitably, the term panic, a perfectly familiar word for a psychological state, began to appear as a synonym. The word panic seems to have been used in psychiatry for the first time in 1879 by Henry Maudsley at the West London Hospital, who described one melancholic patient's sudden efforts to commit suicide: "These paroxysms of anguish or panic, which are a notable feature in some cases of melancholia—paroxysms of *melancholic panic* they might be called—deserve careful notice. They often come on quite suddenly; the patient has perhaps been lying down to rest ... [then] starts up in great agitation, his heart beating tumultuously, his senses distraught, and rushes wildly to the window to throw himself out of it; he is overwhelmed for the time being, driven to desperation, and hardly knows what he does; the frenzy has all the characters of a convulsion affecting the mental nerve-centres. In some cases the convulsive panic is preceded by an anomalous and alarming sensation of distress about the region of the stomach ... [and] is accompanied by an indescribable terror and dreadful feeling of helplessness." Maudsley said that after the paroxysm the patient "trembles from head to foot, is bathed in perspiration and completely exhausted."[75]

Others started to pick up on the presence of panic symptoms in serious psychiatric illnesses. Harvard professor of philosophy William James, who wrote *Varieties of Religious Experience* in 1902, was very interested in psychiatry and corresponded extensively on it. "The worst kind of melancholy is that which takes the form of panic fear," he said, quoting a French patient whose letter he translates: "I awoke morning after morning," said the patient, "with a horrible dread at the pit of my stomach, and with a sense of the insecurity of life that I never knew before, and that I have never felt since."[76]

In 1910 August Cramer at the university psychiatric hospital in Göttingen mentioned the "panic-like" symptoms that overcame some people in situations that provoked anxiety, or, like posttraumatic stress disorder, reminded them of situations, such as railway accidents, that previously had made them anxious.[77] On the other side of the ocean, Harry Paskind, a neurologist in Chicago, called attention in 1929 to "brief attacks of manic-depression" lasting from a few hours to a few days, and often occurring against a background of chronic mood disorder, "accompanied by a feeling of weakness, ready fatigue, head pressure," and abdominal distress. The patients subjectively are sad, hopeless, and briefly inclined to suicide before their symptoms abruptly disappear. "Many patients with manic-depressive depression," said Paskind, "have a peculiar feeling in the epigastrium or pit of the stomach." And often the internist is called in to investigate, said Paskind, almost never the psychiatrist, who specializes in long-term illnesses seen in mental hospitals. There was much anxious vomiting and tightening of the throat, and the patients did not mention pounding hearts but perhaps only because Paskind did not ask them about it.[78]

It was then Oskar Diethelm, born and trained in Switzerland but who had come to Johns Hopkins in 1925 at age 28, who put the concept of panic on the map. In 1932, in articles published on both sides of the Atlantic, Diethelm explained that panic was "not merely a high degree of fear, but a fear based on prolonged tension, with a sudden climax which is characterized by fear, extreme insecurity, suspiciousness and a tendency to projection and disorganization." Diethelm described a woman of 28 years facing a thyroid operation who became "panicky ... knowing that she would have to stay in bed afterward and could not get away even if she should [continue to] feel panicky ... She felt a tightening in her throat, palpitation, nausea and a fear that 'here is something I do not know anything about.'" When she heard that a patient in a neighboring room had been visited by a psychiatrist, "she became afraid of being transferred to a psychiatric clinic. In the evening she became panicky." She tried to read but was overcome by fear. "I got in a panic about having panics," she said.[79] This was the official introduction of panic disorder to psychiatry.

Events in the understanding of these matters were suspended as the Nazis came to power in 1933. Because so many investigators were Jewish, serious research closed down in German psychiatry, a national field that hitherto had been the world's locomotive. Then there was the chaos of war and reconstruction in France and Germany so that, again, interest in arcane matters such as the classification of psychiatric illness—a matter that nonetheless affects the lives of millions of people—came to a halt.

Years passed without any serious interest in extreme forms of panic and anxiety until in 1950 the spotlight shifted to Spain. In 1950 Juan Lopez-Ibor, 43 years old and professor of psychiatry in Madrid, argued that a special kind of anxiety existed that he called "vital anxiety." He did not realize that Josef Westermann had already used the term in 1923 and that his concept was not absolutely original.[80] But what he had in mind was in fact quite

innovative. Lopez-Ibor had studied with the great German psychopathologist Kurt Schneider (older psychiatrists will recognize the name from the
so-called Schneiderian criteria of schizophrenia, such as thought-insertion).
In 1920 Schneider had distinguished between vital depression and reactive
depression.[81] Vital depression was a phenomenon of the entire body: Every
pore oozed depression, and Lopez-Ibor thought vital depression must have
a counterpart in anxiety: Let us call it vital anxiety, or la angustia vital, as
he proposed in a 1950 book. Vital anxiety was serious, even psychotic, and
quite different from neurotic anxiety, Lopez-Ibor argued; it constituted part
of the "thymopathic circle" that otherwise included mania and depression.[82]
A "crisis di angustia" was tantamount to a panic attack. Lopez-Ibor explained
that "What distinguishes the vital anxiety of the anxious timopath from ...
anxious reaction is its unmotivated appearance, and it is the violence of its
manifestation."[83] Thus attacks of anxious timopathy came out of the blue and
swept over the patient with a force having little in common with Freud's anxiety neurosis.

It is now clear that anxiety nestles into the core of the history of the nervous breakdown. And this happened in two ways, each of them searing and
life-changing. Anxiety in the nervous syndrome—together with depression, fatigue, and somatic ailments—was more a chronic illness, often lasting
months and years, and leaving the individual what was once called a nervous
wreck. Anxiety in the paroxystic attack, which is to say panic, was brief and
brutal, leaving the individual psychically exhausted and fearful of the future.

Indeed, in some ways, the only illness worse than panic was melancholia.

6

A Different Kind of Nervous Breakdown—Melancholia

Motto: "*Depressive illness is probably more unpleasant than any disease except rabies.*"[1]

JOHN S. PRICE, NORTHWICK PARK HOSPITAL,
HARROW, MIDDLESEX, 1978

FEELINGS OF LOW mood are not trivial. In 2010 the National Center for Health Statistics of the Department of Health and Human Services asked a random sample of the U.S. population about their mood. In reply to Do you feel hopeless?, 6.8%, or 1 in 15, said yes. In reply to Do you feel worthless?, 5.3% said yes. In reply to Do you feel that "everything is an effort"?, a whopping 16%, or one in seven, said yes.[2] Low feeling is very common. Yet it is not melancholia.

Historically, plenty of people have suffered from low moods. Today, few of us can stay in our beds because we have to earn a living. Yet it was once common for middle-class women, in households that had servants, to take to their beds when feeling down. In 1917, London literary figure Virginia Woolf, age 36, noted in her diary for October 25: "Owing to the usual circumstances, I had to spend the day recumbent." She meant that she was having her period, and always had to lie down. Still, menstruation was not the only reason she went recumbent. Late in 1918 she had a tooth out and spent two weeks in bed, "and being tired enough to get a headache—a long dreary affair, that receded and advanced much like a mist on a January day." "Here is a whole nervous breakdown in miniature," she recorded in July 1926. "Sank into a chair, could scarcely rise; everything insipid; tasteless, colourless. Enormous desire to rest." In November 1931 she was assailed by "a perpetual headache," and "so took a month lying down." On October 5, 1932, she said, "I spent yesterday in bed; headache; infinite weariness up my back: clouds forming in my neck; half asleep."³ So this is the kind of nervous behavior that was congruent with people of her social class at that place and time.

But there are deeper, more alarming notes. On September 28, 1926, "Intense depression: I have to confess that this has overcome me several times since September 6th…It is so strange to me that I cannot get it right—the depression, I mean, which does not come from something definite, but from nothing." (Indeed, melancholia often comes out of the blue.) In June 1929, "And so I pitched into my great lake of melancholy. Lord how deep it is! What a born melancholic I am! The only way I keep afloat is by working."⁴ The metaphor is interesting. She ultimately commits suicide in 1941 by drowning.

What Is Melancholia?

"There is a loss of light in the eyes. They become like fish eyes. And when the patients are treated successfully, the light comes back."

GORDON PARKER, 2012⁵

There are two different kinds of depression, as different as tuberculosis and mumps; it makes no sense to lump both of them together under the general term "depression." The first kind of depression concerns the mood disturbances that occur in the context of nervous disease, and we have already reviewed them. They are nonmelancholic and nonpsychotic, heavily admixed with anxiety and fatigue, laced with obsessive thinking, and often overshadowed by somatic complaints—almost to the point of being invisible. Virginia Woolf had some variety of this, even though she alludes occasionally to things such as "my present fit of melancholy."⁶

The second kind of depressive disorder is melancholia. It is an independent and unmistakable disease entity, often not combined with anything, and fearsome in a far different way than nervousness, for it may lead to despair, hopelessness, a complete lack of pleasure in one's life, and suicide. By the late nineteenth century, the differences between these two depressions lay clear in view and observers often distinguished between them. Subsequently, both swim out of focus; nervous disease is broken up, and what we have emerged with today as "depression" bears little resemblance to these historic ancestors.

Serious depression is a real and terrible illness. William Sargant, professor of psychiatry at St. Thomas's Hospital in London, recalled the back wards in the 1930s and 1940s: "My memory of those days is of patients with melancholia dying of agitated exhaustion after months or years in mental hospitals, and of the rows of depressed patients who had to be kept on special suicidal precautions in mental hospitals and psychiatric clinics alike. Even in the more neurotic types of depression, and despite all the psychotherapy given, suicides were frequent, and patients often took months or years to get well no matter what one tried to do to help them."[7] So in melancholia we are dealing with one of the most terrible afflictions in medicine.

What is melancholia? Like nerves, melancholia too is a disease of the entire body. The endocrine system is intimately involved, and the blackness of affect reaches into the adrenal gland. In melancholia, affect is profoundly down, and stupor and dejection may alternate with periods of agitation and hand-wringing. Oswald Bumke, among the most thoughtful of the German academic psychiatrists of his generation (at a time when Germany was the epicenter of world psychiatry), said in 1908, "The essential characteristic of melancholia is a sadness of mood that is not founded in external circumstances, a strongly depressive affect, from which a gloomy assessment of one's own situation arises, as well as ideas of having deeply sinned in the past and anxious fears about the future."[8] (Bumke was writing as a time when people were still preoccupied with sin; today, melancholic patients often imagine that they have committed some other unpardonable deed.)

But we have to modify Bumke's judgment slightly. It is not so much sadness of the weepy variety as pain that the patients complain of. Melancholia is a disorder of pain. "I can't stand the pain any longer," Edith La Tour, 30 years old, said in a note she left behind in 1934 after she jumped from a twelfth floor room at the Barbizon Hotel for Women in New York. She was said to have suffered a nervous breakdown.[9] (Just to clarify, the term nervous breakdown was the patient term for melancholia; nervous breakdown was never a medical diagnosis.)

Another piece of evidence: In the early 1960s, the young French-born psychologist Rachel Gittelman helped conduct a clinical trial of the antidepressant drug imipramine with Max Fink and Donald Klein at Hillside Hospital (see below). "These were patients whom I will never forget," she later said in an interview. "Severely depressed individuals with retarded or agitated depression. People I wanted to run from because they were in such pain, causing me pain."[10] Yet 6 weeks after medication, "They walked into my office and they were well. I get chills even now thinking about them." They were not sad; they were in pain.

So this is point one: melancholia means a dejection that appears to observers as sadness but that the patients themselves often interpret as pain.

When people look at these patients, they see sadness, though that may not be what the patients themselves are primarily experiencing. "The classical melancholic oozes depression, so that the observer feels depressed himself," said one English physician in 1957.[11] Indeed, Jane S, a domestic servant from Bradford admitted to the West Riding Asylum in Yorkshire in 1872, was the very image of dejection. She had given birth out of wedlock. Said James Crichton-Browne, director of the asylum, "Her fall from virtue had preyed much upon her mind during her pregnancy; and the depression of spirits thus occasioned deepened considerably at the time of her confinement, when she was in poor lodgings…and passed into morbid despondency three days after delivery, when the unexpected announcement of her father's death reached her. She at once formed the idea that her father (who was a very aged man, and really died in the course of nature) had been killed by the shame of her misfortune. She sank into a state of inconsolable grief, wept incessantly, was sleepless, and twice attempted to put an end to her existence and sorrow by jumping through the window. After this she refused all food, complained of insupportable misery and weakness, and repeatedly threatened suicide." Thereupon, she was admitted to the asylum. What is really of interest was her appearance. Crichton-Browne described, "…a thin, pale, careworn-looking woman…seated in the day-room, with her head bowed down, and her hands crossed upon her lap, in an attitude of listless dejection. Her features were fixed in an expression of mental suffering, the angles of the mouth being drawn down, and the corrugators of the upper eyebrows being firmly contracted [this is the Omega sign]. When I spoke to her, she answered slowly and with evident reluctance, turning away from me, as if shrinking from observation and seeking solitude."[12] (This is described as psychomotor slowing.) Was Jane S mainly sad or was she dejected from psychic pain? She had a weepy period, but by the time she reached the asylum her chief complaint seems to have been pain.

Many observers echo this theme. Jean Delay, who was about to become professor of psychiatry in Paris, said of "melancholic mood" in 1946: "Mood is this fundamental affective disposition, rich in all layers of emotionality and instinctuality, that gives to each of our inner lives an agreeable or disagreeable tonality, oscillating between the two extreme poles of pleasure and pain."[13]

The emphasis here is on pain and energy, not necessarily mood and sadness. In melancholia, Delay correctly observed, the mood slides down not necessarily to sadness but to pain. For that reason, patients may land in the hands of the internist rather than the psychiatrist. Said Vienna psychiatry professor Peter Berner in 1972 during a symposium at St. Moritz, Switzerland: "In depressions that present with inhibition, a disturbance of the *élan vital* [core energy] is very pronounced while the affect may be little depressed. Very frequently, these patients consult the internist or the general practitioner."[14]

Today, this note of pain is profound. A psychiatrist in Coral Springs, Florida, writes in 2007 that "Most of my patients suffering from major depression have described their malady as the worst pain they have had to beat."[15] Price at Northwick Park talked of his hospitalized depressed patients' pain: "If one tries to get such a patient to titrate other pains against the pain of his depression one tends to end up with a description that would raise eyebrows even in a mediaeval torture chamber. Naturally, many of these patients commit suicide. They may not hope to get to heaven but they know they are leaving hell."[16]

Melancholic patients often look dejected. There is a characteristic posture, a slump with its dejected shoulders, a facies with its empty eyes and frozen features, that has been familiar across the ages and explains why melancholia is often diagnosable at a glance. Here is Dr. Thomas Robertson, testifying in New York in 1894 at the probation of the will of his patient Frederick Lovecraft, a theater manager who had committed suicide the year before.

"He seemed to be in a very depressed condition," said Dr. Robertson. "He took no interest apparently in anything that was transpiring, when spoken to, he answered in monosyllables, He was exceedingly pale, and complained of insomnia and nervousness. He said he was hardly able to attend to his business." Dr Robertson said that Lovecraft was "suffering from melancholia, following delusions."

"What was the condition of his eyes?" asked a lawyer. "Were they vacant or full of life as in ordinary men?"

"I couldn't tell. I could hardly induce him to look up. He kept his head bowed down. Everything indicated acute melancholia."[17]

Additionally, melancholia patients suffer psychomotor retardation, meaning slowed thought and movement. Bumke: "All movements are conducted slowly, any change of bodily position is avoided, the speech is soft, halting and limited to what is absolutely necessary." As for thought, "the patients have to recollect at length what they want to say, and they complain that nothing at all occurs to them any more." Yet occasionally this slowness gives way to bursts of agitation, and often to extreme anxious excitement. Bumke articulated a point many observers of melancholia had long known,[18] and that Gordon Parker, professor of psychiatry in Sydney and leader of the Black Dog Institute, emphasized in 1996 when he revived the melancholia diagnosis: Psychomotor change, either slowed or accelerated, was a prime characteristic of melancholia.[19]

What else? Suicide. The melancholic at risk of suicide was devilishly difficult to assess because melancholic patients often complain of everything but their mental pain and negation. As neurologist George Riddoch at the National Hospital at Queen Square told the Royal Society of Medicine in 1930 (it was, again, neurologists more than psychiatrists who saw psychiatric outpatients): "The manic-depressive patient, in a state of depression, may come complaining of anything but his depression. The symptoms which he first describes may, for example, be headache, abdominal discomfort, constipation, sleeplessness, or pain in the chest, and the underlying depression may only be admitted after some time, and then with reluctance. It is kept back, perhaps, because the associated suicidal ideas have become intense."[20] Admitting depression would cause others to thwart your desire for suicide.

Bumke said the newspapers in Germany in the 1920s were daily filled with reports of individuals who had made themselves away despite family supervision that "never let them out of sight." "In practice, usually the simple question, how is the patient supervised when going to the bathroom, suffices to evaluate the family's reassurance that he is 'constantly watched.'"[21] That is precisely what happened to Dr. C. J. Miller of Uniontown, Pennsylvania, who was admitted to the St. Francis Hospital in Pittsburg in 1911 "suffering from a complete nervous breakdown." He had requested to be shaved one afternoon and then concealed the razor in his pajamas. "He asked the male nurse,... to accompany him to a bathroom and then sent the man on an errand. A few minutes later a physician saw a stream of blood running on the marble floor from under the door...Dr Miller was found with his throat cut from ear to ear."[22]

There is one other characteristic of melancholia that Oswald Bumke did not know about in 1908: A biological marker exists for it. Melancholia is one of the few illnesses in psychiatry for which there is a blood test: the dexamethasone suppression test. We have already met Bernard Carroll in the preface, the Australian-born psychiatrist and endocrinologist whom everyone calls Barney. In 1968 Carroll discovered that administering a synthetic steroid drug called dexamethasone to melancholic patients uncovered an unsuspected dysfunction of their endocrine system: It keeps their cortisol levels high. Cortisol is the stress hormone. Unlike normal subjects, if you gave them dexamethasone at midnight, their systems did not experience the normal late-night-early-morning reduction of cortisol; this nonreduction correlated with the severity of the illness, and it disappeared after patients were successfully treated for their depression.[23] Later studies found that the endocrine systems of patients with most other psychiatric diagnoses showed normal suppression in response to dexamethasone. Thus, melancholic patients had a distinctive dysfunction of the hypothalamus-pituitary-adrenal axis called "DST nonsuppression." (The hypothalamus is the brain region that directs the endocrine system via the pituitary glad; the thyroid and adrenal glands are among the endocrine organs that lie at the far end of the neuroendocrine axes. In melancholia, the adrenal axis, and, to a lesser extent, the thyroid axis, does not respond properly to endocrine signals.) The marker of cortisol nonsuppression is not biologically unique to melancholia: it occurs in severe physical illness and in some psychiatric disorders that are unlikely to be confused with melancholia, such as anorexia nervosa and dementia. Yet the dexamethasone suppression test, or "DST," has about the same ability to diagnose melancholia properly, without too many "false negatives" and "false positives," that the interictal (between seizures) electroencephalogram has in epilepsy: useful but not perfect.[24] The DST provides evidence that most melancholic patients, whether unipolar or bipolar, have an underlying biochemical homogeneity that is entirely lacking in other psychiatric disorders.[25] (The DST enjoyed a brief popularity in psychiatry as a "screening test for depression"—which it is not—in the 1970s and early 1980s, then lapsed into oblivion, leaving only a few feathers floating on the surface.[26] This abandonment of a promising lead is not a tremendous accolade for clinical psychiatry.)

What was melancholia for physicians was nerves or a nervous breakdown for patients. As we shall see, nervous breakdown was not a doctors' phrase, but for patients, it was a medical calamity. In April 1921 Annette Rankine, wife of William Birch Rankine who developed electric power at Niagara Falls, disappeared. With a history of melancholia, she had probably committed suicide. She had said earlier to her nurse, "If I thought I would never recover from this nervous feeling, I would rather be dead."[27]

Melancholia is such a serious illness that in the past it would automatically qualify as a breakdown. For the headline writers of the *New York Times*, melancholia and nervous breakdown were almost interchangeable: One day melancholia would be assigned as the apparent cause of a suicide and the next day nervous breakdown blazoned as the cause of another. The term melancholia appeared in *Times* headlines three times (the first mention in 1868) before we reach the first headline about melancholic suicide in 1884: "A Brooklyn Suicide: Driven to Kill Himself by Repeated Attacks of Melancholia."[28] Thereafter the drumbeat of suicides attributed by headline writers to melancholia is pretty steady at several per year. (The pace of melancholia mentions then falls off dramatically in the mid-1930s and the last clinical mention in a headline occurred in 1951: "Passenger Lost at Sea: Doctor Says Baltimore Man Was Victim of Melancholia."[29])

In these years, nerves were giving way to affect. Depression would soon inspire the headline writers. In medicine, what everybody recognized before

1920 as the nervous syndrome began to yield slowly in the interwar years to disorders of mood and affect. Mood and affect are mental conditions. Nerves is a whole body condition. The distinction is fundamental. Affect means emotion. The passage from nerves to depression is a major chapter in the history of psychiatry and in our culture's encounters with mood and body feeling.

Melancholia: As Old as Time

Motto: "…considering the ill that trouble of mind and melancholy may in this sickly time bring a family into."[30]
SAMUEL PEPYS, 1665

Most organic illnesses go back in time to the appearance of the first medical records, and doubtless existed far before then. Melancholia is no exception. It is one of the classical evils to which the flesh is heir. The Ancients expanded the definition to many afflictions that we might today consider separately, yet they nonetheless drew attention to the core symptoms of profound dejection and slowing, complete lack of joy in life, and delusional apprehensions of the surrounding world.[31] Galen, a Greek medical writer in the second century after Christ, said, "The melancholic derangements vary, by there being several kinds of false imaginings. In all these, however, one thing seems to be common, which has been stated by Hippocrates: 'If fear or despair continues for a long period, such a thing is melancholia.' For they are all despairing without reason, nor, were you to ask, would they be able to say they are distressed about anything…"[32]

In the early modern period, melancholia remained sufficiently alive, though just barely in the fog of religion, that priests thought it necessary to differentiate melancholia as a clinical illness from demonic possession and bewitchment. How can you tell if your parishioner is ill or bewitched? Francesco Maria Guazzo, a priest in Milan, said in 1608, "The following is the usual practice to determine whether the sick man is possessed by a demon. They [the Church] secretly apply to the sick man a writing with the sacred words of God, or Relics of the Saints, or a blessed Agnus Dei, or some other holy thing. The priest places his hand and his stole upon the head of the possessed and pronounces sacred words. Thereupon the sick man [the bewitched individual] begins to shake and tremble, and in his pain makes many uncouth movements, and says and does many strange things. If the demon is in his head, he feels the keenest pains in his head, or else his head and all his face are suffused with a hot red glow like fire." If the demon is in his stomach, there will be hiccups and vomiting, "so that sometimes they cannot take food." Yet the melancholic will do none of these things.[33] Even in the gloom of the Counter-Reformation, the clinical concept of melancholia survived, so powerfully did it speak to reality.

And patients, or potential patients, knew well what they had. Margaret, Marchioness of Newcastle, an early female scientist and an ambitious writer, described in 1656 at age 30 the turmoil the family suffered during the English Civil War. "But being not of a merry … disposition, I became very melancholy by reason I was from my Lord [husband], which made my mind so restless that it did break my sleep and distemper my health." She clarified: "As for my disposition, it is more inclining to melancholy than merry, but soft, melting solitary and contemplative melancholy. And I am apt to weep rather than laugh, not that I often do either of them."[34] So she describes her melancholia both as a trait, a constant companion, and a state into which a reversal of circumstances might plunge her.

In 1763 English poet William Cowper, at 32 years of age a candidate for a post in the English House of Lords, and a highly nervous candidate at that, was disturbed in his preparations for the examination by yet another attack of melancholy, an illness that ran in the family. Beside himself with agitation, he attempted suicide three times. As he was discovered on the third attempt, any possibility of gaining a parliamentary post vanished, and, says his biographer, "The sense of total failure must have been as overwhelming as the feeling of moral degradation into which, apparently, all other concerns were channeled … In the days that followed his attempts at suicide, whenever he opened a book, he found it filled with allusions to his condition and with details and rhetorical figures that seemed addressed to him. In the streets people seemed to avoid him or laugh at him." Cowper became preoccupied with "the wrath of God punishing the worst of sinners," and his poetry in the midst of this psychotic depression reflects the lowness of his spirits:

> *"Hatred and vengeance, my eternal portion,*
> *Scarce can endure delay of execution,*
> *Wait, with impatient readiness, to seize my*
> *Soul in a moment."*

It is interesting that Cowper was not necessarily sad, or weepy. Rather he experienced his melancholia at a somatic level as pain and numbness. Writing to a friend of how he had spent the previous night, he said, "My ears rang with the sounds of torments, that seemed to await me. Then did the pains of hell get hold on me, and, before daybreak, the very sorrows of death encompassed me. A numbness seized the extremities of my body, and life seemed to retreat before it. My hands and feet became cold and stiff; a cold sweat stood upon my forehead; my heart seemed at every pulse to beat its last, and my soul to cling to my lips, as if on the very brink of departure. No convicted criminal ever feared death more, or was more assured of dying."

In the course of the day, as he anxiously paced his apartment, "a strange and horrible darkness fell upon me. If it were possible, that a heavy blow could light on the brain, without touching the skull, such was the sensation I felt. I clapped my hand to my forehead, and cried aloud through the pain it gave me."[35] We can understand the comparison with rabies mentioned above: Psychotic melancholia is among the most terrible of illnesses and has little in common with the nervous syndrome. (Again, just to signpost this path strewn with "n" words: The nervous breakdown equaled melancholia, which is what Cowper had; the nervous syndrome equaled the five domains of nonpsychotic anxiety, depression, fatigue, somatic symptoms, and a touch of OCD, which is what most sufferers had.)

A poem from these years shows well that Cowper was aware of the difference between his own affliction and the kind of "spleen" and black-bile "humour" that would later be called nerves[36]:

> *"Doom'd, as I am, in solitude to waste*
> *The present moments, and regret the past;*
> *Depriv'd of every joy, I valued most,*
> *My friend torn from me, and my mistress lost;*
> *Call not this gloom, I wear, this anxious mien,*
> *The dull effect of humour, or of spleen!"*

This was full-blast melancholia. And its expression in English romantic poets such as Cowper and Thomas Gray had a dramatic influence on striving young romantic spirits on the Continent. We like to think of melancholia as a predominantly biological illness, and the evidence of biomarkers such as the dexamethasone suppression test and serum cortisol suggest the correctness of that view. Yet there is a cultural component. And when German poets such as Johann Wolfgang von Goethe got their hands on the English romantics, they in turn became melancholic! Or at least they fashioned their subjective illness experiences on the template of those they had been reading about. Goethe said much later in his 1811 autobiography that if German youth at the end of the eighteenth century began to brood upon the transitory nature of passions such as romantic love, it was because the Germans had "an external occasion for these gloomy preoccupations…in the English literature, especially the poetry, whose great merits are accompanied by a serious melancholy, which comes across to every person who tarries at these pages."[37] It was indeed under these influences that Goethe himself wrote in 1774 *The Sorrows of Young Werther,* one of the great classics of Romantic literature—but highly depressive; Werther commits suicide at the end, as in fact Goethe himself had once attempted suicide.

A cardinal characteristic of melancholia is the inability of patients to experience pleasure, called in 1897 by French psychologist Théodule Ribot anhedonia: "insensibility relating to pleasure alone."[38] In 1913 the influential German psychopathologist Karl Jaspers termed it "the feeling of loss of feelings." "The patients complain that they are unable to experience pleasure or pain."[39] (The notion of anhedonia then slumbered for a number of years until in 1974 Columbia psychiatrist Donald Klein revived it in the concept of endogenomorphic depression, the kind of depression not precipitated by external events.[40]) Yet from the patient's viewpoint, anhedonia, conceived as the loss of pleasure rather than the loss of interest, is a core component of the melancholic experience. (As English psychiatrist Philip Snaith at Leeds pointed out in 1992, "A gardener may retain an interest in the flowers he grows but no longer experiences pleasure at their sight or their smell."[41]) In 1821 Fanny Burney, depressed now in her own turn, lamented, "The spirit of enjoyment is gone!—gone!—though the animal spirits still, at times, are revived by social exertions."[42] The blackness of spirits in melancholia that echoes to us across the ages reflects the loss of any pleasure in life.

There are several other important points about melancholia. It is a recurrent illness, not a one-shot affair. "Virtually every patient experiences more than one episode," said Jules Angst, professor of research psychiatry in Zurich, in 1973 apropos of a five-country study of hospital cases.[43]

Melancholia digs deep into the brain and body, putting patients in touch with their most primeval—and often sinister—impulses. Fantasies of murder and suicide are common themes. New York neurologist Landon Gray Carter believed that a vague feeling of distress in the back of the head and neck was a diagnostic sign of melancholia (which it is not); such symptoms in his patients often prompted him to prod a bit deeper. He reported in 1890 a "lady" who had come to see him with such a complaint: "I then asked her whether she had not at the beginning been very much depressed." She said yes, and "with so embarrassed an air as to make me assured that there was something concealed…She burst into tears, and admitted that she also had passed through an attack of melancholia, and astonished me in her turn by telling me that she was the wife of a well-known physician, and that she had concealed all knowledge of her mental condition from her husband, because she was afraid that he would send her to an asylum. This poor woman had absolutely on several occasions felt so strong an impulse to kill her children and herself that she had been obliged to leave the house and get away from them."[44]

Altruistic murder is often at the core of such impulses in melancholia, murdering someone else to save them from an imagined terrible fate. In Houston, Texas, in 2001, Andrea Yates—in the throes of a psychotic depression—drowned her five children one by one in the bathtub of her home to save them from the fires of hell.[45] (That such a tragedy could have been prevented had she been diagnosed in a timely manner and treated with electroconvulsive therapy makes the importance of getting it right all the more urgent.)

A French psychiatry textbook noted in the early 1920s how common suicide was in melancholia, and that "in women it can co-exist with murdering the children, intended to save them from the tortures that await them."[46] And just apropos! Through the forensic infirmary of the Paris Prefecture of Police passed all kinds of melancholic cases, including in March 1921, Angelina-Maria A, age 44 years, housewife, her husband a sommelier in a restaurant. In the telegraphic style of Gaëtan Gatian de Clérambault, the chief psychiatrist, she had "Delusions of persecution. Auditory hallucinations. Patient was also delusional: The malady is filled with consequences. Disordered internal sensations. Melancholic phase with a very marked tendency to suicide and to altruistic murder. For two weeks she had hidden a hammer under her pillow to kill her husband and her child, with the intention of suiciding afterwards by leaping from the window. On March 15, having dispatched the witnesses on a pretext, she began to beat her child with a brush, and tried thereupon to jump out the window. Formal, repeated confession of homicidal intent towards the child with the motive that, if she herself were to die, she would have left the child at the mercy of her own tormentors…Telepathy. Holes in the floor with a fluid rising up. Various odors."[47] Today we would probably say psychotic depression, rather than melancholia, yet such crazed depressions usually are melancholic.

Melancholic patients with the idea of making away themselves and others are often very secretive about their plans because they do not wish to be thwarted. As a result, clinicians may miss the gravity of the diagnosis. Miss Leila Herbert, daughter of the ex-Secretary of the Navy Hilary Herbert, deceived everyone when she committed suicide in 1897 by plunging herself head-first from the window of a house on fashionable New Hampshire Avenue in Washington. She had fallen from a horse and became melancholic in the course of a long convalescence. But on the day of her death, she disarmed the nurses who had been hired to watch over her by being "unusually bright and cheerful, and chatted animatedly with her married sister." Who could have suspected? But then one of the nurses saw a small bloodstain on the patient's bedding. "She inquired what it meant but the invalid endeavored to pass it by lightly. On making an investigation., however, the nurse found that the under bedclothes were saturated with blood, and that Miss Herbert had severed an artery of her wrist with a pair of scissors."[48] As the nurse rushed to the door to give alarm, Miss Herbert took advantage of the occasion to plunge from the window, landing on her skull.

Arthur Zankel, a financier and philanthropist who committed suicide in 2005 by leaping from the window of his New York apartment on Fifth Avenue, was secretive in the weeks before his death. "Everything aches," he told his son Tommy. He asked about falling from the ninth floor, whether the fall would be uninterrupted. He invented excuses for not seeing people and lied to his secretary, said a story in the *Wall Street Journal*, "telling her he would be out for a few weeks because he was having 'a minor surgical procedure.'" The tragedy of his death came as a huge surprise to everyone except his wife, who realized what was going on but thought he was being treated appropriately by his clinicians (the treatments for Zankel's melancholic illness apparently did not include electroconvulsive therapy*).[49] It is, in other words, normal for melancholics to behave slyly about their plans to end their lives, which are often worked out well in advance, in contrast to nervous patients, who too may commit suicide but in a more impulsive manner.[50] Melancholia is nothing if not cunning.

Or for other reasons melancholia may hide its face, even just to maintain the appearances of normality. John Scott Price, a psychiatrist at Northwick Park Hospital in Harrow, England, called such behavior in 1978 the "great cover-up": The depressed patient refuses to "tell others how bad he feels. Most depressives, even severe ones, can cope with routine work—initiative and leadership are what they lack. Nevertheless, many of them can continue working, functioning at a fairly low level... The world leaves the depressive alone and he battles on for the sake of his god or his children, or for some reason which makes his personal torment preferable to death."[51]

---

*Electroconvulsive therapy, or ECT, means procuring a therapeutic brain seizure by applying two electrodes to either side of the cranium; this bilateral placement of electrodes is very effective. ECT is the most powerful treatment that psychiatry has on offer, and more may be learned about its history in Edward Shorter and David Healy, *Shock Therapy: A History of Electroconvulsive Treatment in Mental Illness*. New Brunswick, NJ: Rutgers University Press, 2007.

What emerges from the stories of melancholic patients is how different they are from patients with nervous disease. This is not a continuum of gravity that begins with the mildly nervous and ends with patients curled into a fetal ball, but a discontinuity as two different kinds of illness somehow end up with depression as their name. Melancholia was not neurotic depression. Among the women admitted to the closed ward of the Holloway Sanatorium just outside of London in 1889, there were plenty of melancholics. See if this sounds like nervous illness: Charlotte L, a single secretary of 36, came into Holloway Sanatorium on January 31. She had two medical certificates justifying her involuntary admission to a closed ward. One said, "Is suspicious, restless and sleepless, thinks she has done some crime and ought to go to prison." The other said that "She thinks she has done some great injury to a lady of Torquay."

History of present illness: She apparently suffered overwork in "keeping the accounts of a large house of business. The onset of the attack was marked by extreme depression, loss of sleep and appetite." "Mentally," said a staff psychiatrist, "she is suffering from simple melancholia . . . She has grossly deceived all her friends, that she has led a sinful life (which is untrue)."

Charlotte L spent half a year on the ward and improved steadily, though almost to her discharge in June "she states that her ideas cannot change since her past life has been so unpardonably sinful, and that when her true character is discovered she will be shunned by all good people." Yet these notions, too, passed and in mid-June, at the request of her family, she was discharged "recovered."[52] Holloway Sanatorium had no particular treatments for melancholia and rarely used opium, the only effective medication. But melancholia has a natural history of its own, and most patients recover within 8 months spontaneously.

Some of the melancholic women who came into Holloway in 1889 were suicidal. Mary L, 44, housewife, depressed for a year, was said by the physician who issued her first certificate to be "listless, apathetic, profoundly depressed because of fancied ill-treatment of her husband, thinks she has conspired with others to ruin him, at times is excited at the probable consequences of her awful wickedness and wishes to end her life." The second certificate said she imagined "her wickedness will ruin her husband and the entire world. That the cause of the wickedness is writing a letter. She threatens to drown herself." At admission in February, the nurses were warned, "She is suicidal, but not dangerous to others."

On the unit, "She thinks one of the companions (Miss R) is her brother in female dress, and attacks her whenever she comes into the ward. Of late she has more obstinately refused her food." After the passage of some months she was well enough to travel down to the convalescent home of the sanatorium in the seaside spa of Bournemouth. "She has greatly benefited by the change. Occasionally she goes home for a day in charge of her husband." Thus she slowly became better and in September she was discharged "recovered."[53]

The gap between nervous illness and what was seen at the Holloway positively assails the reader! Emily T, 44 years old when she came into the Holloway in April 1889, was having her fourth attack of melancholia, the first having occurred at age 27. She had been hospitalized for all of them. This time, she had been sick for about a year, and now "was afraid the lady she lived with would murder her. Said she ran after strange men as her brother," said certificate one. Certificate two noted that she "Washes herself with boiling water."

At admission, "The skin both of face and hands and wrists is excessively coarse, thickened and uniformly red from the custom she has of washing them in hot soda [caustic lye]…Mentally she is suffering from melancholia and dementia." (The clinicians took her habit of sitting motionlessly and staring fixedly all day long—possibly a sign of catatonia—as "dementia.") She was generally mute, save for rising at every visit of the doctor to ask "Can I go now?" She also refused her food on the grounds that "It is too fearful to eat in this place!!" She was often tube fed.

By July 1891 she had been at the Holloway, on various wards depending on her behavior, for over 2 years. "She remains weak-minded and depressed, dull and listless. She is reported to be addicted to masturbation." (Many of these female patients, in Victorian Britain, masturbated quite openly, alarming the staff for medical not moral reasons: Masturbation was believed to cause insanity and was carefully noted in the chart. Jane Hillyer, in a private sanatorium in the United States around the time of World War I, also admits to masturbating quite openly: She had the delusional belief that it had "appeared in the papers."[54]) Later in 1891 Emily was transferred to another private psychiatric hospital, and then to another, at which, in August 1892, she was declared "relieved," meaning improved, but not well.[55]

It would be impossible to mistake any of these patients, psychotic and mute, some smearing their feces, for nervous, and the term nervous illness is almost never used in the charts. Yet contemporaries would have widely agreed that they had suffered nervous breakdowns.

Past Physicians' Sense of Melancholia Not So Different from Our Own

Since the seventeenth century, medical writers have described melancholia in a manner quite similar to our own, suggesting that we are dealing here with a relatively unchanging biological type, like diabetes or stroke, rather than—as in the case of many psychiatric illnesses—with a phenomenon heavily influenced by personal beliefs and social attitudes. What changes historically in medical writing is the differentiation of melancholic depression from other kinds of depression. But the basic melancholic prototype has been visible from the beginning.

In 1602 Felix Platter in Basel described a number of "melancholic" patients, who were indeed sad, despairing, and psychotic. One was a peasant woman, "of great beauty," who had given birth, then became melancholic during nursing. "She developed the habit of saying continuously, as she nursed her child and was in medical treatment, 'I can no longer live and be in this world, I must leave it, I must die.' In doing so she mentioned no cause that might have agitated her so greatly. She tried to hang herself with a rope that she had contrived at home, but was freed from death by someone who came along and tore the sling down..."[56] To be sure, Platter includes other cases that sound more directly psychotic than melancholic. Yet he certainly understood the core concept and did not use the term merely as a synonym for madness.

In 1799 James Sims, president of the Medical Society of London, gave a description of melancholy that would not be out of place in a learned seminar today. "In the first approaches of melancholy, the persons become silent and absorbed in thought, dislike being spoken to or roused, and seem always occupied in some grave contemplation. Jests, laughter, and every species of hilarity seem irksome to them." This is a description, of course, of anhedonia, the inability to experience pleasure.

As the illness progressed, said Sims, "Their speech is slow, sedate, solemn, measured, and argumentative; and they are mostly buried in sorrow." In addition to sadness, Sims describes here what later generations would term psychomotor slowing, a fundamental characteristic of melancholia.

At this point, continued Sims, they start to become psychotic, not his term. "They complain of some action that they have done against some friend or relative, or some crime that they have committed, which can never be forgiven by God or man. This action is often totally imaginary."

Yet it gets even worse, said Sims. "They become suspicious of all around them and imagine that they see conspiracies against them in the most trifling occurrences. They think all their friends are become enemies, which induces a taedium vitae, ending often in suicide."

And anxious! Sims painted a picture of melancholic anxiety: "They enjoy but little sleep, and that anxious, waking often in a fright. They become extremely silent, but have great anxiety painted on their countenance, which at the last becomes austere and morose, with eyes betokening treachery and despair." They experience other somatic symptoms that much later generations of doctors would call "neurovegetative" in nature: "They may refuse nourishment, fasting for days, nay, often weeks." They become indifferent to the ambient temperature, huddling close to the fire in summer, "whilst in winter they appear insensible of cold."[57] As a description of melancholia, this is spot on. Few would confuse it with the nervous syndrome.

In the course of the nineteenth century, a much tighter picture of melancholia evolved, one that differentiated it from nonmelancholic depression. But it is necessary to bear in mind an admonition in 1976 of Leo Hollister, an internist with a deep knowledge of psychiatry at the Veterans Administration Hospital in Palo Alto, California, and generally considered the dean of United States psychopharmacology: There is, he said, no given symptom that is pathognomonic, or absolutely characteristic, for any psychiatric illness. "They all overlap, so one cannot go on specific symptoms, which are meaningless." Hollister said it was the *constellation* of symptoms that gives the diagnosis, and this constellation is often referred to as the syndrome.[58] So this is not an exact science, and, aside from the few biological markers that do exist in psychiatry—such as the dexamethasone suppression test—diagnosis remains pattern recognition rather than peering at the laboratory results.

There were several big changes in psychiatric thinking about melancholia during the nineteenth century. For one thing, the medical conception of melancholia as a disease of intellect gave way to views of it as a disorder of the emotions, of affect. Doctors' views are different from actual historic descriptions of the disease itself, which, as we saw above, are full of affective symptoms. But physicians, when they looked, saw more madness than sadness. John Ferriar, an asylum psychiatrist in Manchester and "physician to the Manchester Infirmary," reflected this older view when he wrote in 1819, "A melancholic perceives, not wrongly [as in mania], but too intensely regarding some objects, which induces him to grant them an exclusive attention, and leads him to reason improperly." What does this mean? "A melancholy patient, despairing of his circumstances without foundation, was persuaded with much difficulty to draw up a short statement of his affairs... He placed his debts in one column, and his property in another, opposite. But no argument nor intreaties could prevail upon him to compare the columns, by which it would have appeared that he was master of a considerable sum: his attention was wholly occupied with the list of his debts, and he obstinately averted his eyes from the other column."[59] What Ferriar is describing here is a thought disorder, or perhaps an example of obsessive thinking, but not a mood disorder.

Then the asylum doctors, the alienists, slowly began to pivot and to regard melancholia as a disorder of emotion rather than intellect. Etienne Esquirol, Pinel's successor and staff psychiatrist at the Salpêtrière hospice, later chief physician of the French state asylum at Charenton, was probably the first to conduct this pivot when, in 1821, he proposed the term lypémanie for melancholia, disliking the latter's association with humoralism and black bile. Lypemania was a psychotic "partial disorder" of mind and brain, rather than total insanity, and was characterized by a "sad passion" driving the delusional thinking.[60] Many authors took this up, and the pivot was certainly accomplished by 1852, when Joseph Guislain, professor of psychiatry in Ghent, wrote, "All melancholia expresses the lesion of a sentiment; it represents a painful affect [une affection douloureuse]." Yet "Despite the sadness that strikes these patients, they almost never cry."[61] This is clearly the modern conception of melancholia, and it developed particularly in France in the first half of the nineteenth century—the heyday of the French domination of psychiatry.

In a second development, melancholia and mania came to be seen as the primary disturbances, or original disorders, in a chain of events that would inevitably lead through irrational thought to dementia. There was, in other words, really only one psychotic illness, and various symptoms and syndromes were just stages in an unfolding of that process; it became known as the "unitary psychosis" view (in German, Einheitspsychose). Wilhelm Griesinger, as a young asylum psychiatrist still in his 20s, was its chief initiator—though Griesinger was heavily influenced by the writings of his chief Ernst Albert Zeller. Those who took the unitary psychosis view were analogizing from neurosyphilis, a then common tertiary complication of syphilis: Neurosyphilis was indeed a single disease with a progression through stages, and no two patients might have the same symptoms at the same time because they were at different stages. Hence, psychosis might be like this too, an orderly march through stages from an initial episode of mania or depression to an abject end in the back wards of an asylum. Griesinger wrote in 1845, in the first edition of what was later to become a world-beating textbook, "There is on the whole a constant successive course [starting with melancholia] that can lead to the complete disintegration of psychic life." The therapeutic consequences of this inevitable progression were rather grim: "Insanity is really only during this first group of primary affective mental anomalies curable; with the progression to the secondary [floridly psychotic] disturbances the disease becomes incurable."[62]

We need a footnote here: Connoisseurs of the history of depressive illness may say that the first writer to break up melancholia on a meaningful basis (meaning not on the basis of symptoms but of clinical course) was Karl Kahlbaum, one of the great names in the history of understanding psychiatric illness. It was Kahlbaum who in 1874 coined the term catatonia[63] and whose academic-habilitation essay in 1863 made him among the first to classify illness on the basis of course. At the time, Kahlbaum, age 35 years, was still an assistant physician at the Prussian state asylum in Allenberg, and saw mainly very sick people. He distinguished between melancholia as a "Vesania," meaning insanity affecting the entire mind and brain, and as a "Vecordia," meaning partial insanity limited to the sphere of feeling. Vesanic melancholy, he said, might well pass through a manic stage, and a stage of insanity, to end in dementia. Vecordic melancholy might well not progress. Hence there was a difference between vesanic (terminal) melancholy and vecordic (self-limiting) melancholy. (Kahlbaum used the term dysthymia as well as melancholia. Hence the dysthymia meläna was the typically sad Vecordia.)

Kahlbaum did in fact separate melancholia from nonmelancholia with the term dysphrenia nervosa, which meant organic neurological illness: A subtype of it, nervosa depressa, was nonmelancholic "depression," and Kahlbaum used the d-word.[64] Only when Kraepelin started to rethink the entire question of the psychoses and mood disorders years later did he stumble across Kahlbaum's habilitation, cited it, and made it famous. Kahlbaum's 1863 book itself was not influential.

The name of the game here was to separate melancholia from nonmelancholia, and this Kahlbaum had in fact done but in a manner so confusing and filled with neologisms that few understood it. The first step occurred with a small and often overlooked work in 1867 by Richard von Krafft-Ebing, then a staff physician at the Illenau asylum in Germany and later professor of psychiatry in Vienna and author of the international bestseller *Psychopathia Sexualis*; his little book was intended for use in forensic medicine. Krafft-Ebing said that it was necessary to distinguish between simple psychic depression and the varieties of psychotic depression, of which he discerned two: depression plus hallucinations and "melancholic delusional disorder, which as well might be marked with hallucinations."[65] This was the first formal distinction between depression and psychotic melancholia. But by "depression" Krafft seems to have understood mainly nonpsychotic melancholia, and he uses depression and melancholia as synonyms.

This basic distinction between nonmelancholic depression and psychotic melancholia was then refined in coming years. In 1879 Latvian physician

Theodor Tiling, leader of a private nervous clinic in St Petersburg, tried to drum up business for this kind of open facility by distinguishing between a depressive dysthymia, suitable for such a clinic, and fully psychotic melancholic illness ("I shot the Kaiser!") that was probably the beginning of the progression to madness and dementia and that belonged in a closed facility. The dysthymic were not silent and guarded but easily expressed their opinions to the physicians, and had merely pressures in the head and stomach from their "pangs of conscience." (So in Tiling's dysthymia there was a hint of psychosis.) Dysthymia was recurrent, but did not deteriorate into insanity, Tiling said.[66] (Dysthymia may be conceived as the depressive component of the nervous syndrome, whereas psychotic melancholy occurred in nervous breakdowns.)

Carl Georg Lange, professor of pathological anatomy in Copenhagen and considered Denmark's "first neurologist," evidently did not know of Tiling's work. Lange was much more influential, and in 1886 he formally distinguished between what he called periodic depression and melancholia. "It might at first glance appear singular that such a general and important kind of illness, such as the depressive conditions discussed here, are so little known and that in the literature one finds only slight traces here and there, and that as a result physicians as well have only very vague and unclear ideas of these matters." He saw neurasthenia as a kind of rubbish bin, but made a fundamental distinction between melancholia and "periodic depression." "The pathognomonic features of the illness," he said of periodic depression, were "the heaviness, tiredness, and flaccidity which the patients complain about constantly, the feeling of a great burden that crushes them physically and mentally to the ground, the apathy, that makes them indifferent to everything…Under the influence of this 'mental pressure,' our patients tend to reject all work, all duty and…to surrender to their feelings of misery." In fact, they are still capable of going to work, but report feelings of "mental rigidity, or petrification…as if the protoplasm in their brain cells had truly become fixed." So this was one depression, a kind of running-out-of-gas feeling, as Harvard's Joseph Schildkraut much later would characterize it.[67]

Lange did not use the term nervous syndrome, but periodic depression could well have been yet another term for the depression of that syndrome, given that, in addition to being tired, the patients were also anxious, and tended to obsess about their condition. "This anxiety has no particular foundation; they aren't afraid of this or that, but rather are dominated by a general, indeterminate feeling of anxiety." Men suffered more from an inability to get on with the job at hand and women from a deadening of feeling. Loss of appetite and insomnia completed the picture.

And then there was melancholia. "The depressives never become melancholics," said Lange. "The characteristic aspect of the melancholic is, that his feelings of oppression and anxiety arise from obsessive thoughts, from imaginary persecutions or hallucinations, and that as a result the melancholic considers his desperation to be thoroughly justified." Lange said that melancholia meant psychosis. Among the depressives there was no trace of psychosis: "Their illness consists solely and alone in an anomaly of mood, and they are always completely clear about this, that their mood is not justified by external circumstances."[68]

Subsequent generations would squabble about what exactly constituted depression versus melancholia, but these early works offered the first clear statement that they were different diseases.

The Death of Melancholia

It was Emil Kraepelin who killed off melancholia and prompted its replacement with depression. Normally, we would not assess scientific progress in terms of the successive editions of a textbook, but Kraepelin's textbook, which first appeared in 1883 and started to become highly influential with the fourth edition in 1893, dominated world discussion of the classification of illness. And to understand why the nervous breakdown became less fearsome, we have to understand how melancholia was turned into depression. This happened in Kraepelin's *Psychiatry: A Textbook for Students and Physicians.*[69] In the 1893 fourth edition, the discussion was quite conventional: "melancholia" was a separate illness, and depression was part of "the periodic mental illnesses," a separate category.

It was then the fifth edition in 1896 that abolished melancholia and replaced it with depression. Among the "psychic disorders with a constitutional basis," we find "periodic insanity," and part of these periodically recurring illnesses was "depressive forms." There were also "circular forms" of depression, the depressive conditions alternating with the expansive conditions—classic "circular insanity," in other words, as the French had described it half a century before. Yet the term depression carried the main freight, which melancholia had previously borne.

But this fifth edition did retain "melancholia" in one particular sense: Melancholia was one form of involutional insanity, meaning illnesses that overcame people in mid-life as their sex organs began to shrink up, or involute. This was a serious illness, a crack-up. Patients took much longer to recover than with depression, if in fact they ever did. Of his older patients with melancholia, only 25% recovered completely.[70] Involutional depression or melancholia went on to become a world-beating diagnosis, taken up in the discourse of psychiatry in every land—and even today we occasionally hear the term involutional, for those who fall ill later in life.

Why had Kraepelin substituted depression for melancholia? He never explained exactly, but in the "involutional" section he did say that he was retaining the term "melancholia" only for these illnesses with onset at midlife: "We designate with the term melancholia all pathological sad or anxious mood disorders [Verstimmungen] of the later years, which do not represent part of the course of other forms of insanity."[71]

The Kraepelin story has two more chapters. In the sixth edition in 1899 he created manic-depressive insanity, collapsing a number of previous distinctions about depression in circular insanity and so forth, and lumping every kind of depression and mania, regardless of circularity or periodicity, together in one big pot. Every form of mood disorder became manic-depressive insanity. Note that this is not the same thing as bipolar disorder today, because we have a separate unipolar depression, and although Kraepelin had recognized that separateness in 1896, he no longer did in 1899. (Kraepelin retained involutional melancholia.) He said, by way of explanation for creating what became known as "MDI": "In the course of the years, I have convinced myself more and more, that all these illness pictures [mania, circular and periodic mood disorders etc] are only presentations of a single disease process....It is, as far as I know, entirely impossible to discern any particular boundaries among these individual clinical pictures, that until now have been held separate."[72] (This edition also executed the fateful separation between manic-depressive illness and dementia praecox—later schizophrenia—that has prevailed to this day and that ended the unitary psychosis doctrine: Kraepelin established the idea that these were separate disorders. They did not turn into one another, any more than mumps turned into tuberculosis.)

The great Kraepelinian shift from melancholia to depression was completed in the eighth edition in 1913—the last that Kraepelin personally was able to bring to a conclusion—when he abolished involutional melancholia and made it part of manic-depressive insanity. Georges Dreyfus's 1907 work at Heidelberg convinced him that involutional melancholia had the same course and outcome as other mood disorders, and that it was pointless to keep it separate. Also, the term melancholia was superfluous, said Dreyfus, as the illness picture was part of manic-depressive disease.[73]

Yet involutional melancholia took wings as a diagnosis, even though Kraepelin had tried to withdraw it, and became the catch-all phrase for serious illness in those aged 50 or older. English psychiatrist Eliot Slater recalled the asylum scene in the 1930s: "The involutional melancholic would be a thin, elderly man or woman, inert, with the head lifted up off the pillow [a sign of catatonia]. There were some sort of Parkinsonian-like qualities, mask-like face sunk deep into misery, and speaking in a retarded way. If you could get them to say anything, it would be something about how hopeless things were, how they were wicked, doomed to disease, death, and a terrible afterlife, if there was one."[74] There remained this single trace of the great melancholia edifice.

A diagnosis like melancholia with such a long pedigree could not easily be decreed out of existence, and Kraepelin did make the occasional bow to it. He conceded that psychotic depression might be termed melancholia gravis, to emphasize its pathological fury.[75] Elsewhere in this great work, that by 1913 had swollen to four volumes, he suggested that particularly malignant outcomes might be referred to as melancholic.[76] Yet the term melancholia disappeared as an independent disease entity.

Not everyone was enchanted. Alfred Hoche, professor of psychiatry in Freiburg im Breisgau (the German Freiburg, not the Swiss), disliked the construction of these great disease entities such as manic-depressive illness and dementia praecox because their contents were too disparate. And he deplored the disappearance of melancholia. "It is characteristic," he said in 1910, "of the uncertainty of our current clinical world that such an old and well-established heirloom of psychiatry as melancholia should go into liquidation and fall under the auctioneer's hammer." The whole debate about whether involutional melancholia should be part of manic-depressive illness was pointless, he said, because neither existed.[77] [It is striking how these warnings foreshadowed the criticism of such categories as major depression of the *Diagnostic and Statistical Manual* (*DSM*) of the American Psychiatric Association a hundred years later.]

Yet these warnings were soon forgotten. Kraepelin's advocacy of depression over melancholia proved highly influential. On the other side of the Atlantic, in 1904 Adolf Meyer, who taught psychiatry at Cornell University Medical School in New York City and was already the most influential psychiatrist in the United States (even before taking the chair at Johns Hopkins), cast his ballot for the abolition of melancholia. He told a meeting of the New York Neurological Society that "On the whole, he was desirous of eliminating the term melancholia, which implied a knowledge of something we did not possess... [hard to know what he was getting at here] If, instead of melancholia, we applied the term depression to the whole class, it would designate in an unassuming way exactly what was meant by the common use of the term melancholia…"[78]

Why is it so important, or even interesting, to learn how depression replaced melancholia? Because depression is a less terrible word. Nervous breakdowns that happened to the melancholic were catastrophic events; those in the merely depressed, though subjectively fearsome, sounded less fearful because so many people were calling themselves depressed. Novelist William Styron, in a poignant memoir of his own nervous breakdown, written in 1990, appreciated the importance of this semantic difference: Styron himself had experienced agonies that make the rabies comparison seem realistic, and after his recovery he wrote that "'Melancholia' would still appear to be a far more apt and evocative word for the blacker forms of the disorder, but it was usurped by a noun with a bland tonality and lacking any magisterial presence, used indifferently to describe an economic decline or a rut in the ground, a true wimp of a word for such a major illness."[79]

And so, thanks to Kraepelin, melancholia began to shrink from center stage, giving way to the true wimp, depression. But the term melancholia had acquired huge historical momentum, and would persist decades after Kraepelin and Meyer turned up their noses at it. Henry Yellowlees, physician for mental diseases at St. Thomas's Hospital in London, warned the Section of Psychiatry of the Royal Society of Medicine in 1930 not to make the mistake of adopting the "popular view that melancholia was a caricature of normal depression." "The neurasthenic was a person of active emotional reactions, who bewailed the limitations which his illness imposed upon him; whereas the melancholic was the reverse."[80]

Thus the clinical picture of melancholia remained hard to mistake. Giovanni Mingazzini, professor of psychiatry in Rome and director of the university psychiatric clinic, also headed a private sanatorium for women. He said in 1926, "A good third of the [sanatorium] patients suffer from typical melancholia." He thought the percentage up over time, and also noted that the nature of their self-accusations had changed from having spit on the communion host, to having given the children syphilis (despite not having it themselves) or stolen money from friends.[81] It is for such patients that the term melancholia retains a certain robustness even today.

7

The Nervous Breakdown

NERVOUS BREAKDOWN HAS never been a medical term. It is a patients'
term, just as cerumen has always been a doctors' term for ear wax. Yet patients
once believed profoundly in nervous breakdowns as a psychiatric condition
several pegs higher than nerves, until the great switch to depression. Even
today, the concept of the nervous breakdown has a kind of subterranean existence in the patients' folklore. Yet the nerve syndrome was a quite specific pattern of illness whereas the nervous breakdown was not. The nerve syndrome
entailed anxiety, depression, fatigue, somatic illness, and obsessive concern.
Looking back over historical records, we can see who had the nerve syndrome
and who did not.

Nervous breakdown shares only the term nerves in common with the nerve
syndrome. It is a synonym for serious psychiatric illness of any kind, not a specific disorder. In a short story in *Collier's* magazine in 1935, George, the hero,
tries unsuccessfully to contact Josephine, on whom he has cast a lustful eye. "He
saw no other girls. He went home nights and walked the floor and drank too
many drinks and didn't go to sleep until all hours."[1] The title of the story was
"nervous breakdown," but clearly George did not have a psychiatric illness.

Here, on the other hand, is John F. O'Donnell, the chief of police in
Denver, who shot himself to death in 1949. In a note that he left behind for
his wife and son he said, "I feel like I am going to have a nervous breakdown
and surely do not want to be a burden to you."[2] For Chief O'Donnell, a
nervous breakdown was a nontrivial illness. Dr. John E. Eichenlaub, writing
in *Today's Health* in 1954, said, "You hear a lot of people say that a nervous
breakdown ruins a person for life, that no one ever gets over one."[3] This is
pretty serious business, not at all what George had. (Dr Eichenlaub went on
to dispel readers' fears.)

So clearly a nervous breakdown was not a specific disease but anything going wrong in one's emotional life that was deemed serious, and in today's terms, a nervous breakdown could have been an episode of melancholia, a brief bout of psychosis, an encounter with catatonic stupor, a panic, or a moment of psychotic anxiety. In describing nervous breakdowns we are not therefore identifying a specific disease, but understanding why the term "nerves" has had such staying power in popular culture: It is a tag for distress and inability to cope. But the drama of the story is how this tag, and its cousin the nervous syndrome, slides from nerves to depression.

Doctors and the Nervous Breakdown

Physicians generally speaking have never accepted the notion of the nervous breakdown and when their patients raised it, doctors treated the whole concept condescendingly.[4] Thomas Ross, a specialist in psychoneuroses and former head of an English hospital for the treatment of "functional nervous disorders," said in 1923 that if you asked your patient about his own view of the matter, "the commonest reply is to the effect that his nerves are run down." Of course Ross would hear nothing of this, and suggested telling patients that the nervous system "is more of the nature of a telephone exchange into which messages come and from which they go."[5] This concept was no more scientifically exact than the views of Ross's patients, but illustrates medicine's great impatience in these years with the concept of tired nerves—Ross himself was sympathetic to the ideas of the Freudian school.

Doctors wrote constantly in the popular press about what really constituted a nervous breakdown, hoping to detach readers from obnoxiously unscientific notions about nerves. In 1936 Jacob Markowitz, a member of the department of physiology of the University of Toronto, commented that "There is an extraordinary amount of nervousness in big cities today," and said that, in real medical terms, it would boil down to anxiety neurosis, compulsion neurosis, neurasthenia, melancholia, and hysteria.[6] (After the outbreak of war, Markowitz became something of a hero in treating desperately ill men—he himself had also been taken prisoner—in a Japanese prisoner of war camp.[7]) It is ironic that many of the supposedly scientific diagnoses that doctors in the 1930s wished to thrust upon their patients, such as hysteria, were themselves later discredited. Medical efforts to substitute truth for folly have themselves a long and embarrassing history.

But in the patients' world, the nervous breakdown was omnipresent and medicine had to deal with it. During World War II, many draftees gave histories of "nervous breakdowns" to Army psychiatrists such as Samuel Kraines, who normally taught at the University of Illinois College of Medicine. Should they be deferred? Yes, said Kraines. The histories the patients gave of "breakdowns"—which he put in quotation marks—savored of insomnia, great fatigue, inability to concentrate, and depressive feelings. Kraines diagnosed this as manic-depression and said the men would crack under combat.[8]

Thus doctors often came into contact with the concept of nervous breakdowns, but always in the tales of their patients, received with an arched medical eyebrow.

Did physicians nowhere accept the notion of breakdown and crisis? Yes, in France. The French term for nervous breakdown is "crise nerveuse," and there is a tradition in French psychiatry of diagnosing "crises," analogizing from the fever crisis in internal medicine as the moment when the patient takes a turn for the better. Etienne Esquirol inaugurated this kind of analogy in 1816, saying, "Why wouldn't the doctrine of crises be applicable to mental alienation [psychiatry]? Does madness not have causes, symptoms, and a course that are distinctive? Why should it not be judged as other diseases?"[9] In 1860 Bénédict-Augustin Morel, chief physician of the Saint-Yon asylum near Rouen (and originator of the doctrine of degeneration in psychiatry), spoke of the "crisis"—possibly an eruption of erysipelas, a bacterial infection, in a manic patient—as the first prognostic sign of a favorable outcome.[10]

In French psychiatry it was then neurologist Jean-Martin Charcot who abducted the crisis concept, borrowed from the study of fevers, and imported it into psychiatric pathology in the form of the "hysterical crisis," a theatrical display of great passions as the supposed episode of hysteria found its climax.[11] Because of Charcot's great influence, this kind of crisis reached its apogee in French psychiatry late in the nineteenth century, and lingered on in official diagnostics as the "crise émotive," something resembling a panic attack.[12]

But French psychiatry is very distinctive in this regard. Psychological medicine elsewhere had little use for crises and certainly not for breakdowns, regarded as unscientific metaphors.[13]

The Rise and Fall of the Nervous Breakdown

The term nervous breakdown itself had a relatively brief life. It surfaced only late in the nineteenth century. Ella Adelia Fletcher, a popular health writer, deplored in 1900 the reckless expenditure of "nerve-force" that led to "a form of disease which is so much more acute in the United States than anywhere else in the world, that it has received the generic name Americanitus." And the specific form of Americanitus was "nervous collapse." "The living death of a nervous wreck is one of the most pitiable spectacles that we ever encounter, and destroys the happiness of more homes than actual death ever does."[14] So, here is the nervous breakdown before our eyes.

In American periodical literature a slow trickle of articles on nervous breakdown begins before World War I. In 1909, for example, James Jackson Putnam, a distinguished Boston neurologist, with a large psychotherapy practice, cautioned against nervous strain and tension.[15] After World War I, nerves and nervousness took increasing prominence in the national discussion—including contributions in 1918 such as "Why the Jew is Too Neurotic."[16]

References to "nervous breakdown" in headlines of the *New York Times*, searchable in a database, do not begin until 1905. "C Oliver Iselin Ill: Suffers a Nervous Breakdown," was the initial headline (Iselin was a noted yachtsman).[17] Thereafter, most nervous breakdown stories oscillated between suicides and people who abandoned public life because they could not function anymore. The 5-year period 1925–1929 was the highpoint of such stories, with 34. References to nervous breakdowns then decline steadily across the 1930s and peter out after 1944. Subsequently, there would be only a handful; the last clinical nervous breakdown story ran in 1961: "$100,000 Bail Asked in Miami in Event Frenchman Returns to U.S.—Wife Says He Had 'Nervous Breakdown.'"[18] The nervous breakdown arc thus clearly tracks across the first four decades of the twentieth century. Previously, headline writers chose terms such as mental derangement; afterward they used the term depression.

It is of interest that the *Times* treated "nervous disorder" as a synonym for nervous breakdown, using it, however, far less frequently. The mother who shot her child and killed herself in 1909—the first mention in a headline— had a "nervous disorder."[19] Thereafter it was used interchangeably with nervous breakdown in describing suicides. Al Capone's nervous disorder made it impossible, said his doctor, for him to appear in court in 1941.[20] The last reference to nervous disorder was in 1947 ("Turkish Patriarch ... Said to Be Victim of Nervous Disorder"[21]). So newspaper editors did not care very much for "nervous" terms, certainly not after the Great Depression.

But among people in the real world the nervous breakdown was indeed a hot topic, becoming by the 1920s the standard designation for any serious psychiatric affliction. Julian Huxley, the well-known evolutionary biologist and science writer, suffered a "nervous breakdown" in 1913 following a romantic misadventure; the symptoms sounded like melancholia and there was a history of melancholic illness in the Huxley family.[22] Huxley simply reached for the popular term of the day to describe his distress. Similarly, Vienna playwright Arthur Schnitzler, who also had a lifelong history of psychiatric illness, described in his diary the "nervous collapse" that he experienced in the early 1920s, including "deepest despair" and "bitter tears." In the grips of melancholic illness, he would lie in bed and sob.[23]

In 1936 novelist F. Scott Fitzgerald experienced a "crack-up" that sounds more like a kind of time-out than an extended breakdown. But it caused him plenty of misery. At age 39—he wrote of himself in the third person: "… It was his nervous reflexes that were giving way—too much anger and too many tears." He described the symptoms as follows: "I had a strong sudden instinct that I must be alone. I didn't want to see any people at all." He describes anhedonia: "… For a long time I had not liked people and things, but only followed the rickety old pretense of liking. I saw that even my love for those closest to me was become only an attempt to love." He experienced insomnia, "hating the day because it went toward night," and loss of judgment, in a famous line: "At three o'clock in the morning a forgotten package has the same tragic importance as a death sentence…and in a real dark night of the soul it is always three o'clock in the morning, day after day." He went to a rented room "in a drab little town" and tried to puzzle out "why I had developed a sad attitude toward sadness, a melancholy attitude toward melancholy and a tragic attitude toward tragedy." This might be constructed as illustrating Jaspers' dictum about serious illness as beginning with "the feeling of loss of feelings." Fitzgerald likened himself to a worn old plate that just suddenly cracks.[24]

Many had experienced crack-ups and breakdowns. "Have you ever had a nervous breakdown?" social researcher Katharine Bement Davis asked 1000 American women in 1929. One hundred and ninety-six had actually had a breakdown, and a further 104 had "almost" or "nearly" had one. "This together amounts to 30 per cent of the entire 1000," Davis observed.[25] Clearly, among the public the concept of nervous breakdown was ringing a massive bell.

But then the diagnosis nervous breakdown underwent a drift from meaning serious-illness-but-not-insane to becoming a circumlocution for insanity. This was a kind of bait-and-switch that befell the notion of nerves in a number of settings, as, for example, in the private nervous clinics that insisted they did not accept psychotic patients but in fact often did so, assuaging family members with the notion that their afflicted relative, who was totally psychotic, just suffered from nerves.[26] This drift had started with nerves relatively early. At the turn of the century, T. Seymour Tuke, the third generation of that famous Quaker dynasty, was a staff psychiatrist at Chiswick House, a private nervous clinic in a London suburb. In 1901 he deplored "the tendency to gloss over what is in reality actual insanity and unsoundnesss of mind by calling it by euphemistic epithets." He said he had "personal knowledge of cases that have been called and treated as 'nerve cases' that have been without doubt cases…of insanity and certified."[27] By 1940 "very nervous," at least in the cosseted little world of Swiss private psychiatric clinics, had come to be identified with frank insanity. What kinds of patients did the La Soldanelle clinic in ritzy Chateau d'Oex admit? Patients with organic diseases, to be sure, such as anemia and rheumatism were accepted, as well as psychiatric patients with "weakened nervous systems." But "Contagious patients and the very nervous are excluded."[28] The coded language is clear.

Might you be having a nervous breakdown? asked the *Ladies Home Journal* in 1941. What are some of the symptoms? "In the throes of an acute nervous attack, no matter how organically healthy the victim might be, the heart *does* beat abnormally fast, the hands do clench and stiffen, the breath comes with difficulty, and the brain may falter and go temporarily blank."[29] We would later recognize this as a panic attack, but in 1941, it sounded like insanity, with the brain going blank and the hands clenching uncontrollably. This would not, unlike nerves, be a diagnosis that people would seek out.

In understanding the departure of the term nervous breakdown there are, accordingly, various forces. Some were pull forces. Psychiatry pulled nerves off center stage and rushed on depression as an understudy. Patients themselves pushed nerves off stage because it had come to mean insanity, which nobody wanted.

Yet even today if you put the term in people's mouths, they will respond positively. Several national-level random surveys of the American population, most recently by the National Opinion Research Center of the University of Chicago, asked respondents if they felt "an impending nervous breakdown." In 1957, 18.9% of the population said yes; in 1976, 20.9% said yes and in 1996, 26.4%. These respondents might all have been diagnosed as depressed by their physicians, yet the public clung sufficiently to the breakdown concept that, when prompted, in the 1990s a quarter of Americans confessed to fearing one![30] (One survey of people's associations with the term "nervous breakdown" concluded that the term "appears to maintain a unique linguistic value to laypersons."[31] Here again, of course, the investigators were putting words into people's mouths.)

Yet on the whole, by the end of the 1950s the oomph had gone out of the nervous breakdown concept. Popular magazines ran articles on it only to debunk it in favor of depression. "There is no such thing as a nervous breakdown," said *Good Housekeeping* in 1960. "Mrs Thompson" didn't have nerves. "She had a depressive reaction."[32]

8

Paradigm Shift

KRAEPELIN'S INFLUENCE IN renaming melancholia "depression" was enormous. But that alone would not suffice to explain why, an ocean away and a hundred years later, everybody became depressed. Mediators were needed to carry the doctrine of depression to the discipline of psychiatry, and then to individual patients. Those mediators were the American psychoanalysts, many of them distinguished migrants from Europe, and they gave pride of place to neurotic depression. Other mediators extracted depression and anxiety from the pool of nerves and yoked them together, making mixed depression-anxiety the favored disorder.

To gain some perspective: In the first third of the twentieth century, in a great paradigm shift that transferred behavioral disorders from neurology to psychiatry, the spotlight shifted from nerves, a diagnosis that implicated the whole body, to mood, a diagnosis that implicated mainly the mind. Mental illness triumphed over nervous illness, and depression became the main mood diagnosis. In 1908, Oswald Bumke, a psychiatrist then at the university psychiatric hospital in Freiburg, Germany (later to become professor of psychiatry in Munich), scolded the family physicians who never suspected depression in their wealthy patients whom they sent from spa to spa and sanatorium to sanatorium for the treatment of nondisease (symptoms without organic causes). The family doctors, who doubtlessly suspected the symptoms were of psychological origin, focused on the symptoms themselves; Bumke, more interested in mental than in physical symptoms, focused on what he believed the underlying cause to be: "depression," as manifest in symptoms such as tiredness or an anxious preoccupation with their bodily health.[1] For clinicians of Bumke's generation, depression was a familiar concept.

In understanding the rise of depression there are two questions that have to be sorted out: Why the depression diagnosis becomes so common and why depressive symptoms become divorced from the nervous syndrome and take on a life of their own as an affective disorder. Because events on both tracks happen around the same time, the narratives interblend, but they are separate stories.

To foreshadow, it was American psychoanalysis that first put depression in the spotlight. The analysts took the neurosis diagnosis, which had been around for a century or more, and made the commonest of the neuroses depressive neurosis. This became the workhorse of everyday psychoanalytic practice. Most psychiatrists were not psychoanalysts, but because of the prestige of psychoanalysis, analytic formulations became the meat and drink of everyday psychiatry. This explains why depression triumphed as an affective disorder: The analysts were interested in affect; they were not interested in fatigue, insomnia, or any of the rest of the nervous syndrome.

But quite outside of psychoanalysis, attention became focused upon mood as well. As mainline psychiatry shifted attention from nerves, hysteria, and neurasthenia, its glance fell upon the mood disorders depression and anxiety, and in particular that they were usually hooked together. In the community, the main psychiatric complaint was mixed anxiety-depression. Beginning in the 1920s and culminating in the 1970s, this mixed disorder became the commonest psychiatric illness. It was in fact the core of the former nervous syndrome, with fatigue, the somatic symptoms, and the obsessiveness stripped away.

The triumph of the American analysts' neurotic depression, and of the nonanalysts' mixed anxiety-depression, put an end to anything nervous. Nerves and the like were common terms term until World War I, then began to seep away from medicine. Outside medicine, people would still use the term nervous breakdown—as indeed they do today—but within medicine nerves became passé, old-fashioned. Thus changes in fashion in medical diagnoses eclipsed a fundamental reality for millions of people: Their problems were not really owing to their depressed or anxious mood, depressed or anxious although they may have been, but to a disorder of mind, brain, and body together. This disorder had previously been called the nervous syndrome. It now took on a different cast entirely.

Just two words up front: Long before Freud, the term depression was alive in popular culture. Late in eighteenth-century England, young Fanny Burney, in addition to recording her own panics (see pp. 60–61), noted as well her father's downcast mental state. In 1792 she wrote in her diary of "My dear father … lower and more depressed about himself than ever. To see him dejected is of all sights, to me, the most melancholy."[2]

The 29-year-old English parliamentarian—later Prime Minister—William Gladstone noted in his diary in 1838 of the day's sessions in the House of Commons, "Through the debate I felt a most painful depression." Later that year, attending someone's funeral: "The Cemetery beautiful and soothing. I am tempted to desire to follow. I ought to be happy here, having the means to be useful: yet I live almost perpetually restless and depressed."[3] These examples could be multiplied many-fold. Mental depression, as we understand the term, was a solid concept in people's vocabulary from the late eighteenth century on.

Second, for physicians, depression and melancholia were in one pool, nerves in another. We have seen this in earlier chapters. Nervosity, nervosisme, and cognate terms designated garden-variety distress, not depression. Depression was considered a "difficulty in the exercise of the intellect"—as one English asylum doctor put it in 1854—and was seen as part of melancholia before the doctrine of the two depressions arose (see Chapter 6).[4]

The term neurosis itself had been in common use since the late eighteenth century to mean any disease of the central nervous system. It was only with Parisian internist Auguste Axenfeld in 1863 that neurosis (névrose) came explicitly to mean disorder without a lesion.[5] In German-speaking Europe, in 1879 Richard von Krafft-Ebing, professor of psychiatry at the time in Graz, coined the term psychoneurosis to mean a behavioral disorder in an individual who was not genetically predisposed, not degenerate, in the language of the day. "For those mental disorders that affect individuals with healthy brains let us use the designation psychoneuroses; for those that arise on the basis of predisposition, the expression psychic degeneration will serve."[6] Thereafter, neurosis and psychoneurosis did yeoman service in the description of nonpsychotic disorders, which was the situation up to Freud.

Restoring the Notion of Two Depressions

Kraepelin's manic-depressive illness (MDI) was a powerful concept. It abolished the notion that there were two depressions—melancholia and neurasthenia—and said that all the clinical pictures of depression and mania boiled down to more or less the same thing, "MDI." Yet like nerves, the concept of two separate depressions as illnesses as different as measles and tuberculosis had a good deal of face value and did not die out with a snap of the Kraepelinian fingers. The continued coexistence of melancholia alongside neurasthenia, neurosis, spleen, and the rest of it meant that there must be two depressions: a terrible psychotic illness leading to suicide versus a kind of blues that, although unpleasant, were not the end of the world. Even though Kraepelin had admitted a "psychogenic depression,"[7] his doctrine of manic-depressive illness said that there was just one depression. Something had to be done about that.

In 1913, Karl Jaspers, a student of Kraepelin's in the Heidelberg university psychiatric hospital, identified reactive depressions in his influential book on psychopathology. "Reactive depressive conditions are especially frequent," he said, differentiating understandable reactions to events from incomprehensible attacks of psychosis that seemed to come out of the blue.[8] This put an alternative to manic-depressive illness on the table, making a second depression conceptually available, in other words.

This second depression was quickly taken up. In 1920 Kurt Schneider, a 33-year-old assistant physician at the university psychiatric hospital in Cologne who had just returned from military service (he had studied in Tübingen and was not a Kraepelin pupil), proposed a division of the depressive illnesses that would endure right until 1980, and represented the most powerful illness dichotomy that psychiatry had to offer until the advent of *DSM-III*: It was Jaspers' *reactive* depression versus *endogenous*, or vital, depression. (Kraepelin himself had suggested the category endogenous psychosis.) Every psychiatric reader of this book who trained before 1980 will recall from his or her residency the distinction between reactive and endogenous depression— reactive taught as a reaction to an unhappy event and endogenous as a kind of physical depression that seemed to well up within the body without an external cause. This is not exactly what Schneider meant. Schneider wrote, "In considering depressive conditions let us begin with both of the characteristic types in their extreme forms: the pure unmotivated 'endogenous' and the pure reactive depressions ... In the endogenous depressions disturbances of vital feelings have a very much greater role." Schneider was referring to "disorders of body feeling and life feeling," a physical concept dating back to the notions of vitality of the nineteenth century. With reactive depressions, by contrast, "The primary issue is disturbances of psychic feeling." Both endogenous and reactive depressions could be triggered by external events. Take, for example, the death of a loved one. Patients with endogenous depression experience the loss at a different "emotional layer" than do patients with reactive depression: vital body feelings versus emotional sadness. It was thus thoroughly possible for a vital depression to be precipitated by external events, just as a reactive depression was triggered—merely that they would be experienced differently, at a total body level or at an emotional level.⁹ (Vital depression did not even necessarily mean sadness, said one of Schneider's colleagues, but probably represented an endocrine disturbance.¹⁰) This was a concept of huge power, one that had doubtlessly dawned slowly on Schneider, even as a kind of visceral insight, as he treated the men invalided back from the trauma of trench war at the front. It is rather unfortunate that it became misunderstood in American psychiatry, because its "disproof," showing that endogenous depressions had as many unhappy external events as reactive depressions, opened the way to *DSM-III* and the disaster of "major depression."¹¹

Now let us consider how the Freudians conceived depression.

Neurotic Depression

Sigmund Freud's literary career in Vienna lasted from about 1890 to 1930, and in these years he launched the doctrine of psychoanalysis as a way of understanding "mental" illness, an illness he saw as arising in the mind rather than the brain, and of treating it—his technique of psychoanalysis used free association and dream analysis. Freud himself had little interest in depression. For him, unlike hysteria, phobias, and so forth, depression was not one of the classical neuroses, and he doubtless felt what Jerome Frank at Johns Hopkins articulated much later, that it was almost impossible to do psychoanalytic work with the morbidly depressed patient "who interacts sparsely with others, is dull and unproductive [unwilling to confess interesting fantasies], sees the world in an impoverished and stereotyped way, and really wants to be left alone."¹² So Freud wrote little about depression with the exception of "Mourning and Melancholia" in 1916, in which he laid the groundwork for future analytic writing on depression by explaining it as the threatened loss of a beloved "object," which usually meant the mother.¹³

The rise of psychoanalysis was to have deep consequences for total-body views of psychiatric illness. Simply put, the psychoanalysts did not believe in the body as the locus of disease. They situated "mental illness" in the mind, and ascribed its origins to unconscious conflicts within the psyche. In 1926 Freud noted that "A physician experiences in a medical faculty approximately the opposite of what he needs in preparation for psychoanalysis. His attention is directed to objectively determined anatomic, physical and chemical facts, whose correct appreciation and suitable treatment determine medical approaches." Psychoanalysis, by contrast, is "the science of the psychic unconscious."¹⁴ Amazingly, for therapists who had been educated as physicians, many analysts did not believe even in touching their patients, especially the females, fearing interference with the transference relationship and loss of control over themselves in these sexually highly charged consultations. Freud said, "The attempt to reciprocate the tender feelings of the patient is not entirely without danger. The analyst may not have sufficient self-control and suddenly find himself further along the road that he might have envisioned."[15] Thus, avoid physical contact in order to avoid conveying to your patient that her erotic ambitions with you might be realized. The intention here is of the best. Yet it was a fatal development that such antiembodiment views, so to speak, were brought to the study of depression at the same time that the diagnosis was growing by leaps and bounds.

The first member of Freud's circle to write about depression as a neurosis, rather than about melancholia or manic-depressive illness, was Berlin psychiatrist Karl Abraham, who noted in 1911 at the Third Psychoanalytic Congress in Weimar that there was a hole in the psychoanalytic coverage: "While the conditions of nervous anxiety have been treated in detail in the psychoanalytic literature, the depressive conditions have not found similar consideration. And yet depressive affect is just as widespread in all forms of neurosis and psychosis as anxious affect." He noted that both conditions often occurred in the same individual. Both were also linked, he said, to the process of repression: "One of the earliest results of Freudian neurosis research is that neurotic anxiety stems from sexual repression. This is neurotic anxiety separated from fear. By the same token we are able to separate the affects of mourning or dejection [Niedergeschlagenheit] from affects originating in the unconscious, which is to say, neurotic depression based on repression."[16] This was the beginning of neurotic depression as a diagnosis separate from the other big depressive illnesses.

Abraham's essay remained widely unknown. Somewhat bizarrely, the figure who planted the diagnosis neurotic depression firmly in the medical imagination was the senior London neurologist Farquhar Buzzard, at a conference in 1930. Buzzard did not care a fig for psychoanalysis, but needed a term to differentiate psychotic depression from other, less serious depressions, and so he chose neurotic depression. " ... There is no evidence," he said, "that features which distinguish neurotic from psychotic forms of depression have received due recognition." And what might those features be? He proposed one: "Am I right in thinking that the neurotic throws the responsibility for his troubles on others while the psychotic is ready to shoulder it himself?" Buzzard mentioned other differentiating features as well, asserting that "psychotic depression is always associated with physical disturbances," whereas neurotic depression is not. In psychotic depression, by which he meant melancholia, not formal psychosis, there was a much heavier family history of illness, and so forth.[17] Neurotic depression as a diagnosis took off from here.

There the Anglo-European story rested. The next chapter in the neurotic depression story would be written in the United States, by émigré European analysts. One keeps in mind that the depression of psychoanalysis was a neurosis, not a mood disorder.

It was owing to the great prestige of the émigrés that neurotic depression as a diagnosis took off in the United States in the 1930s and 1940s, at a time when Europe was convulsed by war and the Holocaust. In 1927, Sandor Rado, a Budapest analyst then at the Berlin Psychoanalytic Institute, took up again, at the Tenth Psychoanalytic Congress in Innsbruck, the question of neurotic depression, in contrast to melancholia, to which he devoted most of his disquisition. "Neurotic depression is a kind of partial melancholia of the (neurotic) ego," he said.[18] This brief squib might perhaps have had little impact had Rado not, in 1931, been summoned by New York's Abraham Brill (who was Austrian) to lead the newly established New York Psychoanalytic Institute, the very epicenter of psychoanalytic influence in the New World. Rado became immensely influential in the United States and in 1944 was appointed professor of psychiatry at Columbia University. In 1951 he had another go at depression, this time a more extensive treatment, calling it "a desperate cry for love, precipitated by an actual or imagined loss which the patient feels endangers his emotional (and material) security."[19] Rado is generally seen as having imported the study of depression, of any variety, to American psychiatry.

But as for specifically neurotic depression it was Otto Fenichel who became the major figure. Born in Vienna in 1897, Fenichel graduated there in medicine in 1921, joined the Vienna Psychoanalytic Society, then in 1922 moved to Berlin and began a training analysis with Rado at the Berlin Society. Just before emigrating from Germany to Norway in 1933, Fenichel completed his *Outline of Clinical Psychoanalysis,* which was translated into English and published in 1934 in New York—in a measure of the prestige Freud's doctrines were acquiring in the United States—by a major trade publisher, W.W. Norton. Here Fenichel had a good deal to say about neurotic depression: "Neurotic depressions occur in all varieties of neuroses," he wrote. "The mildest cases need no special technique: the solution of the basic infantile sexual conflicts in the course of the analysis of the main neurosis automatically brings about a concomitant harmony with the super-ego."[20] Fenichel moved from Europe to Los Angeles in 1938, and in 1945 brought out a revised and expanded edition of his 1934 text under another title; in this edition the discussion of neurotic depression acquired still greater amplitude. "Neurotic depressions are desperate attempts to force an object to give the vitally necessary [narcissistic] supplies, whereas in the psychotic depressions the actual complete loss has really taken place and regulatory attempts are aimed exclusively at the superego." Furthermore: "In the phenomenology of depression, a greater or lesser loss of self-esteem is in the foreground." In neurotic depressions, "The patients try to influence the persons around them to return their lost self-esteem."[21]

By this time, neurotic depression had gone from almost 0 in Europe to 60 in the United States. During World War II, psychoanalysis received a major boost by capturing the psychiatric services of the United States Army, with analyst William Menninger as chief military consultant; the classification of psychiatric disorders that the Army issued in October 1945 bore witness to this influence. Here is what the Army, guided by a committee Menninger had convened, had to say about the "neurotic depressive reaction": "The anxiety in this reaction is allayed and hence partially relieved by self-depreciation through mental mechanism [sic] of introjection ... Dynamically the depression is usually related to a repressed (unconscious) aggression."[22] Thus, if any of the troops developed a neurotic depression after demobilization, Dr. Menninger had laid out what they could look forward to.

This Army document, "Bulletin 203" as it became known, provided the basis for the first edition in 1952 of the famous DSM series of the American Psychiatric Association. Neurotic depression had by now become a concept with great momentum.

The DSM series became, for better or worse, the distinctive U.S. contribution to world psychiatry. Begun in 1952 as an offshoot of the diagnostic school of the Swiss émigré Adolf Meyer, professor of psychiatry at Johns Hopkins University, the series accelerated in size and in impact over the years, becoming by the end of the twentieth century the cardinal international guide to psychiatric diagnosis. At present, as a revised version, DSM-5, lies in the wings, even the daily newspapers are filled with accounts of what the next edition may or may not contain—and why it is so vitally important for the average citizen. It therefore was a sign that a diagnosis such as neurotic depression had acquired a key to the temple, that DSM-I in 1952 dilated upon the psychodynamics of it all: The Manual said of the "psychoneurotic disorders" in general, "The chief characteristic of these diagnoses is 'anxiety' ... controlled by the utilization of various psychological defense mechanisms." Of "depressive reaction" in particular it was stipulated, "The anxiety in this reaction is allayed, and hence partially relieved, by depression and self-depreciation," which was largely the language of the Army bulletin for neurotic depression.[23]

DSM-II, which appeared in 1968, was even more explicit about the neurotic part, and said of "Depressive neurosis: This condition is manifested by an excessive reaction of depression due to an internal conflict or to an identifiable event such as the loss of a love object or cherished possession."[24] This was really Psychoanalysis 101, and even if neurotic depression was not the commonest depressive diagnosis in the United States (see below), it was the most prestigious: People who received psychoanalytic diagnoses were a cut or two above the run of the mill and could afford to see analysts, or at least to consult psychoanalytically oriented psychiatrists (who were the majority).

When Silvano Arieti's three-volume textbook of psychiatry appeared in 1966—almost entirely delivered into the hands of the psychoanalysts—the big chapter on "The Psychodynamics of Neurotic Depression" by New York analyst Walter Bonime represented a kind of apex of the diagnosis in American psychiatry: It really does not get any better than this. "The depressive is an extremely manipulative individual who, by helplessness, sadness, seductiveness, and other means, maneuvers people toward the fulfillment of demands for various forms of emotionally comforting response."[25] (It was under the influence of this doctrine that analyst Gregory Zilboorg decided that the physical complaints of his patient George Gershwin were owing to neurotic depression—rather than to the brain tumor that ultimately killed him—and instructed the family to ignore behavior such as putting his fork in his ear at a dinner party, "apparently unable to locate his mouth"; these gestures should remain without comment, Zilboorg advised, in order to deny him the attention he was obviously seeking.[26])

To understand why depression became such a huge diagnosis, we thus have the role of psychoanalysis, the thread that begins with Karl Abraham and passes through the émigré analysts, to make depth psychology such a popular conveyor belt for neurotic depression. It is almost unimaginable to us today that psychoanalysis once represented the very heart and soul of psychiatry. Robert Cancro, chair of the department of psychiatry at New York University, said in 2002, looking back, "While this may sound facetious, it is not. The belief that repressed, unconscious conflicts were the basis of all psychopathology was held with near-religious zeal."[27] Nowhere was this zeal hedged more ardently than in the offices of the fashionable psychiatrists on the Upper East Side of Manhattan or Westwood in Los Angeles. Nathan Kline, who floated back and forth between high-end psychotherapy and the budding discipline of psychopharmacology, had a private practice in Manhattan located in one of the "mental blocks" on streets such as Park Avenue, so-called, as Kline said in 1973, "because there are so many psychiatrists located there."[28] This was the world of neurotic depression.

Was psychoanalysis really all that important in U.S. psychiatry in those days? Yes, it was. In 1955 the pro-psychoanalytic Group for the Advancement of Psychiatry surveyed departments of psychiatry in U.S. medical schools about their programs for educating budding psychiatrists. Of 26 training programs contacted, the 14 that replied "all indicate that their training program is based on psychodynamic theory." Of the teaching staff in these programs, 56% were psychoanalytically trained "and another eleven percent had a personal analysis without formal psychoanalytic training."[29]

Psychoanalysis was pervasive in U.S. psychiatry, and in American society, in those years. Why did everybody become depressed? Psychiatry had something to do with it.

Mixed Anxiety-Depression

Motto: "The arguments for supposing that anxiety and depression share a common cause are persuasive."[30]
DAVID GOLDBERG, INSTITUTE OF PSYCHIATRY,
LONDON, 1996

After neurotic depression, the second mood diagnosis to emerge from the ruins of the nervous syndrome was mixed anxiety-depression. From the 1920s on, it surged in popularity, not being dependent on exotic theoretical schemes that assigned the ills of humankind to anomalies in early childhood sexual development. And empirically it was obvious that most depressions were accompanied by anxiety—and vice versa.

Mixed anxiety-depression was the true inheritor of nerves; today, it is by far the commonest presentation of either anxiety or depression. In a nationwide poll in Great Britain in 2000, over 10% of women and 6% of men suffered from "mixed anxiety and depressive disorder," the most frequent of the neurotic disorders, followed at a distance by generalized anxiety disorder, depressive episode, and then, way down, obsessive-compulsive disorder, phobias, and panic.[31] In 1981 psychologist John Overall, one of the pioneers of psychopharmacology, told a committee of the FDA's Early Clinical Drug Evaluation Units, an entity that sponsored many trials and had a databank of 2700 depressed patients, "I would assure you that 90 percent or more of the patients had mixed anxiety and depression along with other symptoms. It is very difficult to find depressed patients who do not have anxiety."[32] We are talking here much more about the anxiety accompanying nonmelancholic depression than that of melancholy (although melancholics can be anxious too). Alan Schatzberg, another leading figure in psychopharmacology, then at McLean Hospital, a psychiatric facility in Belmont, Massachusetts, associated with Harvard University, said in 1990 that "63 percent of depressed patients met criteria for a lifetime DSM-III-R anxiety disorder and 52 percent met criteria for a current diagnosis."[33]

But it was not just the more seriously depressed hospital patients who were anxious. Those individuals in the community who never came within shouting distance of psychiatric care for their symptoms also had mixed anxiety-depression, as David Goldberg and Peter Huxley at the University of Manchester discovered in 1980, in a classic study of mental illness in the community, identified in a sample of primary care patients (They did a transatlantic study, but these particular data are from Philadelphia.) "Minor affective disorders—that is to say, anxiety states, minor depressive illnesses, and states of both anxiety and depression—account for the vast majority of illnesses seen in a primary care setting... Anxiety and worry is the most widely distributed symptom, depression and fatigue follow closely behind. The idea that depression represents a more differentiated form of disorder contained within the population of patients with anxiety states, is not borne out by the data." What the authors described was the nervous syndrome: 82% of the patients had anxiety and worry, 71% had despondency, sadness, and fatigue, 52% had somatic symptoms, and 50% had disturbed sleep.[34] (I do not want to get ahead of the story, but I cannot resist pointing out that Goldberg, a leading epidemiologist later at the Institute of Psychiatry in London, went on to ridicule the "comorbidity" concept, because, after depression and anxiety were separated in *DSM-III* in 1980, they were considered comorbid when they occurred together: "Comorbidity has some meaning if we are referring to combinations of diabetes and schizophrenia, or even of depression and alcohol dependence, but it is surely stretching the concept to absurdity to allow one or two symptoms from correlated domains to produce the phenomenon."[35])

The polarity of the depression, whether bipolar or unipolar (today "major depression"), does not seem to make much difference to the presence of anxiety. The depression of bipolar disorder is melancholia, just as a portion of the unipolar patients with "major depression" are melancholic.[36] There is no difference between the melancholias of either unipolar or bipolar disorder. And the polarity does not seem to matter in terms of anxiety: In a study of patients with both kinds of depression, Paula Clayton at the University of Minnesota found that around 75% of all depression patients were worried, 60% or more reported psychic anxiety, around 30% reported panic attacks, and so forth. There were no important differences between those with major depression and those with the depression of bipolar disorder..[37]

It is possible that mixed depression-anxiety is in fact the natural form of mood disorder—or that the nervous syndrome of which mixed anxiety-depression is a part—is the natural form. Mixed anxiety-depression seems to have a genetics of its own. In a 1996 study of 1029 female twin pairs, Kenneth Kendler and co-workers at the Medical College of Virginia found that twins with severe depression were almost always anxious: "More than 75 percent of twins with severe typical depression had, at the same time, an anxiety syndrome diagnosable as either GAD [general anxiety disorder] or panic disorder. In this epidemiologic sample of women, severe depression rarely occurred *without* major symptoms of anxiety."[38] (If both twins have the same illness, particularly both from the same egg, the odds increase that it is genetically determined.) Around the same time, in a study of 446 adult twin pairs, Gavin Andrews and team at the University of New South Wales in Sydney were not able to isolate genes specific for either anxiety or depressive neurosis, but did identify "a genetic contribution to neuroticism," meaning a mixture of the two.[39] In 1996, Andrews described a genetically based "general neurotic syndrome,"[40] which is tantamount to the nervous syndrome. In 2002 Assen Jablensky and Robert Kendell, two leading psychopathologists, concluded "that the genetic basis of generalized anxiety disorder is indistinguishable from that of major depression."[41] In genetic terms, mixed anxiety-depression was a single disorder, not two separate entities that happened to be "comorbid."

Thus, mixed depression-anxiety was unquestionably the commonest form of either depression or anxiety and is, in fact, the diagnosis that corresponds to the "nerves" of yesteryear. (In a study in 1988 in a Virginia clinic of 47 patients with "nerves" compared to controls, the nerves patients had more anxiety and depression than the controls, and more somatic symptoms as well; they also reported fatigue twice as often.[42])

Historically, just as nerves were sliding into yesteryear, we find clinicians commenting on the frequency of mixed-depression anxiety. Kraepelin himself never endorsed anxiety as a disease, but acknowledged its frequency in manic-depressive illness, saying in 1909: "We find anxiety most frequently in the depressive phases of circular insanity [manic-depressive illness]."[43] Edward Mapother, superintendent of the Maudsley Hospital in London, seconded this in 1926: "Anxiety neurosis has achieved a persistent acceptance even among the large majority who reject Freud's views as to its causation. There seems no particular objection to isolating it if it be regarded as merely one of the numerous subdivisions of the manic-depressive group."[44] Thus, anxiety was considered part of manic-depression.

In England there certainly were community physicians with upper-middle-class practices who described mixed anxiety-depression without using the term. In 1933 J. W. Astley Cooper, with a practice in Middleton St. George in Durham County, who frequently sent his patients to expensive private nervous clinics, called the profession's attention to "rest in the treatment of neuroses." He considered many patients "neurotics of the anxiety type." But what else did they have? They presented with "all the indications of mental and physical exhaustion—namely, tremors, loss of appetite, loss of weight, restlessness, insomnia, loss of interest (in everything but their own troubles)." He considered them cases of "mental and physical exhaustion," but another analysis might have called it mixed anxiety-depression. (In any event, they responded wonderfully to the enforced inactivity of the Weir–Mitchell rest cure.)[45] Likewise, Thomas Ross did not use the term mixed anxiety-depression. Yet of the 45 patients with symptoms of depression admitted to the Cassel Hospital for Functional Nervous Disorders in 1927–1928, 69% had symptoms of anxiety.[46]

The foundation stone of the modern doctrine of depression and anxiety as a single illness was laid by Aubrey Lewis in 1934. Lewis, then an assistant medical officer at the Maudsley, had studied carefully in 1928–1929—not with rating scales but with close personal observation—some 61 patients in Adelaide, Australia with melancholia. The paper on the subject that he wrote in 1931, and published 3 years later, is one of the most influential in the history of mood disorders. Notable was Lewis's declaration that "The relation of depression to anxiety is intimate."[47] Given that Lewis went on to become arguably the most influential psychiatrist in the world—the more so after the destruction of German psychiatry following 1933, and after Kraepelin's death in 1926 and Freud's in 1939—this was an opinion of enormous weight.

We are not going to follow the depression wars that took place in the mid-twentieth century, the endless squabbling over how to classify depression. Yet from these debates several clinical realities emerged. One was that mixed anxiety-depression was a meaningful type of depression. This is important because it shows the survival of the nervous syndrome at some kind of gut level, even though diagnostic officialdom was, in 1980 with *DSM-III*, about to separate anxiety and depression completely. Fridolin Sulser, a psychopharmacologist at Vanderbilt University, was of Swiss origin and had graduated in Basel in 1955. At a conference on the role of serotonin in psychiatry in the

1990s, he professed himself puzzled: "I was taught by Manfred Bleuler [in Zurich] 30 years ago that anxiety is a core symptom of depression. If this is true ... how can fluoxetine [Prozac] be a good antidepressant if from animal data it is thought to increase anxiety."[48] The point was a delicious one, given that Prozac is not a very good antidepressant. But Sulser put anxiety squarely in the center of the depression table.

Bleuler and Sulser were part of a powerful European tradition of seeing anxiety as central to depression, although there were other kinds of depressions as well. Parisian psychiatrist Jacques Launay, who with Henri Baruk created in 1958 the first French psychopharmacological association, the Société Moreau de Tours, gave anxiety pride of place in his typology of depressions in 1965. He postulated, "depressive states with a predominance of anxiety and neuropsychic irritability [éréthisme]," the main characteristic of which was "a more or less permanent feeling of malaise, with interior tension, emotional incontinence, affective hypersensibility, physical anguish such as feelings of tightening of the throat ... "[49] Even though in these years American psychiatry was taking the baton from Europe, this continental stream remained influential.

In England, Max Hamilton at Leeds, creator of depression and anxiety scales named after him, was probably the most influential thinker in disease classification (especially after Aubrey Lewis died in 1975); Hamilton believed that there were really two kinds of depressions: endogenous (meaning melancholic) and anxious. He told a conference in 1973, "I myself am very skeptical about all these pseudo categories of psychotic versus neurotic; endogenous versus reactive, and so on. Most of these terms, when carefully examined, turn out to have very little clear meaning and I tend to avoid them. But in the rating scale, the factor analysis ... clearly groups the symptoms of what is sometimes called endogenous depression, such as guilt, suicide, [psychomotor] retardation, loss of insight, on one side, and on the other it puts anxiety, agitation, somatic anxiety and so on."[50]

Across the Atlantic, John Overall, a psychologist in the Department of Psychiatry at the University of Texas Medical School at Houston, figured prominently among American psychopharmacologists and disease classifiers. Overall was particularly interested in depression, and in his own subtyping, anxious depression was the most numerous "phenomenological class," ahead of agitated, retarded, and hostile depression.[51]

These are really just snapshots from a much larger clinical literature showing that mixed depression-anxiety, the descendant of the nervous syndrome, was very much alive in international psychiatry in the 1960s and 1970s.

But there was some pushback. Several influential psychiatrists believed that anxiety and depression were in fact quite different disorders, and their voices contributed to the fateful decision in 1980 to tear apart the conjoined twins.

In England during the 1960s and 1970s a tremendous battle was fought over whether anxiety and depression were the same illness or separate (a battle muddled by the failure of the participants to exempt melancholic depression from the discussion). The main protagonist of the view of the separateness of anxiety and depression was Martin Roth. Born in 1917 and trained at the Maudsley, in the 1950s Roth became the virtual founder of the field of geriatric psychiatry.[52] In 1956 he took the chair of psychiatry at Newcastle on Tyne, and in 1959 launched a diagnosis that he rather clunkily entitled "the phobic anxiety-depersonalization syndrome," a combination of phobic anxiety and depersonalization that eventuated upon a personal calamity or severe illness and became known as "Roth's calamity syndrome."[53]

At Newcastle, Roth and colleagues became involved in factor analyses, trying to sort out what symptom overlap existed between anxiety and depression. There was little, they argued. There was "a significant negative correlation between anxiety and a diagnosis of endogenous depression."[54] Quite so. Yet this did not respond to the issue of an overlap between non-endogenous depression and anxiety. That lay ahead. In 1972 the investigators factor-analyzed depression and anxiety broadly conceived: The anxiety symptoms clustered at one pole of the analysis and the depressive symptoms at the other pole, "confirming that within an affective material there are two distinct syndromes corresponding to anxiety and depression."[55]

Roth was knighted in 1972 and became professor of psychiatry at Cambridge in 1977. In the years ahead, his views, enunciated from the towering heights of psychiatry, would be highly influential, although they remained largely unreplicated. Some workers, such as Hagop Akiskal, then at Tennessee and later at the University of California at San Diego, affirmed them[56]; others, such as Frank Fish at Liverpool, threw cold water on the supposed differentiation as artifacts of suggestion.[57] Despite Roth's prestige it is fair to say that a majority of clinical opinion supported the view that mixed anxiety-depression was a disease of its own quite distinct from pure anxiety and pure depression.[58]

For insiders, the supposed difference between anxiety and depression became largely a matter of convenience. Ross Baldessarini at the McLean Hospital wryly recalls that when he first came to work at McLean, "There was a young colleague here running an outpatient psychopharmacology clinic. Within about a one-month period, he had two site visits on two grants projects. It turned out that a couple of the visitors came to both visits. At lunch on the second visit one of them called the PI [principal investigator] aside, and said, 'I've been scribbling some numbers on the back of an envelope about the patient flow through your clinic,' and he said, 'the numbers don't add up. Can you explain them? Last time we visited, you had a project on major depression, today we're talking about anxiety disorders. How come?' The PI blushed and said, 'Some of them are the same people. You can move them one way or the other, depending on the needs.'"[59]

Until *DSM-III* in 1980, the supposed difference between anxiety and depression lived on mainly in the world of pharmaceutical advertising, where diseases were found to fit the compounds on hand, rather than the other way around. The benzodiazepines, launched in 1960 with Librium, are actually quite suitable agents for mixed anxiety-depression. But they would be spun either toward anxiety or depression, depending on the needs of commerce. The Upjohn Company, for example, wanted to introduce its benzodiazepine alprazolam (Xanax) in 1981 as an antidepressant and was blocked from doing so only by the absence of an inpatient study.[60] So they ended up with a marketing hit for panic disorder! (more on this in Chapter 9). Big bucks were riding on the question of whether anxiety was a separate disease: If separate, different agents would be needed to treat it. If the same, the patient could be spared one prescription. The entire issue became degraded by commercial considerations.*

*After the disaster of *DSM-III*'s major depression in 1980, a campaign began to insert "mixed-anxiety-depression," called "cothymia" by Peter Tyrer,[61] in the official diagnostic roster; and the campaign seemed to have succeeded in an early draft of *DSM-5* in 2012. Yet, incredibly, in May 2012, the *DSM-5* Task Force elected to delete the historic diagnosis on the grounds that not quite enough was known about it.[62]

The Big Run-Up in Depression Begins

Carried aloft by the two great wings of neurotic depression and mixed anxiety-depression, from the 1920s on the frequency of diagnosed depression soared.

A red light: It is unlikely that the frequency of serious depression, which has deep genetic roots in brain biology, ever changes over time. Why would it? Genetic influences shift very slowly, if at all, and there is no reason to think that patients who would have had a positive dexamethasone suppression test—which identifies organicity in melancholia—would be more numerous today than in 1790. A number of clinical observers believe this too, and view claims of an increase in depression with skepticism (although they did not always say this loudly in public, as the pharmaceutical industry had a great deal invested in the idea of an increasing epidemic of depression enveloping us all). Paul Kielholz, professor of psychiatry in Basel who, with his powerful personality, had a great deal to do with spreading the notion of epidemic depression (in forming the International Committee for Prevention and Treatment of Depressive Illness in 1975), was privately of the opinion that serious depression did not change historically. His friend and colleague Raymond Battegay recalled in an interview with David Healy, "Kielholz was always of the opinion that the major depressions remain constant over time because they are predominantly hereditary diseases. What increased were the depressions resulting from a more and more stressful human environment."[63] Gerald Klerman's article in 1986 in a volume edited by Munich psychiatry professor Hanns Hippius firmly implanted in the profession the idea that the *incidence* of depression was increasing (although all he had to go on was the *diagnosis* of depression.[64]) Yet ever since the eighteenth century, people have believed that they lived in a stressful environment, and the idea that increasing stress causes increased depression would be comparable to the notion that rising stress in the nineteenth century caused increased nervousness: Certainly doctors were impressed that nerves and stress were always on the rise. But this is meaningless.

As early as World War I, depression became a significant diagnosis. In 1912 the *New York Times*, in one of its earliest uses of the term depression in connection with suicide, noted the death of Professor Robert Syms in the Manhattan State Hospital of "depressive insanity." Professor Syms had been ill on several occasions and initially was taken to Bellevue Hospital in Manhattan "suffering from melancholia and mental depression."[65]

Thus did depression begin its strut. In 1926 Farquhar Buzzard spoke at a meeting of the Section of Neurology and Psychology of the British Medical Association. "Dr Buzzard believed that this psychosis [manic-depressive 'psychosis'] was very common, if not the commonest, mental disorder; it was rarely recognized, except by experts; but its recognition was a matter of great practical importance in relation to prognosis and treatment. It was as common as migraine … "[66] Today we think migraine afflicts around one in 10 people. That would have made the depression of Emil Kraepelin's manic-depressive illness common indeed among Buzzard's upper-middle-class practice.

At the Maudsley Hospital the percent of inpatients with a diagnosis of "depression" in selected years from 1924 to 1938 totaled 38% and of outpatients 25%.[67] Again, these are sizable figures.

At the Basel university psychiatric clinic between 1945 and 1957, the number of patients "with depressive manifestations" increased more than five-fold, as Paul Kielholz told a Montreal meeting in 1959. "It is particularly marked in respect of female patients with reactive depressions, melancholias and involutional depressions."[68] Psychoanalysis was all the rage in Switzerland in these years, yet these are not Freudian diagnoses, and the Basel department of psychiatry was not a hotbed of depth psychiatry. So clearly, something had changed in the Swiss medical gaze to make all these patients, who previously would have received other diagnoses, now appear depressed, or to give these female patients in particular, who previously might have just been considered unhappy, medical labels.

At psychoanalytic centers as well, the frequency of depression diagnoses increased enormously in these years. At the C. F. Menninger Memorial Hospital, a psychoanalytic redoubt in Topeka, Kansas, 8% of patients had depression as their syndrome diagnosis in 1945 and 30% in 1965. (The patients received a character diagnosis as well as a syndrome diagnosis.)[69] At the Massachusetts Mental Health Center, which increasingly became a bastion of psychoanalysis after World War II, there was a huge shift from "manic-depressive illness," a Kraepelinian diagnosis of mainline psychiatry, to depressive reaction, a diagnosis that demanded psychotherapy. Cases defined as manic-depression declined from 71 in 1945 to 25 in 1965, and over those years the number of depressive reactions rose from 6 to 110. (Of these patients 82% were female and 51% were below the age of 30. The hospital abolished its ECT service. "The admission of young, bright, and verbal patients who are suitable for psychotherapy is encouraged.")[70]

Depression, as a diagnosis easily given, increased in other settings as well. Willi Mayer-Gross was not a psychoanalyst, but in 1959 this refugee who imported German science to English clinical psychiatry saw which way the wind was blowing: away from neurosis and toward depression. "Illness seems to manifest itself nowadays ... very much more by means of depression than by neurosis, so that depression is common enough in general practice if one cares to look for it."[71]

By World War II depression had become the standard term for any accumulation of symptoms involving fatigue, anxiety, and so forth. But this was a depression that was far from melancholia. In fact, many of the patients who got the diagnosis did not even seem depressed. As John Dewan, a psychiatrist trained in England but teaching at the University of Toronto, said in 1952, "An outstanding feature of mild depression is that the patient rarely complains of feeling depressed and often does not appear particularly despondent." The patient was not slowed in thinking and acting. He might admit that his mood was "down" if questioned about it, "but attributes this to discouragement with the persistence of his other symptoms. Early and continuous complaints are fatigue, difficulty in concentrating and lack of interest." Insomnia, lack of appetite, and loss of weight accompanied the description of "feeling 'neutral,' as if a 'pall' had settled over him." There would be various pains and gastrointestinal upsets. "The patient is inclined to explain his illness on the physical disturbances." There were seldom any physical or laboratory findings. "It is sometimes difficult to differentiate between anxiety states and mild depressions when features of both may be present," said Dewan.[72] That Dewan would implicitly assume the underlying diagnosis was depression shows what vast strides the diagnosis had made in these years.

In the 1950s depression began to expand from a doctors' diagnosis to become a folkloric diagnosis, in the sense that this is what most people believe they have and they have the symptoms to prove it. In England and Wales in 1956, only 2.9 patients per 1000 population received the diagnosis of depression from their family doctor[73]; very few, in other words. A systematic review of the literature in 2004 on the occurrence of depressive illness found the 1-year prevalence of "major depressive disorder," "dysthymic disorder," and "bipolar disorder I" combined to 6.8% *per 100 population*, in other words, more than 20 times higher than the earlier English doctors' diagnosis rate.[74]

Clearly in the 1950s and 1960s, many patients did not realize they were depressed; they were unfamiliar with the term. A. M. W. Porter, a general practitioner in a small town in the county of Surrey, England, told his colleagues in 1972, sure, patients learn sooner or later to say that "It's my depression again, doctor." Porter continued, "But there has to be a first time when the patient has not been conditioned to say 'I am depressed, doctor.' This is a 'doctor phrase' rather than a 'patient phrase' and results from the constant reiterated question, 'do you feel depressed'? The new patient will present with one or more of a great variety of physical and mental symptoms."[75] The inference is that it was only the physician who stamped upon this odd-lot the label "depression."

Years later, patients had made the d-word part of their vocabulary. Psychiatrist John Marks said in 1987 that "in his experience in Liverpool, 'depression' was a term commonly used because patients had learned that it was an acceptable label: if they complained about their real problem—marital or financial for instance—no-one paid attention."[76] Depression had finally become part of the patients' medical folklore, and they had all become depressed.

In the belief that they were doing God's work, psychiatrists did quite a bit of public information work to assist patients, as well as their colleagues, to this understanding. Psychiatric efforts were unabating to convince people that depression was really a very widespread illness and was vastly underdiagnosed. In 1977, under the chairship of Gerald Klerman, 51 years old—Klerman was among the master figures in postwar American psychiatry and then at Harvard—the National Institute of Mental Health (NIMH) initiated a huge five-city study of depressive illness called the Collaborative Program on the Psychobiology of Depression. Klerman at this point had barely completed the migration from psychoanalysis, where he had begun, to psychopharmacology, where he was to end, dying prematurely of diabetes in 1992 in the middle of a large study of Xanax for panic disorder. In 1977 he and Myrna Weissman had described "the chronic depressive in the community: unrecognized and poorly treated"[77] and now it was time to do something about that. "The depressions, like all severe mental disorders," the investigators of the NIMH psychobiology project correctly noted, "are conditions of the whole organism."[78] Unfortunately, influenced perhaps by a residuum of the investigators' interest in psychoanalysis, the findings of the project focused much more upon down-mood than they did upon the nervous condition of the whole body.

Articles from this large project peppered the literature for the next decade, alerting everyone to the omnipresence of depression. In 1982, for example, Martin Keller, at the Massachusetts General Hospital and Harvard, said there was not one but two depressions—not, alas, melancholia and nonmelancholia—but major depression, an acute illness, and an underlying chronic depression, a separate illness.[79] These depressions would require being separately diagnosed, and, as it subsequently unfolded, separately treated, needing two prescriptions instead of one. The eyes of marketing agents in the pharmaceutical industry grew wide with expectation (and Keller, himself a considerable scientific figure, consulted widely and became a wealthy man[80]). Much later, Myrna Weissman, who in the meantime had married Klerman, placed the NIMH study in perspective. She said it had "brought depression to the forefront."[81]

9

Something Wrong with the Label

HOW DID EVERYONE become depressed? A depression needed to be created that could be applied to everyone. The drafters of the third edition of the American Psychiatric Association's (APA) *DSM* series did this in 1980 by creating major depression.

At the same time, the drafters completed the demolition of the nerve syndrome, which had been slowly unraveling. The analysts had removed neurotic depression from the nervous syndrome; psychiatry removed anxiety from the larger nervous picture with the diagnosis mixed anxiety-depression. And *DSM-III* completed the job by separating completely anxiety and depression, and fragmenting anxiety into a volley of meaningless microsyndromes. Fatigue was left completely out of the picture and ceased to be a psychiatric ailment. And obsessive thoughts had long vanished from the nervous picture into the vast anxiety basin, where they would tumble about with social anxiety, posttraumatic stress, and the like.

Like moving pieces of furniture from the room, all the furniture was removed from the nervous room except depression. Of the unitary diagnosis of nerves, a disease of the entire body, nothing was left except major depression, an expandable diagnosis that could be applied to almost the entire population—and a series of minianxiety diagnoses pseudospecific for different settings in which anxiety might arise: parties (social anxiety disorder), trauma (posttraumatic stress disorder), public places (agoraphobia), and so forth. The shattering of the nervous syndrome was complete.

DSM: *The Beginning*

In February 1973 the Board of the American Psychiatric Association decided that in the forthcoming edition of the World Health Organization's *International Classification of Diseases*, scheduled for 1979, some minor terminological clarifications were necessary in the input of American psychiatry, including issues such as "problem-oriented records" and how, exactly, to classify levels of disabilities. These were not big problems, but they would necessitate another edition of the APA's *Diagnostic and Statistical Manual*, the second edition of which has appeared in 1968[1]; the Board asked the APA's Reference Committee to get cracking, and in April the Reference Committee asked the Council on Research and Development to appoint a Task Force to revise *DSM-II*.[2] The research council, composed of psychoanalysts, viewed the entire classification question as secondary. "They didn't think diagnosis important," said Washington University psychiatrist Samuel Guze later. "No one wanted to give it the time."[3] So in January 1974 they chose a junior figure, Robert Spitzer, to head the Task Force. There was no indication at this point that a major upheaval lay ahead.

Spitzer was an interesting choice. Born in White Plains, New York, in 1932, he earned his MD degree from the New York University School of Medicine in 1957, then interned at Montefiore Hospital, where he caught the eye of Sidney Malitz, a senior figure at the New York State Psychiatric Institute, which is the department of psychiatry of Columbia University; Malitz persuaded him to train at "PI," as it is called. As was customary at the time, Spitzer also trained in psychoanalysis and, because he was plagued by chronic depression, he entered analysis with Abraham Kardiner and then Arnold Cooper. (Spitzer was ultimately cured of his depression by the drug Wellbutrin.) Something misfired in his encounter with psychoanalysis and Spitzer turned upon it snarling; in 1961 he became a research fellow in what is probably at the far end of the spectrum from psychoanalysis: the biometrics department at PI, headed by psychologist Joseph Zubin. Spitzer later said of Zubin, "He created a department where the atmosphere was, anything that's valid, you have to be able to measure it, that was the Zeitgeist. Within that Zeitgeist, I flourished."[4]

While in the Biometrics Department, Spitzer developed an interest in the classification of psychiatric disorders and began collaborating with Sam Guze, Eli Robins, and others in the department of psychiatry of the medical school of Washington University in St. Louis, which was then the prime locus of biological thinking in U.S. psychiatry. Spitzer had attracted the attention of the APA leadership as a result of his campaign to rid the *DSM* of the diagnosis of homosexuality, culminating in a historic vote in 1973 to depathologize gayness, and so he was a natural choice in 1974 to head the Task Force that was to draw up the U.S. contribution to the international classification of diseases (ICD), due 5 years later.

On the plus side, Spitzer was an engaging, lively—indeed, almost charismatic—individual with a strong will to put through his own ideas. He infuriated fellow Task Force members with what seemed authoritarian, unilateral decisions on vital issues, such as the diagnosis of major depression. It was this very force of character that produced *DSM-III* as the vision of the future of world psychiatry, a dramatic departure from *DSM-II* with its vague psychoanalytic constructs and lack of guidance for making diagnoses. On the minus side, Spitzer had had relatively little exposure to clinical psychiatry and did not have that deep intuitive understanding of psychological illness that many senior clinicians acquire. One noted U.S. specialist in psychopathology confided to the author, "Spitzer knew nothing about psychopathology. I wrote some papers on first rank symptoms [of schizophrenia] in the early 1970s and he invited me to his house in Westchester to discuss them. He asked me to describe them, as he might incorporate them into the proposed *DSM-III*. He typed my answers rapidly into the first desk-top computer I'd ever seen. As he did so, he muttered 'too hard …too subtle …too complicated.' He had no understanding of clinical psychiatry."[5]

Also on the minus side was that Spitzer's very determination to impose his own ideas made him a difficult figure to work with—and ultimately ensured that after *DSM-III-R*, the revised version in 1987 of *DSM-III*, the helm would be given to someone else. As Carolyn Robinowitz, a senior administrator at APA, wrote to the organization's medical director Melvin Sabshin in June 1979 of efforts to educate psychiatrists in the use of the new manual, " …Dr Spitzer has had an immense degree of effort and dedication to the process of developing a new nomenclature. The problem in that, however, has been that Dr Spitzer has not necessarily thought through how one goes about educating psychiatrists or other mental health professionals and is so exceedingly sensitive to any negative input (to which he responds as if there were an attack on his knowledge, integrity, etc.) that it is difficult to deal with him. He tends to respond with more personalized …attacks and accumulates data as if he were doing battle over a legal or political issue."[6]

Doing battle is a good metaphor. Spitzer saw himself engaged in a political not a scientific exercise in drawing up *DSM-III*. The point was to win, not to establish scientific exactness, and, above all, to triumph over the hated psychoanalysts. In a later interview he dismissed *DSM-II* as "based on psychoanalytic concepts." We wanted "a fresh start," he said.[7] Spitzer was determined to drive the diagnosis neurotic depression, the bread and butter of the analysts, from the scene, and in 1978 and 1979, when the horse trading at the bargaining table was most intense, he negotiated a number of political concessions that made little scientific sense. In April 1978 Donald Klein, one of the main players on the Task Force and a senior colleague of Spitzer's at PI, wrote to him, apropos Klein's suggestion that the depression diagnosis hysteroid dysphoria be included: "You and I have agreed that there are a number of categories included in DSM III in which we have little confidence concerning their reality but feel that at least this will afford the field an opportunity to decide whether they are there or not. I think the same logic applies to Hysteroid Dysphoria," a diagnosis that Spitzer dismissed with the back of his hand.[8] This is not how we usually do science.

The first fateful decision was taken soon after Spitzer became director. It was the decision in September 1974 to separate the committee that dealt with depression from that which dealt with anxiety. It is difficult to put it this way but I cannot think of any other way to say it: The fact that they separated depression and anxiety into two entirely different disease basins shows that they did not know what they were doing. A note from that month stated, "The grouping of the following conditions was made by the secretary [Spitzer] and does not represent product of Committee discussion." Group V was dedicated to "affective disorders," group VII, which at that point did not have a title, to "hypochondriasis, sexual disturbances, conversion reaction, and anxiety state."[9] This insured, for bureaucratic reasons, that there would never be a mixed anxiety-depression diagnosis.

A veteran clinician would probably have protested the separation. Spitzer seems to have made the separation almost as an afterthought. In 1975 he signaled that he disapproved of the concept of "mixed, anxious-depressed neurotics …because within that group will be included some people who have the full endogenous depressive syndrome, some who just have a dysphoric personality …and some who have just an episode of depression."[10] The separation must have seemed natural to him: He had been brought up in the world of psychoanalysis, and even though he tried to put it behind him it was probably a leftover psychoanalytic reflex to see depression, a matter of uninterest to Freud, and anxiety, the core symptom of psychoanalytic theory, as separate. In fairness to Spitzer, however, it must also be said that from the early 1950s on, the pharmaceutical industry had been flogging anxiety as an independent disease entity, not necessarily independent from depression but certainly independent from nerves and from the whole concept of sedation (see Chapter 10). Yet whatever the motivations for Spitzer's thinking, the consequences were enormous: In the decades ahead, depression and anxiety would in academic disease classification be seen as separate diseases requiring separate treatments.

In New York in September 1974, at the first meeting of the Task Force, Spitzer gonged that he was going to lead the group far beyond the timid mission that APA had originally conceived for it: They were going to abolish the terms neurosis and psychosis (though they left intact the firewall between schizophrenia and manic-depressive illness that Kraepelin had constructed). " ... 'Psychosis' and 'neurosis' are useful possibly as adjectives," the minutes of the first meeting said, "but not as classificatory principles. The term psychosis has become vague in usage." And neurosis, said the Task Force, has come to characterize "a more or less steady state," whereas Spitzer and colleagues wanted terms that would be adequate for episodes. As well, Spitzer intended to move "what has been known as depressive neurosis" from the neuroses to "the affective disorders." Thus, a page was turned on a century of previous psychiatric history.

How about cause? Until then, American psychiatry had known only one main cause of psychiatric illness: Freudian doctrines about unconscious conflict. With a stroke, this entire tradition now ended. The Task Force professed to be agnostic about cause: "Etiology should be a classificatory principle only when it is clearly known."[11] But the only etiology that counted had been Freudian, and the Task Force ultimately came up with a system of "disorders," rather than neuroses, that perfectly accommodated biological thinking: What could the cause of all these various disorders be if not brain biology? Spitzer's Task Force was about to break the stranglehold of psychoanalysis upon American psychiatry.

Thus the *DSM* revision began with firmly fixed scientific principles. But what began as science ended as politics. Donald Klein looked back somewhat ruefully: "When we started out with DSM, it was quite hard-nosed. If you didn't have data for a diagnosis, then screw it. Then Spitzer said if there's a group in favor, we'll take it."[12] Somehow, neither the public nor the profession ever quite understood that this is what happened.

Depression

It was Spitzer who devised all the committees, each specific for a different set of disorders, and appointed all the members. He also made himself a member of each committee, thus ensuring that he would be the spider at the center of the web.

If not neurotic depression, then what? The committee on "Schizophrenic, Paranoid, and Affective Disorders" was nominally chaired by Nancy Andreasen, a Washington University graduate now at the University of Iowa (which was becoming a psychiatric powerhouse); it included Paula Clayton, also at Washington University—replacing Robert Woodruff of the St. Louis school who had just committed suicide. Also on the committee was Jean Endicott, a psychologist at PI, and Janet Williams, a PI social worker who was initially Spitzer's girlfriend, then his wife. Thus the depression committee very much embodied the whole Washington University–PI axis that was the backbone of the Task Force.

But the key decisions were made at the level of the executive committee, not the individual disease committees. The main players on the executive committee were Clayton, Andreasen, Endicott, and Rachel Gittelman and Donald Klein, who were married to each other, he of PI, she a child psychologist at Long Island Jewish Hillside Medical Center; both kept trying, more or less in vain, to pull the Task Force in the direction of science and away from Spitzer's authoritarian control.

In the 1970s, as stated, Spitzer, together with the Washington University nosologists, had laid out a whole classification of disorders that culminated in the Research Diagnostic Criteria (RDC) of 1978, a subtle document including both major depressive disorder (with numerous subtypes) and "minor depressive disorder with significant anxiety"—another way of saying mixed anxiety-depression.[13] (Major was already a familiar adjective in psychiatry and Michael Shepherd of the Maudsley Hospital had referred to "the major depressive illnesses" at a conference in Montreal in 1959.[14]) It might have been expected that the momentum would continue and that the RDC would become the intellectual framework of *DSM*. Yet this is not exactly what happened.

At the beginning, in the Task Force's first draft of proposed diseases in August 1975, under "mood disorders," the basic classification that Spitzer, Endicott, and Robins had been hewing away at in the RDC, the Task Force had "major mood disorders" versus "minor mood disorders," and each had its major depression or minor depression.[15] So far, so good.

But the Task Force was constantly stung by the reproach that the insurance companies would never pay for anything "minor," so minor depression had to go—and therewith the doctrine of two distinct depressions, which we have been calling melancholia and nonmelancholia, went as well. In their next draft, in

March 1976, the Task force forgot about major and minor and distinguished between episodic (meaning acute) and intermittent (meaning chronic) mood disorders, adding, probably at Don Klein's insistence, demoralization disorder, in which Klein was a big believer.[16] The two depressions had become not major and minor as before, but acute and chronic ("intermittent"). This acute–chronic distinction, together with a severity scale, was maintained for the next several drafts.

Meanwhile in the real world, news was starting to trickle out that the Task Force had big changes in mind for the profession. The first public airing of the new scheme took place at a meeting in St. Louis in 1976, and here the analysts began to scream. At a meeting of the Assembly, the American Psychiatric Association's House of Delegates, in May 1976, these voices became loud, and Howard Berk, an analyst in Forest Hills, New York, became chair of an oversight body the Assembly created to ride herd on Spitzer and his crowd. In April 1977 Berk wrote the district organizations that, in essence, Spitzer was out of control and that the APA Assembly would definitely need to review the draft *DSM* before it was forwarded to the World Health Organization as "the official nomenclature of the United States."[17] So, there were big stakes.

The analysts' fierce opposition created an unexpected political problem for Spitzer: acute versus intermittent depression corresponded to none of their categories. And Berk was whipping up the Assembly in the direction of rejecting the entire draft. In November 1978 Washington, DC analyst Paul Chodoff, tongue in cheek, called Spitzer "the chief assassin and gravedigger of the concept of neurosis."[18]

Within mainline psychiatry Spitzer was simultaneously being pulled in opposite directions. Impressed by research that showed the number of stress factors in endogenous depression was the same as that in reactive depression,[19] some psychiatrists started to argue that there was no difference between endogenous and reactive, and that endogenous depression should be abolished. Lyman Wynne, a Task Force member from the University of Rochester, told Spitzer in February 1978 that endogenous should be dropped from the vocabulary: " …I would wager that 'endogenous' means lack of precipitating factors to most psychiatrists. On the other hand, when life events are carefully assessed, the alleged lack [of such events] for the 'endogenous' cases has repeatedly evaporated."[20] And Paula Clayton added in February 1979, "I wholeheartedly concur with Lyman's suggestions." Many patients with the diagnosis endogenous depression had very low Hamilton depression scores, she said: "Clearly severity does not necessarily correlate with 'endogenicity.' I am very much in favor of the term endogenous being dropped from DSM-III."[21]

By contrast, Don Klein was pulling hard in the other direction, of shoring up endogenous in such a way as to differentiate it truly from nonendogenous depression. Klein had in mind the symptom of "autonomy," meaning that the patient does not get better on good news. In April 1978 Klein told Spitzer that the crucial question was not whether the depression came out of the blue, but whether "Once the episode is underway, it is autonomous, that is unresponsive to changes in the initiating circumstances. If the patient with a depressive episode regains his job the illness continues."[22] (Mood autonomy became the basis of Klein's doctrine of endogenomorphic depression that he floated in 1974; later, he emphasized "non-precipitation" rather than autonomy. Endogenomorphic depressions could be either endogenous or nonendogenous, but had a special responsiveness to medication.[23])

Thus Spitzer was torn between the advocates of one depression versus two, and for the duration of the drafting was buffeted by the two camps.

In January 1978 the term "major depression" returned to the draft classification. But what did this mean, given that "chronic affective disorders" was also in the roster? In March, Spitzer made a crucial decision: How to classify a woman featured in a training exercise who had episodic depression? Is she "major" or is she "chronic"? He decided that she was "major." "The Cross sectional symptomatic picture of Major (full syndrome) takes precedence over the course." Yet the analysts would not agree. "Most analytic types would regard this patient as a good example of a Chronic Depressive Personality, despite the fact that one can with perseverance count up four or five associated symptoms."[24] (The Task Force was now listing symptoms, and saying that a patient would have to score a given number to qualify for the diagnosis.) Herewith Spitzer was saying that whatever the patient's past history of illness, it was the current picture that counted, and if a patient had over three symptoms on the list, the diagnosis would automatically be major depression. "I now have a picture of Kraepelin and Bleuler staring at me hauntingly in my room," Spitzer added.

In April 1978 this decision was solidified: all "episodic affective disorders" would be called "major affective disorders" and all recurrent major affective disorders lasting more than 6 months would be called "chronic." So any acute episode clearly not part of a recent history of depression would be major depression.

We are witnessing here, under the pressure of politics, the slow evolution of the sophisticated depression scheme of the Research Diagnostic Criteria into a single diagnosis: major depression. But we are not quite there yet because the classification still contained "chronic affective disorders," and Spitzer wanted to characterize them as "minor," despite the yowls of the insurance companies, to indicate that "the full depressive syndrome is not present."[25] (This puts to rest the charge, often heard later, that Spitzer abolished minor depression at the insistence of the insurance companies.)

Was there trouble ahead? In May 1978 Spitzer told the Task Force that "Part of our problem is that there is some feeling that it may be too easy to get into Major Depressive Disorder in DSM-III." RDC requires 2 weeks; our current draft requires only 1.[26] In fact the published version in 1980 would require 2 weeks, but at this point Spitzer only vaguely sensed "the plague of affective disorders," as Don Klein put it, that was about to descend on psychiatry. It was, in fact, far too easy to get into Major Depression. And there was nothing else.

The final piece of architecture fell into place in July 1978 when Spitzer suggested rechristening Chronic Minor Depressive Disorder (CMDD) "dysthymia." "CMDD" was "doomed to fail," he said, "and rightly so ... It is clumsy, and a four-word diagnostic term is hardly very appealing. Of more importance, there are not only insurance problems with the use of the term 'Minor' but there are also conceptual problems. This diagnostic entity can be devastating, and the term 'Minor' certainly does not suggest this."[27] (Unknown to Spitzer, who found the word dysthymia in Leland Hinsie and Jacob Shatzky's *Psychiatric Dictionary*, dysthymia had a long history in medicine and "distimia" was in current use in Italy as a synonym for mood disorders.[28])

Now this sounds very much as though the concept of two depressions had been somehow preserved, doesn't it? We have a major depression, which you can "get into," as the phrase went, with four of the eight listed symptoms, and we have a chronic depression called dysthymia that, Spitzer insisted, could be devastating. Yet in the events that followed, dysthymia was downgraded to being a new name for neurotic depression, a kind of depressive personality that, although it kept the term depression current, previously had not even been considered a mood disorder but rather a neurosis. (Tom Ban, veteran psychopharmacologist at Vanderbilt University, later said of dysthymia patients, "They don't have a depressive disease in which the mood transforms their experiences."[29])

The analysts had been simmering with discontent for the previous 2 years. In March 1979 this discontent came to a boil as analyst Roger Peele, assistant superintendent of Saint Elizabeths Hospital, a government psychiatric facility in Washington, DC, proposed to Spitzer the revival of "neurotic disorders," which would cover many of the proposed *DSM-III* diagnoses as a kind of umbrella. Peele's note had a collegial tone, yet there were teeth in it: "Preservation of 'neurotic disorders' provides us with a greater unanimity within the profession, avoids a major clash within the Assembly and a possible Assembly-Board struggle. It would also head off, I would submit, a referendum that would ill serve DSM-III even if DSM-III won."[30]

Spitzer panicked at this head shot. Without consulting with other Task Force members, 2 weeks later he wrote the committee of the American Psychoanalytic Association that liaised with the Assembly of the American Psychiatric Association a humble letter requesting a "neurotic peace treaty." The *DSM-III* draft would insert "neurosis" at various strategic points.[31] Would this be enough to satisfy them?

Spitzer's letter of concession certainly was not enough to satisfy members of the Task Force, who were furious at this authoritarian end run. Don Klein wrote Spitzer 3 days after receiving Spitzer's memo confessing what he had done: "I must admit that I was flabbergasted by this memo....I was particularly concerned about the seemingly autocratic procedure ...The Task Force already has taken a clear stand upon the utility of the term 'neurosis.' Your current stand is, as far as I can see, entirely your own creation and was taken without their consultation with the Task Force or its agreement." Terrible time pressure, sure, said Klein, but not even a telephone call! "I am left with the nagging feeling that this was an attempt to create a fait accompli, so that the Task Force has its hands tied."[32] The point here is that yet another fateful decision in the *DSM* process was entirely Spitzer's alone, and not that of a group of psychiatrist Wise Persons.

The psychoanalysts held out for something more than a bunch of vague references to neurosis strewn throughout the text. They evidently wanted dysthymia to be renamed neurotic depression, and Spitzer conceded.[33] The revised draft of April 25, 1979 said that "chronic depressive disorder" had been renamed "Dysthymic disorder (Neurotic depression)."[34]

So neurotic depression, the blues of bored suburban housewives in the 1950s, had survived as the second depression. Everything else was major depression. This was actually quite a stunning achievement. Spitzer had collapsed the two depressions of melancholia and nonmelancholia, in use in psychiatry for over two centuries, into a single depression, called major depression, and ensured that it was the only diagnosis you could get into unless you were seeing a psychoanalyst and could qualify for neurotic depression. Major depression, often simply called "depression," went on to become the diagnosis of one-tenth of the United States population—one out of every 10 on that subway car was depressed—and it all happened at the Psychiatric Institute.

Melancholia, Kind of

In *DSM-III* major depression had various subtypes. One of them was melancholia. This was a result of the buffeting Spitzer received from the different camps. In February 1979, he got an impassioned letter from Bernard Carroll at the University of Michigan. Carroll, an Australian "double doctor" (endocrinology and medicine) by origin and then 39 years old, had proposed the dexamethasone suppression test in 1968 and was in the vanguard, together with Edward Sachar, Don Klein, and Max Fink, of biological thinking in psychiatry. "My emphatic view is that it is a serious mistake to have only one basic depressive typology or category ...I believe that there should be two categories of depression. These should be endogenomorphic [Klein's 1974 idea] and non-endogenomorphic depression." Carroll explained that each category might have its own severity scale. "I am sincerely suggesting these changes to you with the greatest possible sense of urgency. I honestly believe that you will be buying yourself (and the rest of us) a lot of grief if you allow the unitary category of major depressive disorder to remain."[35]

At this late stage in the drafting, such a missive was as welcome to Spitzer as rat poison, and he replied dismissively.[36] But it made him aware that he would have a problem if he ignored melancholia.

Around the same time, in early February 1978, Carroll and colleagues at the Mental Health Research Institute of the University of Michigan published a letter critiquing the concept of "endogenous depression," as articulated in the Research Diagnostic Criteria, which, of course, Spitzer had edited.[37] He may have got the wind up over this as well.

Two weeks after replying to Carroll, Spitzer resolved to act. He wrote to the "Affective Mavens," as he called the inner circle, "We are in big trouble!" Our severity typology misses the point of whether the cases of major depression are endogenous or not. "There needs to be some way of subtyping Major Depressive Disorder that would enable this distinction to be made." Spitzer went over the factors that, he believed, constituted endogenous depression, such as loss of pleasure in activities, nonreactivity, inappropriate guilt, and psychomotor slowing.

"What to call this syndrome?" he asked the committee, taking for granted that they would agree to include it. Here, again, he went over the obvious

candidates—endogenomorphic (con: "implies the absence of a precipitating event"); vital depression (con: "Does this mean a lively depression?");
and anhedonic syndrome (con: "the syndrome includes features that are not
symptomatic of anhedonia").

Then Spitzer came to the last candidate on the list. "Sit down for this one,"
he advised Task Force members.

It was melancholia.

Spitzer noted that Dartmouth (later UCLA) psychiatrist Peter Whybrow
had suggested melancholia to the Task Force several years previously as
preferable to major depression, but people rejected it "because it was out-
dated. Its resurrection now is a suggestion of Bernard Carroll and Michael
Feinberg." This is an interesting comment, given that Carroll in his letter had
not proposed this, and the Carroll letter in *Lancet* did not envision such a
resurrection either.

What positive could be said about melancholia? Spitzer noted that Freud
had used the term, an argument that usually sufficed, in those days, to justify
just about anything. And then: "Perhaps one of the strongest arguments in
favor of the term Melancholia is historical continuity." (It was, indeed, one of
the jewels in the crown of psychiatry.)

And con? "The term is antiquated and will cause a lot of guffaws."[38]

Spitzer proposed melancholia as a subtype of major depression
(a "fifth-digit code"). The published version of *DSM-III* included the melancholia subtype of a "major depressive episode," with at least three of six features (largely those he had enumerated above).[39]

But the melancholic subtype that emerged from Spitzer's pen, weeks
before the draft *DSM-III* was to go to the press, was a pale shadow of the
historic melancholia, with its crushing burden of intolerable pain. As your
three melancholic features, you could have loss of appetite, early morning
wakening, and symptoms worse in the morning than in the afternoon. You did
not need to have psychotic guilt about having killed all your children (when
in fact you had not); or agitated pacing alternating with stupor and brooding
about your sinfulness; or thoughts so slowed that you were unable to think, to
concentrate, to read a book, and to remember by the bottom of the page what
you had seen at the top. As Thomas Ban has pointed out, in research studies
of the patients diagnosed with major depression, only 30% definitely fulfilled
criteria for Kraepelin's depressive states in manic-depressive illness, and only
14% for Kurt Schneider's vital depression.[40] Spitzer's melancholic subtype was
not real melancholia, and the uselessness of the subtype contributed further
to erasing the real version from the collective memory of psychiatry.[41]

Carroll commented on Spitzer's melancholia: "So what Spitzer did was to take this metaphysical concept that he had and to disembody it from the patients it happens in."[42] This was a world historic defeat for psychiatry.

Anxiety

The anxiety section of *DSM-III* ended up as a real dog's breakfast, not to put too fine a point on it, because of the politics of the Task Force. The result was the further fragmentation of a concept that had begun as an organic part of the nervous syndrome, had transitioned to an ionic bond with depression in the diagnosis mixed anxiety-depression, and was now dismantled. Jean Endicott chaired the anxiety committee, though Don Klein seems to have been the driving force.

Readers of this book are familiar with panic as a paroxystic form of anxiety. This well-established concept was essentially extinguished by psychoanalysis, which had little interest in such fine differentiations; and aside from the brief awakening that panic experienced at Oskar Diethelm's hand in 1932, panic went off the radar in psychiatry until Klein and Max Fink began trials in the early 1960s with the new antidepressant drug imipramine (Geigy's Tofranil), the first member of the chemical class of tricyclic antidepressants, at Hillside Hospital in Glen Oaks, Long Island. The work Klein published with Fink was important and led to the understanding that drugs such as chlorpromazine were not just antipsychotics. But on his own, Klein observed on the ward a number of "extremely anxious patients" who had received no benefit from either sedatives or antipsychotics. "Such people, often feeling quite well, are doing something innocuous, such as walking down the street or having a meal, when suddenly they are struck by the worst experience of their life: they become suffused with terror, with a pounding heart and inability to catch their breath; the very ground underfoot seems unstable, and they are convinced that death from a stroke or heart attack is imminent." Symptoms worsen, and eventually such patients are admitted to a place such as Hillside. "The happy thought struck us that perhaps these patients might benefit from imipramine. The logic behind this was not exactly coercive: it was more a case of our not knowing what else to do for them." Slowly, these patients with "panic attacks," soon to be called agoraphobia, began to get better. Imipramine did not work on any other type of anxious patients, but it had a slow but powerful effect on the panic patients.[43] Klein did a double-blind study of 28 of these patients at Hillside, publishing the results in 1964. (Preliminary findings had appeared in a paper published with Max Fink in 1962.[44]) Klein had, in effect, established panic as an independent illness separate from anxiety. The paper concluded that "The use of patterns of drug response as dissecting tools, allowing the discovery of specific … similarities within psychiatric subpopulations is emphasized." [45] The discovery of "pharmacological dissection," that drugs could be used as a pharmacological torch to carve out illness entities in psychiatry, gave Klein an impressive reputation.

In 1967 Klein described the effectiveness of imipramine in panic with subsequent agoraphobia, meaning that "Their activities become progressively constricted until they are no longer able to travel alone for fear of being suddenly rendered helpless while isolated from help." [46] But there could also be agoraphobia without panic attacks. The diagnoses had started to multiply.

Bear in mind that *DSM-II* in 1968 had only one anxiety disorder, anxiety neurosis; obsessive-compulsive neurosis and phobic neurosis were separate diagnoses. [47] Under "anxiety disorders," the anxiety committee for *DSM-III* in its draft of August 1975 produced five separate conditions: panic disorder, generalized anxiety disorder, phobic disorder, obsessive-compulsive disorder, and somatic preoccupation disorder.

How did generalized anxiety disorder (GAD) get in there? Once panic was in, the question arose of differentiating it from anxiety, which was to be a separate diagnosis. James Sheehan at Harvard recalled hearing of a dinner involving the members of the anxiety committee. " … They decided that, while they could identify this panic disorder, they should invent another disorder that would be a benzodiazepine-responsive disorder. So the pharmacological dissection was that panic disorder is the tricyclic responsive syndrome [imipramine] and generalized anxiety was going to be the benzodiazepine [Valium-style drugs] responsive syndrome. It sounded like it had a good ring to it—GAD—somebody said 'gee that sounds wonderful, these people are generally anxious when they don't have panic attacks.' But nobody really went out to see where one ended and the other began." Sheehan recalled that as he heard of this discussion, "I thought this doesn't make sense to me because I don't think there are two distinct syndromes and that really the anxiety neurosis concept is probably closer to the truth and maybe even hysteria is closer … It was chaos at the time." [48]

GAD was said to be a residual category, a place to put the anxious patients who were not panicky, phobic, or preoccupied with their bodily symptoms. "Don insisted on panic disorder and generalized anxiety disorder," said Paula Clayton later in an interview. "GAD got there because they weren't going to give Don hysteroid dysphoria." [49] Hysteroid dysphoria was a coinage of Klein that ultimately became the diagnosis of atypical depression. Spitzer, however, had no patience with hysteroid dysphoria and refused to grant it to Klein, who was a sufficiently powerful figure that he had to be placated with something else, hence GAD. The horse-trading here is delicious.

Klein, it must be said, did *not* regard GAD as a residual category. He told Spitzer that it was the only disorder in the anxiety basin that was not autonomous. For panic disorder and so forth, "Although something may kick it off, we really expect the syndrome to continue even if the precipitant disappears. That's not the case with Generalized Anxiety Disorder. Here implicitly we really do not expect autonomy."[50] [This issue has not really been resolved even to this day. In any event, *DSM-IV* did not take it on, and *DSM-5* differs from *DSM-IV* only in the most trivial ways, hiving off packrat behavior into a separate category ("hoarding disorder") for example.]

All this subdividing did not sit well with other committee members. Isaac Marks, a well-known specialist in anxiety at the Maudsley Hospital in London, found the distinction between generalized anxiety disorder and panic to be without foundation. In June 1977 he wrote Spitzer, "The evidence for the importance of panic attacks as a basis for classification is shaky at the present time and needs much better replication …"[51] And Michael Gelder, professor of psychiatry at Oxford who, unlike Marks, was not a committee member yet had been consulted, told Spitzer in May 1978, "As you know, I do not accept the existence of the diagnosis of panic disorder. Panics are symptoms of the agoraphobic syndrome and they may be present in some cases and absent in others."[52] (Klein hotly denied that this was true: "I have seen many patients with panic disorder who do not have agoraphobia." It was such exchanges that led, in the draft of March 30, 1977, to the inclusion of the diagnoses "agoraphobia with panic attacks" and "agoraphobia without panic attacks," a distinction that Klein subsequently found to be without a difference.)[53]

Simultaneously, the anxiety committee began to splinter the phobias into separate diagnoses: agoraphobia, social phobia, simple phobia, and mixed phobia had all cropped up by March 1976.[54]

There was more. An "atypical anxiety disorder" was added in December 1976,[55] making the number of separate anxiety diagnoses now nine. Then, as we have seen, in March 1977 the "with and without panic attacks" qualification appeared. Then at the very end, on the final draft of November 15, 1979 just as *DSM-III* went to press, "post-traumatic stress disorder, acute versus chronic or delayed," was shoved into the anxiety section.[56]

To think that in 1968 we had started with one anxiety disorder, and now there was a veritable cascade. And people were asking themselves, is this science?

Did any of this concern depression? We saw above Spitzer's resistance to mixed anxiety-depression. Then something strange happened. In a close to final draft, in January 1978, Spitzer allowed that " . . . All of the manifestations of Anxiety Disorders can occur in individuals with Affective Disorders, although the converse is not true."[57] This would seem to demolish much of the firewall between anxiety and depression that he himself had constructed. And perhaps that is the reason this statement was not included in the published version.

After *DSM-III* was launched in 1980, there was a good deal of dissatisfaction with the splintering of anxiety. At Sheehan's Psychosomatic Clinic at Massachusetts General Hospital, one of Harvard's teaching hospitals, there was a succession of patients who "presented . . . for treatment of spontaneous panic attacks and phobic symptoms." Of 100 consecutive such patients:

- Panic disorder, 100% of them
- Generalized anxiety disorder, 100%
- Agoraphobia, 100%
- Simple phobia, 100%
- Conversion disorder [classic hysteria], 100%
- Atypical somatoform disorder, 100%
- Dysthymic disorder (atypical depression), 92% (depressed feelings, but no "vegetative" signs of depression)

Sheehan concluded that "Simultaneous assignment of the majority of the patients to all of these diagnostic categories suggests that these categories, as distinct entities, do not reflect the natural order. They do not 'cut nature at the joints.'"[58]

Juan Lopez Ibor, professor of psychiatry in Madrid, was more blunt. "Generalized anxiety, as currently defined, might be described as a waste basket of conditions."[59]

Envoi

DSM-III was big. It gave psychiatry a public profile much larger than ever before, and attuned people to psychiatric diagnosis as a kind of normal event, much like any other illness, rather than as some nightmarish visitation. But the line between the beneficial destigmatization of illness and the epidemic spread of an illness attribution is a thin one. At some point, medicine stops and culture takes over. Spitzer agreed subsequently with an interviewer that *DSM-III* and its successors had become "cultural events." "It is amazing. I guess it defines things. . . . I guess it defines what is the reality."[60]

Much after the circumstances described in this chapter took place, Max Fink, one of the pioneers of biological psychiatry, commented on the shift from manic-depressive illness to major depression. "When it was manic-depressive illness, it was a small number of people. When it became major depression . . . 50 percent of the people are depressed. That's absurd. That means there's something wrong with the label."[61]

Yes, sir. One of the reasons everybody became depressed was that there was indeed something wrong with the label.

10

Drugs

*"We are troubled on every side, yet not distressed; we are
perplexed, but not in despair. Persecuted, but not forsaken;
cast down, but not destroyed."*

II CORINTHIANS, 4, 8–9

HISTORY HAS ALWAYS known antidepressant remedies. In an era of faith, the faithful held to the Word as an augury of recovery: "cast down, but not destroyed." But in a secular era and certainly by the middle of the twentieth century, pharmacological remedies were required.

Indeed they were urgently indicated, for the diagnosis of depression itself was starting to spread. Because of Kraepelin and Freud, by 1940 depression had become a common term for serious psychiatric disease. An editorial in the *Lancet* called depression "perhaps the most unpleasant illness that can fall to the lot of man."[1] Depression was thus, while not terribly common, a considerable public health issue.

What is puzzling in this story is that around 1940 depression began an inexorable, irreversible climb from awful but unusual to epidemic status. With the 1960s, depression started to become epidemic.

Sedatives and Nervous Disease

One reason for the upswing in depression in mid-twentieth century was the cheering of the pharmaceutical industry. The drugs of the first generation of psychoactive medications were indicated for nervous disease, but thereafter the firms switched to depression because here were clearly the markets of the future.

The early drugs represented an effective treatment for nervous disease. Their effect was sedation, and sedative drugs in medical practice go back to opium and to members of the belladonna family that have been known since

Ancient times. Sedation means the process of calming, or allaying excitement. It does not necessarily involve the obtunding of consciousness, although large doses of sedatives may do that. Sedation means easing the pain of being, soothing the griefs and worries of existence, and calming the depressive and anxious agitation of the nervous syndrome. Although we all have worries and anxieties, we do not all have a pathological syndrome called nervousness. Historically, it was those with nerves who benefited from the early psychopharmacological treatments, beginning with the bromides at mid-nineteenth century. The first sedative made by chemical synthesis, chloral hydrate, was used clinically in 1869. A succession of sedatives from the organic chemical industry followed. None had huge currency because they either tasted foul or had an unpleasant odor.

The game changed at the turn of the century with the introduction of a new class of sedatives called the barbiturates. The first, Veronal (barbital), was ushered into the university psychiatric clinic at Jena, Germany, in 1903. Less addictive than opium and less dimming of consciousness than belladonna alkaloids such as scopolamine (commonly used as an anesthetic), the barbiturates calmed and soothed and sedated the cares of many. Of course they had side effects, including the risk of overdose; in particular, they could be accumulated and used to commit suicide. Yet there are many ways to commit suicide, and sinking an entire drug class for this reason was unnecessary pharmacocide (to coin a phrase).

The barbiturates achieved instant acceptance. "Veronal at present is very popular," said Francis Boyd, lecturer on therapeutics in Edinburgh, in 1910.[2] A torrent of barbiturates, often in combinations with other agents, poured onto the market. By 1932 Indonal, a combination of barbital and cannabis indica (a cousin of marijuana), was on sale in Britain, as were Veronidia (barbital and passion flower) and Alepsal (belladonna, phenobarbital, and caffeine).[3] These were effective sedatives and hypnotics, and were found in medicine chests around the western world.

The medical press was filled with advertisements for the barbiturates as hypnotics and sedatives: Merck in Darmstadt flogged Veronal Sodium as suitable for rectal applications and as an essential companion in travel.[4] In 1931, Dehaussy Laboratories in Lille, France, offered "Sedoneurol" (phenobarbital) to "calm without depressing" for the indication of "nervous instability." Likewise, Buisson Laboratories in Paris proposed the abovementioned "Veronidia" as an "ideal sedative in nervous hyperexcitability, in all of its manifestations: various neuroses, palpitations, phobias, insomnia, anxiety neurosis, etc."[5]

So the uptake of barbiturates for nervous diseases of various kinds was considerable, without, as far as one can tell, reaching the level of cocktail party chitchat, as was later to happen with the "antidepressants." I realize this is a difficult judgment call for historians to make, since these people are all dead and we do not really know what drugs they mentioned as they convened socially. Yet there are hints: Virginia Woolf, for example, a prominent member of the London literary circle, took Veronal, but mentioned it only casually to her lover Vita Sackville-West (Woolf had just suffered one of her periodic nervous illnesses and believed Veronal had plunged her into it).[6] Marcel Proust, the Parisian novelist, initially took the nonbarbiturate Trional, then around 1909 switched to Veronal, apparently swallowing the tablets in great numbers, discussing this only with a handful of intimate confidants.[7]

In 1936, 99,000 pounds of phenobarbital alone were sold in the United States; sales for all barbiturates equaled 2,200,000 doses a day.[8] Some barbiturates, such as butabarbital (Soneryl), had a short half-life and were useful as sleeping agents; others, such as phenobarbital, with longer side chains had more lasting half-lives.[9] Their calming and sedating effects were much demanded in psychological medicine, where agitation and "excitement" of an unpleasant sort are the order of the day. "Sedation" today is in bad odor, and the preferred concept is "anxiolysis."

Thus, the effectiveness of the barbiturates lay in sedation. Arthur Foxe, a veteran Manhattan family doctor with an office on West 54th Street, said in 1943, "Sedatives hold their eminent position by virtue of their assistance in bringing about a more peaceful withdrawal from worldly affairs."[10] We would never encounter such a phrase in the pharmaceutical advertisements of today, yet Dr Foxe had touched on a truth: This sort of withdrawal is often called for, to calm the agitated spirit, rather than the use of antidepressants.

Despite the horror stories that have come down to us in the textbooks, the barbiturates in their day enjoyed a reputation as safe and effective agents, particularly as hypnotics. In 1957, Louis Lasagna, a pharmacologist then at Johns Hopkins—and later acknowledged as the dean of American pharmacology—reexamined "objections raised to barbiturates and other older hypnotics," finding most of them overdrawn. This was 3 years before the introduction of Librium, the first of the benzodiazepines. Lasagna wrote that "Barbiturates and chloral hydrate remain the prime reliance of most physicians in managing the sleep disorders of their patients. When *properly* used, these older drugs are remarkably safe and effective, and produce untoward effects infrequently."[11]

To be sure, there is a difference between sedation and the relief of anxiety: Sedation means controlling a high arousal state, whereas anxiolysis relieves an affective state characterized by excessive tension. A high arousal state may be present without the accompanying mood disorder of anxiety.[12] Yet in the real world of medical practice, meliorating anxiety often does mean sedating the patient in some way. Notwithstanding the commercial hype surrounding the Valium-style drugs, the benzodiazepines, in the 1960s, their antianxiety and antidepressant action accomplished much the same thing as the sedation of the classical barbiturates.

Is the Rise of Drugs for Depression Responsible for the Later Epidemic?

But depression was part of the nervous package as well. The barbiturates were effective not just in the treatment of insomnia and anxiety, which were two of the pieces of the nervous syndrome, but also enjoyed success in the treatment of depression. English family doctors and patients alike looked back with fondness upon "the green medicine" for "mild or moderate emotional disorders"—a mixture of hyoscine (scopolamine) and phenobarbital in peppermint water. Said family practitioner Ian Tait in retrospect of his practice in a village in Sussex, "Long after the early antidepressants became available [late 1950s] the green medicine was often used as a first treatment. It very often worked. The pressure to prescribe antidepressants really came from the hospital." Once discharged from the hospital, patients would invariably return with prescriptions for medications that none of the family doctors had ever used. "I certainly remember patients coming back and asking if they could go back on the old green medicine again, known and trusted and without significant side-effects."[13]

The evidence for the effectiveness of the barbiturates for depression and anxiety is considerable. Several Midwestern universities had departments of psychiatry that, unlike most American psychiatry at the time, were fortresses of psychopharmacology. It was at the University of Wisconsin that Richard Bleckwenn in 1930, associate professor of neuropsychiatry, found the new barbiturate sodium amytal of the Eli Lilly Company useful in a number of conditions, including depression. "It can be said without reservation that no drug in common use...will produce the degree of mental rest and physical relaxation in so short a time or over so long a period apparently without danger to the patient as does 'Sodium Amytal.'" He said of "manic-depressive psychosis": "In the depressed stage of this disease, the favorable response takes the form of a greater willingness to eat and take fluids...They are more active, more talkative, have less constrained and less awkward attitudes, and certainly the course of their depressions [is] materially shortened."[14] At the University of Iowa, another powerhouse of biological thinking, in 1949 Jacques Gottlieb referred to sodium amytal specifically as an "effective anti-depressant," and advocated it in combination with the amphetamine Benzedrine in the treatment of depression.[15]

As late as 1967 the World Health Organization accepted the barbiturates for the treatment of "depressive disorders."[16] By these years people had long stopped talking about nerves and sedation. But the barbiturates were effective in treating complaints that previously would have been deemed nervous.

The benzodiazepines (Valium-style drugs), introduced in 1960, did change the sedative picture, because they were not marketed as sedatives. In other respects, it is not at all clear that the benzodiazepines were superior to the barbiturates. Donald Klein and John Davis wrote in 1969 that "There is no very convincing evidence that these drugs [the "minor tranquilizers" including the benzodiazepines] are superior to short-acting sedatives, such as amytal, for the relief of manifest acute anxiety." All, however, were superior to placebo, the authors said.[17] The barbiturates were thus effective drugs and the "new antidepressants" argument for the rise of depression cannot be sustained: Depression and anxiety did not become a treatment focus in the 1960s and after because of the advent of miracle new drugs: The barbiturates too were quite efficacious. It was not the march of the antidepressants that prompted an epidemic of depression.

If the barbiturates and amphetamines were successful before the 1960s in the treatment of the components of nervousness, why did their success not occasion the epidemic spread of these diagnoses—just as the marketing of the "antidepressants" today has contributed to the spread of "depression"? The diagnoses of the pre-1960 era, such as mixed depression-anxiety, did not spread epidemically because the entire diagnostic and therapeutic concept of psychiatry, based on psychoanalysis, was opposed to them. Psychiatrists, whether analysts or not, were most often trained under the Freudian paradigm, which valued psychotherapy above all else and maintained that illness stemmed from anxiety over unconscious conflicts. Psychiatrists were often obliged to prescribe medications in order to reach patients otherwise unsuitable for psychotherapy, or unresponsive to it. But they did so reluctantly and with an absence of conviction. The setting in which a drug is given does influence treatment response. Heinz Lehmann found at the Douglas Hospital in Montreal that patients given phenobarbital in a group therapy session became very lively. If you gave it to them individually, they became sleepy.[18]

The New York State Psychiatric Institute, the epicenter of postwar American psychiatry, was heavily oriented toward psychoanalysis. Phillip Politin—an analyst—and Paul Hoch, who was trained in Budapest and was not an analyst but was sympathetic, were in charge of the female service; they had been using sodium amytal to carry out narcotherapy, inducing patients into a semistupor and then hoping they would cough up revealing unconscious material. In 1948 they noted that the success of this approach had been uneven: "War neurosis responded well to this treatment but the civilian neuroses do not show the remarkable effects observed in the war neuroses... This method is not a substitute for intensive psychotherapy or prolonged analysis."[19]

So there we had it: The true convictions of analytically schooled American psychiatry lay on the side of psychotherapy and against what many analysts contemptuously referred to as "pills." Under such hostile conditions, drug treatments, and diagnoses responsive to pharmacotherapy, would not flourish. The physicians would not grant nervous diagnoses but rather would label their patients with anxiety neurosis. And the patients would not clamor for the drugs or the diagnoses because—and this is a cardinal rule of medicine that is as old as the hills—patients are always intent upon producing symptoms that their physicians will find convincing. If the doctor believes that I have neurotic anxiety, then I will give him neurotic anxiety (so that he will believe I do not have hysteria).[20]

Before World War II, other classes of drugs as well showed benefit in the treatment of nervous illness and its depressive component. Opium was used for melancholia by the Ancients, and its modern service in depressive illness goes back to the eighteenth century.[21] In 1936 the amphetamines began to be indicated for depression, and methylene blue, an early ancestor of the antipsychotic phenothiazine drug class, showed promise as well. Here is not the place to explore these byways in the history of psychopharmacology, which have been detailed elsewhere.[22] The point is that drugs effective in depressive illness have a long history and certainly do not begin with the introduction of the first official "antidepressants," the tricyclic compound imipramine (Geigy's Tofranil) in 1957.

Neurotransmitter Chatter

What made depression epidemic was flogging it to the public as a concept with a firm scientific basis. This occurred in two steps: First, the rise of what one might call neurotransmitter chatter, as opposed to the solid science of neurotransmission in the brain; and second, the marketing to the public of drugs for depression on the grounds that they rested on an unshakable foundation of neuroscience. In the end, the public was gulled into believing that a disorder of mood called depression was as common as the common cold, but that, unlike the cold, its treatment was based on a firm platform of science.

After World War II, psychiatry began its transformation from a discipline based on Freud's concepts and on psychotherapy to one based on biological neuroscience and pharmacotherapy. In 1949 the National Institute for Mental Health (NIMH) opened its doors, pouring hundreds of millions of dollars into research on disorders of the mind and brain. Led by towering figures such as pharmacologist Seymour Kety, the NIMH became a great bastion of scientific research in world psychiatry, and pioneered domains such as the genetics of psychiatric illness.

Elsewhere within the vast National Institutes of Health, laboratories led by Bernard Brodie and Julius Axelrod in the mid-1950s were laying bare the mechanics of the reuptake of neurotransmitters: A neurotransmitter, once discharged by the end bulb of a neural cell, or neuron, stays in the synapse between the neurons until it is reabsorbed; the process is called reuptake, a return to the upstream neuron that discharged it. For key neurotransmitters such as serotonin, dopamine, and norepinephrine, it was believed that delaying, or inhibiting, the process of reuptake would lengthen the amount of time the neurotransmitter dwelled in the synapse, thus maximizing its potential to do good: This grounded the assumption that increasing the synapse time of these monoamine neurotransmitters would combat illnesses such as depression. Whole theories of depression were spun about the neurotransmitters. In 1965 Joseph Schildkraut at Harvard proposed the norepinephrine theory of depression, attributing the illness to a shortage of the catecholamine neurotransmitters, of which norepinephrine is one[23]; and serotonin theories of depression had been circulating ever since the work of the Scottish pharmacologist John Henry Gaddum in the early 1950s.[24]

The early 1960s were alive with vibrant debate about serotonin and nor-epinephrine and their role in illness. Arvid Carlsson, a pharmacologist then at the University of Lund, recalls taking his group's ideas about the role of dopamine and noradrenaline in the brain to a Ciba Foundation symposium in London in 1960.[25] The Brits, still caught up in ideas about electrophysiology rather than neurochemistry, dismissed the Swedish group's beautiful graphs showing brain concentrations of norepinephrine after the administration of drugs.[26] Five years later it was game over. At a symposium at the Wenner-Gren Center in Stockholm in February 1965, Carlsson brought beautiful photographs showing the presence of norepinephrine in the nerve terminals of the rat.[27] The paper was respectfully listened to—helping to win Carlsson a Nobel Prize in 2000. And the British electrophysiologists had either fallen silent or become converted to the hypothesis of the chemical transmission of the nerve impulse.

In 1963 Alec Coppen and colleagues put one group of depressed patients already being treated with a monoamine oxidase inhibiting agent (MAOI) on tryptophan, an amino acid that is a precursor of serotonin; this group got dramatically better than a control group that did not receive the tryptophan supplement.[28] This was the first research to suggest that serotonin might be important in depression. (Subsequent research on tryptophan did not produce such brilliant results.[29])

Now this was hugely important research, but the field largely failed to move beyond these concepts. English psychoharmacologist Merton Sandler later reflected somewhat ruefully about these developments: "In the 1950s there were so many major discoveries, the tricyclic antidepressants, the monoamine oxidase inhibitors, the neuroleptics, lithium—and then nothing!"[30] Instead, the buzz words of the field were hijacked by the pharmaceutical industry. Chatter about shortages of neurotransmitters became part of the commercial buzz. This is not to disparage the importance of neurotransmission, a fundamental means of communication within the nervous system! Reuptake of neurotransmitters is real, and its inhibition does have demonstrable clinical effects. But neurotransmission is only a small part of the vast world—a world of hitherto unknowable size—of neurochemistry and neurophysiology. And it is not necessarily the central chemical mechanism in psychiatric illness. Nor has any psychiatric illness been convincingly attributed to a shortage of any particular neurotransmitter.

We may analogize to the world of computers: How does your desktop computer work? Let's unravel the code. But if we unravel only the code that controls communication between the keyboard and the central processor, we have not really answered the question. Knowing how the keyboard communicates with the rest of the thing is important but not necessarily central. Similarly, in the brain there are vast domains of transmission between neurons that we understand little of, to say nothing of chemical events taking place within the neurons and the other brain cells; hypotheses about serotonin and norepinephrine clarify little of this. Even at the height of his involvement in neurotransmitter research, Alec Coppen, at the Medical Research Council's Neuropsychiatric Research Unit at Carshalton in Surrey and one of the chief players in the serotonin story, was able to step back reflectively and say that "We must face the very real possibility that we are far from the primary disturbance in depression [in studying neurotransmitters]. The changes may all be secondary to other abnormalities which have not been taken into account at all."[31]

The point is not to retrospectively judge who was wrong and right in the scientific debates of the 1960s, but to show how exciting they were, and how avidly they were pursued. The whole discipline of psychopharmacology and clinical neuroscience was being opened up, and researchers around the world were on the edge of their seats.

But there were reflective observers who saw peril in all this excited discovery, and they were not just psychoanalysts who feared endangerment of their bread and butter with the implosion of the Freudian edifice. Yale epidemiologist Alvan Feinstein, generally considered one of the cleverest minds of his day, said in 1972 that "The concept of pharmacologic action is a fashion of this era. It represents whatever particular patterns of physiologic, biochemical, and mechanistic thought exist at any given point in time." The problem, said Feinstein, was that for many effective treatments we had no idea how they worked. Take acupuncture. "What shall we do with the fact that acupuncture works, and yet, we haven't got the foggiest idea of its pharmacologic mechanism except that it may move yin molecules to yang molecules."[32] In other words, there was more to the brain than neurotransmitter reuptake. Yet these words fell upon fallow ground.

By 1976 people had progressed to the belief, as Marie Asberg and colleagues at the Karolinska Institute in Stockholm put it, in "the existence of a biochemical subgroup of depressive disorders, characterized by a disturbance of serotonin turnover."[33] This appeared in the journal *Science*, adding full weight to what Thomas Ban, professor of psychopharmacology at Vanderbilt University, later referred to as "the whole biobabble about receptors."[34]

These beliefs in the reuptake activity of certain neurotransmitters in depression were even divided up on the basis of country. "The Anglo-Saxon countries were the 5-HT [serotonin] countries," said Peter Waldmeier in retrospect, a scientist at what was then Ciba-Geigy (later Novartis). "The more German-speaking countries, including the Scandinavian countries, were more catecholamine [norepinephrine and dopamine] countries." Alec Coppen, who advocated a serotonin hypothesis, was a dominant figure in the United Kingdom, whereas Arvid Carlsson, and Norbert Matussek in Munich "were noradrenaline [norepinephrine] people," Waldmeier said.[35]

The neurotransmitters serotonin, dopamine, and norepinephrine are called monoamines, and theories about which monoamines caused which illnesses would dominate psychiatry for the next 30 years, despite a lack of evidence about a shortage of any of these chemicals in the brains of ill individuals. This dubiety began to build from the mid-1960s. In 1973 George Ashcroft, an Edinburgh pharmacologist, showed that in some depressions, notably the bipolar variety, levels of the serotonin metabolite 5-hydroxyindolacetic acid (5-HIAA) were not lower than in controls. "These findings are against the amine hypothesis which postulated in depression a lowered concentration of transmitter amine at synaptic junction," he wrote.[36] Ashcroft's work progressed further. He later told David Healy in an interview that administering the precursor tryptophan to neurological patients would produce a rise in serotonin in the cerebrospinal fluid. "Then we did it in a range of psychiatric patients and showed, to our horror, that there was no failure of production of 5HT [serotonin] in depression. People with depression or recovered depressives had exactly the same maximal synthetic capacity as people without depression." So, in depression more must be going on "than just the release of the transmitter."[37]

At a conference in Marbella, Spain, in March 1976, the doubts started to pile up. Coppen expressed skepticism that there might be two groups of depressives, a serotonin-deficient group and a norepinephrine-deficient group. "If this were so, you would expect a different response rate to a good all-round drug like amitriptyline or imipramine [early tricyclic antidepressants], which presumably affects both systems equally, than you would to a drug like maprotiline, which seems to be mainly an inhibitor of noradrenaline. Yet there seems to be almost no evidence of any difference in the clinical response rate between depressives treated with [the two drugs]."[38] This was one of the early statements of uneasiness—and from an investigator who had championed the serotonin hypothesis!

Many more followed and in 1985 William Potter's group at the National Institute of Mental Health provided a definitive scientific burial: If you take the most powerful serotonin reuptake inhibitor you can find, and the most powerful norepinephrine inhibitor, their effect on serotonin and norepinephrine levels was equal.[39] Potter later said, "Each drug, after several weeks of administration, influenced both norepinephrine and serotonin metabolism," and a Lilly scientist (where Potter later became scientific director) told him, "It was the most important clinical paper he had ever seen; it has had a large impact in the way people think by supporting a shift in focus from single neurotransmitters to interacting and coupling systems."[40]

Today, these theories are widely disbelieved. Shortages of the standard monoamine neurotransmitters and receptors turned out to have little role in depressive illness except in pharmaceutical advertising and in the explanations that doctors give to patients. In an interview in 1998, Ross Baldessarini, a senior research psychiatrist at the McLean Hospital, flicked the exaggerated interest in neurotransmitter deficiencies and surpluses dismissively from the table: "We have [pursued fads] in much of biological psychiatry, including grossly overvaluing our partial understanding of the pharmacodynamics [effect on the body] of some drugs as a putative route to clarifying the pathophysiology [mechanism] of psychiatric illnesses." Baldessarini indicted "largely fruitless efforts to support a dopamine excess hypothesis of schizophrenia or mania, a norepinephrine or serotonin deficiency of major depression, a serotonin deficiency hypothesis in obsessive-compulsive disorder, and so on." Baldessarini said these emphases had kept the field stuck on the study of "old mechanisms and old theories."[41]

But if science was stuck, the public was stuck as well. For decades, people clung to Prozac-style remedies in the view that their nervous troubles stemmed from a lack of serotonin or norepinephrine. Even though the drugs work on some anxious and agitated patients, in the area of affective disorders, drugs that inhibit the reuptake of serotonin, the selective serotonin reuptake inhibitors (SSRIs), do not work very well, and even less well on the millions of people who take them because their basic problem is unhappiness, not illness. The SSRI-type drugs, the Prozac-type drugs, failed over 50% of their licensing trials. One scholar considers them virtual placebos.[42]

So how did this public health disaster come about, putting much of the population on pharmacological agents from which they would derive few of the benefits but many of the side effects?

It happened because the pharmaceutical companies badly needed these neurotransmitter reuptake theories in their communications with the medical profession and with the public.

In the early 1970s the pharmaceutical industry was not at all interested in this research and saw little promise in the pursuit of drugs that inhibited the reuptake of anything. It was in 1969 that pharmacologist Archibald Todrick at the Crichton Royal Hospital in Dumfries, Scotland, established that the tricyclic antidepressant clomipramine inhibited the reuptake of serotonin.[43] This was a continuation of his important findings showing that the tricyclics acted both on norepinephrine and serotonin. But only in 1990 did Geigy begin mentioning this in its ads for clomipramine, a drug they marketed as Anafranil and, by this time, were also indicating for obsessive-compulsive disorder. Thereafter, however, the floodgates opened, not just for Anafranil but for everything else.

Among the earliest attempts to market antidepressants with neurotransmitter chatter was Geigy's ad campaign for its tricyclic drug desipramine (Pertofrane) in 1974. Desipramine, a metabolite of imipramine, had been on the market since 1965 ("a rapid lift from the hell of depression"[44]) and had trouble distinguishing itself from the slew of competing tricyclic antidepressants. In 1974 the company emphasized that desipramine was not a "tranquilizer" but was indicated "specifically for depression." How do we know? "It is hypothesized that in depression there exists a deficit of specific CNS neurotransmitters known as biogenic amines (e.g. norepinephrine and serotonin)," and that desipramine reduced the "deficit…by blocking their reuptake and permitting these neurotransmitters to accumulate in the synaptic clefts. Result: amelioration of depression."[45] This is the first known piggybacking of a pharmaceutical product on a theory of disease-specific neurotransmission. Further ads offered large drawings of the synapse, showing norepinephrine's reuptake being blocked by Pertofrane. Psychiatric readers of the medical journals running these ads who had not been at the conference at Marbella and had not followed insider discussions could not have failed to be impressed.

In 1973, the Angelini Company launched trazodone, a chemically novel compound, in Italy as an antidepressant, Trittico, and by 1976 were flogging it for "nervous exhaustion" (esaurimenti nervosi). When Mead Johnson & Company acquired the American license in 1982, they decided to take it, rebranded as Desyrel, in a different direction: "It does not act by CNS stimulation, but rather, selectively inhibits serotonin uptake in the brain."[46] Trazodone, which has only a weak effect on serotonin, was billed as the first selective serotonin reuptake inhibitor, the first SSRI! (The drug performed poorly as an antidepressant but has recently undergone a revival as a hypnotic, or sleeping agent, and is now widely prescribed.)

The avalanche of marketing neurotransmitters to gain market share roared louder. In 1983, 4 years after its launch in the United States, Ciba started hyping its tetracyclic antidepressant maprotiline (Ludiomil) as a norepinephrine reuptake blocker: There was an impressive artist's drawing showing serotonin and norepinephrine molecules in the end bulb of a neuron awaiting their discharge into the synapse, much as fairies await the advent of Midsummer to come and dance on the lawn.[47] Much more colorful art, designed to grip the prescriber's mind as powerful science, was to follow.

There were inconvenient scientific findings. How curious, said biological psychiatrist Edward Sachar, head of psychiatry at the New York State Psychiatric Institute, in 1979, that the recently discovered tetracyclic mianserin is effective in depression, yet has "no effect on reuptake of serotonin or noradrenaline."[48]

In the background, doubts grew stronger. In 1978 Seymour Kety, the dean of neuroscience in the United States and by now head of biological psychiatry at the Mailman Research Center of McLean Hospital in Belmont, Massachusetts, said that "The simplistic notion of 'one neurotransmitter— one function' is no longer tenable, and we are beginning to recognize that complex psychological functions can only be the result of complex interactions among neuronal circuits and the transmitters that mediate them and modulate them."[49]

Across the Atlantic, other lights scoffed as well. At a conference in London in 1979, Laurent Maitre, a scientist in the research department of Ciba-Geigy, said that "it is very doubtful that there is a correlation between 5-HT [serotonin] uptake inhibition and clinical effects." He was dubious about analogizing research on the inhibition of reuptake in platelets, where much previous work had been done, on a one-to-one basis to the brain.[50] At a meeting in Monte Carlo that same year, Alain Puech, a pharmacologist in Paris, called attention to the absurdity of the notion of influencing just one neurotransmitter system: "It is inconceivable that modifying one monoaminergic [serotonin, dopamine etc] system can be done independently, because all the circuits are linked in a chain. Thus, every time there's a change in one neurotransmitter system, there is very probably at least one other neurotransmitter system that is modified."[51]

Such reservations echo down massively from these years. A meta-analysis in 2009 led by Kathleen Merikangas at the National Institute of Mental Health found no evidence of a link between the region in the genome that controlled the reuptake of serotonin and the incidence of depression.[52] Science raced on, from studying reuptake in the "presynaptic" neurons, to studying actions on the membranes of the postsynaptic neurons, to "second messenger" biochemical events involving protein kinases within the neurons themselves, to happenings within the cell nucleus, which is where we are today. But little of this science reached the ears of the community psychiatrists, internists, and family physicians who were prescribing the Prozac-style antidepressants.

Neurotransmitters and American Culture

What is happening here is the turning of a massive crank, to make the concept of depression scientifically acceptable to physicians, and thus indirectly appealing to their patients. Yet another crank was simultaneously grinding as well: the media crank that sold the neurotransmitter doctrine of depression directly to a mass audience. From the 1970s onward, the public was increasingly exposed to the concept of neurotransmitters as the scientific basis for confidence in the antidepressants and the whole doctrine of depression, on the logic that if it responds to Prozac, it must exist. A search of the *New York Times* digital database for the years 1955 to 2000 revealed the following number of hits for the word "neurotransmitters": 1955–1960, 0; 1961–1970, 1; 1971–1980, 17; 1981–1990, 108; 1991–2000, 171.[53] The number of references is not large, but the trend is clearly skyward.

Among the three main neurotransmitters in affective disorders, serotonin got the greatest play in the *Times*: 18 mentions in 1955–1960, rising to 67 in the 1980s and 168 in 1991–2000. Dopamine and norepinephrine displayed similar trajectories with fewer hits. There is no doubt that by 2000 readers of the *New York Times* had been fully exposed to the latest science on serotonin. Other important developments remained, however, quite uncovered, and a search on the dexamethasone suppression test, which would have revealed the state of the art on psychiatry's only biological marker, turned up only three mentions for the entire period from 1955 to 2000. The coverage, therefore, reflects what readers wanted to see rather than what neuroscientists thought important—and readers wanted to know that powerful scientific developments had uncovered the key to their dysphoria, which everyone was happy to define as "depression."

Thus, just as popular culture was turning toward neurotransmitters as the explanation of what ailed everybody, academic culture was turning away from them. In 1985, Eugene Paykel, among the most distinguished international figures in the field as professor of psychiatry at the University of London and editor of the *Journal of Affective Disorders*, asked rhetorically at a conference: "Is the amine hypothesis of depression dead?" meaning the hypothesis that viewed depression as a disorder of serotonin and norepinephrine. "Diabetes comes down very clearly," he said, "to a relative deficiency in insulin. Fifteen years ago depression was like that; we thought it was a clear-cut deficiency of noradrenaline or serotonin in a particular neurotransmitter system in the brain. But it's not as simple as that."[54] Was the whole line of inquiry dead?

Three years later, in 1988, the response of the pharmaceutical industry to this massive scientific dubiety was to launch Prozac (fluoxetine), the first of the drug class that shortly became known as SSRIs, the most popular drug class in history. "The first highly specific...highly potent blocker of serotonin uptake," screamed Lilly in its launch ad in the *Journal of the American Medical Association* in June.[55] Using a model of drug action that had been largely discredited, Lilly and the other SSRI manufacturers went on to promote a drug class—and reap billions of dollars in profit—that captured the imagination of the public and the medical profession not just in the United States but in the whole world: Depression, a disease suffered sooner or later by half of the entire population (it was argued),[56] could be cured with a drug that made your serotonin right again! Is it any wonder that depression spread epidemically within the medical profession as a diagnosis and within the public as a supposed disorder? You are wondering why everyone became depressed? This is why.

The Return of the Two Depressions (and an Anxious Postscript)

Motto: "A patient whose high numbers are for things like sleep and fatigue has a different kind of 'depression' than somebody who mainly endorses hopelessness, anhedonia, and guilt."

HERBERT PEYSER, SENIOR PSYCHIATRIST, NEW YORK CITY,
POST TO A PSYCHOPHARMACOLOGY LIST-SERVE,
JANUARY 8, 2010

BEFORE 1980 THERE had been two depressions, melancholia—also called endogenous depression—and nonmelancholia, called a number of terms such as reactive depression and neurotic depression.[1] *DSM-III* flattened this distinction, abolishing the clinical distinction between the two with the homogenizing term major depression. To be sure, *DSM-III* reinserted the term melancholia in the discussion as a subtype of major depression, but only in letter, not in spirit. In the decades after 1980 melancholia returned, but to a landscape of mood disorder that had been leveled and laid waste by the concept of "depression." In a world where everybody is depressed, nobody is melancholic.

The Return of Melancholia

Motto: "Melancholics rarely complain of 'depression.'"[2]
MICHAEL ALAN TAYLOR (1999)

Emil Kraepelin had sent the diagnosis of melancholia into a death spiral. The psychoanalysts had little interest in the concept, aside from venerating a single essay of Freud, and the only people interested in keeping melancholia alive as a notion after the 1930s were the British who, with their admixture of Heidelberg science and homegrown common sense, had turned into shrewd psychopathologists. The textbook that Willi Mayer-Gross, a Heidelberg refugee, published in 1954 together with Eliot Slater and Martin Roth gave pride of place to involutional melancholia as the serious melancholic illness that often affected people at midlife and afterward.[3]

But world psychiatry after World War II marched to an increasingly American beat, and the Americans had little use for the antique term melancholia. The glossary of Alfred Freedman's *Comprehensive Textbook of Psychiatry,* the world's leading textbook first published in 1967, had scads of psychoanalytic terms but claimed of melancholia: "Old term for depression that is rarely used at the present time."[4] In Europe after World War II, endogenous depression was the serious variety and melancholia was deemed as "contaminated by Freud and the 19th century novels that degraded it to grief," as Tom Ban, who trained in Budapest in the early 1950s, put it. "For Kraepelinians, grief and depression were not the same, and they excluded each other. Anyone who had an identifiable precipitating factor could not be labeled as having a depressive state."[5] In 1978 Pierre Pichot, one of France's leading psychopharmacologists, found the term "mélancolie" useless and urged that it be abandoned.[6] So on both sides of the Atlantic, melancholia was toast.

Yet melancholia as an illness has such a distinctive clinical profile that images of it remained in the minds of experienced clinicians: the expressions of utter hopelessness and despair, the slouched shoulders, and the tight little smile intended to conceal firm plans of suicide. And then a week later the patient is found swinging from the underside of a bridge. This was a special horror that engraved into the collective memory of the profession the engram that there was, after all, such a thing as melancholia, and that it was different from every other illness entity in psychiatry. So even though official academic psychiatry had long lost interest, a subterranean stirring of curiosity remained.

Yet the crucial event in reviving the concept of melancholia as not just a severe form of depression but a different illness was Roland Kuhn's discovery in the mid-1950s of a drug specific for what Kuhn was calling "vital depression" but was in fact melancholic illness. The drug was the first tricyclic antidepressant (TCA), imipramine, marketed by the Geigy Company in Switzerland in 1957 and in the United States in 1959 under the brand name Tofranil.

For Kuhn, an experienced psychiatrist, the effect of imipramine on hospital depression was nothing less than extraordinary. On August 11, 1956, he wrote to Robert Domenjoz, chief of pharmacology at Geigy, on the workings of the drug. "In the beginning, the effects are sedative. The patients sleep better and are calmer during the daytime." Yet the sedation, Kuhn said, was less intense than with the antipsychotic drug chlorpromazine, and "during the day, the patients feel less sleepy and are less lethargic. In many cases, the hallucinations become softer and seem to retreat into the distance. Illusions and delusions lose their threatening character. The train of thoughts often runs more smoothly and the patients become more relaxed when dealing with other people." In contrast to chlorpromazine, Kuhn continued, imipramine "has an obvious effect on depression. The vital depression visibly improves. The patients feel less tired, the sensation of weight decreases, the inhibitions become less pronounced, and the mood improves.... The patients also become more open to psychotherapeutic efforts and it even becomes possible to establish psychotherapeutic contact with people who have very severe depressions, with whom one could not have a meaningful conversation prior to the treatment."[7]

The chart of the first patient treated with imipramine at the Münsterlingen Mental Hospital, Paula G, 49 years old, has survived. The entry for January 21, 1956: "For three days now," Kuhn wrote in the chart, "it is as if the patient had undergone a transformation. All of her restlessness and agitation have vanished. Yesterday, she herself observed that she had been in a complete muddle, that she had never acted so dumb in all her life. She did not know what had caused her behavior, but she was just glad to be better again ... The patient is also different now from before the depressive phase. She is no longer so aggressive and quarrelsome. She is energetic and friendly, likes to read and work. Her sleep is now also markedly better."[8]

Kuhn's observations mark the opening of a remarkable new chapter in the history of the treatment of mood disorders, and emphasize at the same time that his patients at Münsterlingen had a very special kind of depression in which they were psychotic, unreachable, and gravely disabled. Imipramine's launch sent the message that these kinds of depressions were now treatable with something other than electroconvulsive therapy (ECT), which had been introduced in 1938. Indeed, several of Kuhn's patients had failed to respond to ECT.

Vital depression did not readily catch on as a term, but neither did melancholia in these years. The term that psychiatry used for these serious, often psychotic, mood disorders was endogenous depression. And opinions drifted back and forth about whether endogenous and reactive depressions were just two different levels of severity or quite different illnesses.

Bernard Carroll, his training Australian but his scientific career passed largely in the United States, was at the University of Michigan as he attempted to shore up his initial discovery in 1968 that melancholic depression had a biochemical marker in the form of the dexamethasone suppression test (DST, see p. 84).[9] Patients with what Carroll called "serious depression" and "endogenous depression" failed to suppress the secretion of cortisol after the administration of a dose of the artificial steroid dexamethasone the night before; the adrenal glands of patients with lesser depressions and other psychiatric disorders suppressed cortisol secretion normally. This is the most fundamental biological finding in psychiatry, and it would be pleasant to argue that Carroll did much to reestablish the concept of melancholia as a distinctive entity. But things did not work out that way. Carroll began using the term melancholia only around 1981,[10] and his work on the DST, that by rights should have merited him great honor, was forgotten in psychiatry in the 1980s in a dismal episode that Max Fink and I have described elsewhere.[11] The bottom line is that Carroll's work was elbowed aside right about the time that melancholia began its great resurgence.

What caused the resurgence? It was partly the inclusion of the diagnosis of melancholia in *DSM-III* in 1980 and partly the progression of scientific curiosity.

The APA's *Diagnostic and Statistical Manual* did reimport the term melancholia into psychiatry, albeit as a subcategory of major depression, simultaneously abolishing endogenous depression. This put melancholia again on the radar, although, as we saw in a previous chapter, in an attenuated form. You would qualify as melancholic if you had low appetite, awakened early in the morning, felt really guilty about something, and good news did not make you feel better. This is a pale shadow of the real McCoy, with its psychotic desperation, deep psychic pain, and massive changes in bodily function. *DSM-III* was also silent on other kinds of information useful in making the diagnosis, such as past history, family history, biological measures, and nonverbal behavior.

From the outset, it was clear that the *DSM* criteria of melancholia did not aptly characterize the illness. If, for example, you were looking for "a distinct quality of depressed mood," as the *Manual* specified, you might miss melancholia in your patients. Robin Priest, a psychiatrist at St. Mary's Hospital Medical School in London, remembered a patient, "a chubby person," whose symptoms were "of melancholic depression, some of them delusion." "I've committed the most awful sins," she told him. "I'm riddled with disease."

But from the live interview he got a rather different impression. "She had a ready smile and after each proclamation of disaster she would grin, giggle or in some way suggest that she was far from feeling miserable." Priest took her statements to be fictitious, "falsehood at an unconscious level" and "self-deception of a hysterical nature." Having missed the diagnosis of smiling depression, he took no particular action.

"The outcome was tragic. I forget exactly how many days afterwards … she was found dead, floating in a nearby pond. The consultant, a Scotswoman, was horrified at my diagnosis of hysteria."[12]

So although clinical diagnosis is often pattern recognition, and the classic melancholic pattern is instantly recognizable, not all cases are classic and if you have only *DSM* "phenomenology," as it is called, you might tragically miss the diagnosis.

Research started to be conducted using the new *DSM* criteria. In 1981, Craig Nelson and Dennis Charney, both at Yale, singled out lack of reactivity to good news as the most characteristic symptom of the melancholia subtype of *DSM*'s major depression (psychomotor change also ranked highly).[13] These were pretty generous criteria: A study of 800 women at midlife in Gothenburg, Sweden, in 1984 found 6.9% of them *currently* had major depression: 2.9% had melancholia and 4.0% had nonmelancholia.[14] (Informed observers, mindful of the tremendous difficulty of gaining true prevalence rates, estimate the *lifetime prevalence* of unipolar melancholic and psychotic depression in the community to be about 2–3%.[15])

How else was melancholia different? It was discovered, or rediscovered, to be quite unresponsive to psychotherapy and placebos. This was actually something long known. In 1930 Henry Yellowlees, medical superintendent of The Retreat at York and lecturer in psychological medicine at St. Thomas's Hospital in London, told the Section of Psychiatry of the Royal Society of Medicine that, in the words of the secretary, "Melancholia was a psychosis, and it was, *ipso facto,* not amenable to psychotherapy. Neurasthenia, on the other hand, was amenable to psychotherapy in general, and was often especially amenable to [psycho]analysis in particular."[16] This insight was then forgotten in the decades ahead as melancholia went out of style and psychotherapy became the treatment of choice for many conditions in psychiatry. In 1988 Duane Spiker and David Kupfer at the Western Psychiatric Institute in Pittsburgh revived this classical truth, finding the response rate to placebo in psychotic depression zero.[17]

Then there was the revival of sheer scientific curiosity about melancholia, stimulated perhaps by the discovery that some depressions were unresponsive ("treatment resistant") to conventional antidepressants. Many of these resistant depressions responded to ECT, and ECT in the 1980s was beginning a comeback.[18] It is actually quite remarkable that ECT needed a comeback because the treatment, launched in 1938 and entailing the induction of therapeutic convulsions with electricity, is the most powerful therapy that psychiatry has to offer. It was almost driven off the boards in the 1960s by the flower children (and by a systematic campaign of the Church of Scientology). Yet ECT did hang on because some patients will respond to nothing else and will kill themselves if they do not get shock treatment. In the 1980s common sense conduced to a revival of ECT, and this reanimation of convulsive therapy doubtlessly spurred a revival of curiosity about melancholia.

There was also growing awareness that melancholia responded better to the TCAs than to the Prozac-style drugs that, from the late 1980s, began to run the board in psychiatric treatment. In 1996 Paul Perry at the University of Iowa, in a review of controlled trials, found that the TCAs were "consistently more effective than the SSRIs" in "endogenous/melancholic depression."[19]

Thus, research began to edge away from the *DSM* subtype and toward a restoration of the concept of two depressions, one of which would be melancholia independent of major depression, although the term was not yet current. Danish investigators were leading figures in this work. As early as 1979 Per Bech and Ole Rafaelsen at the Psychochemistry Institute of the university psychiatric hospital in Copenhagen, both major figures in international circles, had proposed at an academic meeting a "Bech-Rafaelsen Melancholia Scale." They published a comparison with the famed Hamilton Depression Scale, the field's standard, in 1980.[20] Eight years later, Bech, by now in the department of psychiatry at Frederiksborg General Hospital in Hillerod, felt the evidence on the dissimilarity of outpatient and inpatient depression was sufficient that they should be treated as "two different diagnostic entities."[21] These Danish neuroscientists disliked the term depression. Tom Ban, who knew Rafaelsen well, said of him later, "Ole was quit explicit that the word depression should be dismissed because people on the street associate it with something different from psychiatrists. Psychoanalysts extended it in a way that one can use it practically for any somatic complaint, and biologically oriented psychiatrists use it inevitably to mean that depression is a disorder of arousal or of the EEG [electroencephalogram]."[22]

The term melancholia itself was not used, yet small groups of researchers not yet in the grip of *DSM* began to return to such aspects of melancholic depression as slowed thought and movement ("psychomotor slowing"). In 1982 Robert Gibbons and John Davis at the University of Illinois medical school and David Clark of the Rush Presbyterian St. Luke's Medical Center, all in Chicago, who reanalyzed data on 65 patients previously studied in several

Scandinavian centers, said there were two very different kinds of depression: In one type, the patients were at the outset deeply depressed, yet responded well to the TCA antidepressant imipramine. Their symptoms were psycho-motor slowing and a loss of interest in sex. In a second group, the depression was less severe at the outset yet responded less well to imipramine; in this group psychomotor slowing and sexual inertness were not important.[23] The first group would have been considered melancholic.

Against this background of rising interest in melancholia, both within and without the *DSM* framework, in 1995 Gordon Parker placed a full-bodied melancholia definitively on the radar and quite outside the *DSM* framework of major depression, a diagnosis that Parker despised. Parker, then 53 years old, was professor of psychiatry at the University of New South Wales in Sydney (and later director of the Black Dog Institute for Mood Disorders, founded in 2002, its namesake the Churchillian figure of melancholic illness). Parker said that "psychomotor disturbance" was the main characteristic distinguishing melancholia from nonmelancholic depression, meaning mainly that thoughts and actions were slowed, but sometimes speeded up. There were also "endogeneity" symptoms such as insomnia and weight loss that constituted a kind of "mantle" about the core of psychomotor disturbance. He based this conclusion on a careful multivariate analysis of 407 patients at the Mood Disorders Unit of the Prince Henry Hospital, the forerunner of the Black Dog Institute, and this conception of melancholia has had great staying power.[24] In 1996 Parker edited a volume on melancholia, arguing that although there are few homogeneous entities in psychiatry, "melancholia is one such entity and capable of being clinically circumscribed." It was Parker's achievement to introduce the terms melancholia and nonmelancholia to describe the two depressions, the terms most in vogue today.[25]

Gordon Parker's research is of particular interest because it took the emphasis in depression off mood, rather, harkening back to the nervous diagnosis of the nineteenth century. If slowness of thought and movement were the key to depressive illness, the patients' mood did not matter so much. Daniel Widlöcher, professor of psychiatry at the Salpêtrière Hospital in Paris, had begun this line of inquiry in 1983 and Parker explicitly built upon it. (In 1983, Widlöcher criticized the conventional wisdom: "Current clinical opin-ion considers mood change as the primary disturbance, and that retardation is an expression of sadness and loss of interest. According to [the conventional] viewpoint, depression is primarily a painful experience and there is no need to invoke retardation as an independent behavioral pattern." Widlöcher's view, by contrast, was that retardation "is a core behavioral pattern."[26])

It is interesting that Widlöcher was at the Salpêtrière, where Charcot once strode the wards, because past memories are being reawakened here. Walter Brown, a long-experienced psychiatrist at Brown University in Providence, Rhode Island, once described the depressed patients who respond well to medication—as compared to the many who do not: "We don't have good clinical language for characterizing these patients, for articulating the ways in which they differ from those who don't so clearly require and benefit from medication, but like patients who need ECT, we often know them when we see them. We find them among the melancholic depressed and among the bipolar depressed. The 62-year-old with the now-forgotten involutional melancholia is among them."[27] It was precisely among those veteran clinicians who believe that psychiatry is an art as well as a science that the discipline's collective memory of melancholia came flooding back.

"Not unexpectedly," said Barney Carroll, by now chair of psychiatry at Duke University, at a conference in Germany in 1982, apropos *DSM*'s failure to differentiate, "These historical themes continue to reassert themselves— they will not simply go away." "Melancholic, vital, biological endogenomorphic, psychotic, or autonomous: these illnesses probably have a major biological basis."[28] That is why they appeared historically and continue today.

By the dawn of 2000, the field of psychiatry was in tumult. The extent to which rational diagnosis and treatment had been sold out to the pharmaceutical industry was starting to become apparent, and the drafting of a new version of *DSM*, due in 2013, was the first time in history that a technical issue in psychiatry was followed in the mass media, the subject of prominent articles in the daily press. The field seemed on the cusp of change. In 2006 Michael Alan Taylor at the University of Michigan and Max Fink at the Stony Brook campus of the State University of New York published a major overview of melancholia, essentially reintroducing it to the field. "Melancholia is a severe disorder of mood, often fatal, that has been described for millennia in medical texts and by poets, novelists, and playwrights," they said. The field had lost sight of it because of *DSM-III* and because "intrusive actions of the pharmaceutical industry encouraged a weakening of criteria to justify the use of antidepressant drugs in the largest number of persons. The safety and efficacy of the older, no longer patentable agents … were maligned through aggressive marketing that relied on unsound industry-sponsored comparison studies. Academic psychiatry went to the highest bidder."[29] Wow! This was a harsh judgment in explaining the eclipse of melancholia, but not necessarily untrue.

Fittingly, it was in Copenhagen in 2006 that a conference considered melancholia "beyond DSM, beyond neurotransmitters."[30] The time had truly arrived to take a second look at the epidemic of depression that *DSM* and the neurotransmitter doctrine had created, and to attempt to put the field once more on a scientific basis. But there is a difference between talking the talk and walking the walk. Whether the field of psychiatry will shake free and walk toward a substantial reconsideration of its diagnostics and therapeutics remains to be seen.

"Depression" Rides Supreme

Whereas melancholia designated a small population of people with life-threatening illness, the diagnosis called simply "depression" was applied to millions. Before *DSM-III* in 1980, psychiatry had always had two depressions, and now it had only one, and that depression, which began life in 1980 as "major depression," was a scientific travesty, a poor limp thing of a diagnosis that did not necessarily mean that the patient was sad at all—which is what a depressive mood diagnosis is supposed to convey—but was unhappy, aggrieved, tired, anxious, uncomfortable, or had nothing at all really wrong; the doctor had put her on antidepressants because he or she could think of nothing else to do.

Most depressions—referred to in the literature simply as "depression"—are community depression and not melancholia. And the diagnosis of this type of depression has recently experienced a substantial increase. Between 1985 and 1995, the percentage of office visits to psychiatrists for depression increased from 29.5% to 46.8%. Bipolar disorder rose from 6.1% to 9.1% of the total, making the final amount of depressive illness by 1995 well over half of psychiatric practice. Visits for "other mental disorders" declined from 16.9% of the total to 6.2%, suggesting that depression was becoming a kind of residual category.[31] In 1987, three experts on depression noted that "one of every four Americans will suffer from a significant depressive experience in the course of his or her lifetime."[32]

The increase continued. Between 1991–1992 and 2001–2002 the prevalence of major depression in a random sample of the U.S. national population more than doubled, up from 3.3% to 7.1%.[33] And so depression has become a mass illness. Within a given year, 1 in 10 Americans today will have a mood disorder, the great majority of them major depression.[34] Similarly, the consumption of psychotherapeutic medications has more than doubled in a decade, according to the Center for Mental Health Services of the federal government, from

174 million prescriptions in 1996 to 372 million in 2006. Prescriptions for "antidepressants," a term that can only evoke a smile, rose from 80 million in 1996 to 192 million in 2006.[35] In the period 2005–2008, according to the National Center for Health Statistics, 11% of all Americans over 12 years of age took antidepressant medication—1 in 10! And 25% of women aged 40–59 did so.[36] Exclamation marks fail. Who can stop this terrible epidemic of depression!

Certain subpopulations, such as late-adolescents, have been hard hit indeed. In 2005–2007, 8.3% of Americans aged 12–17 years had a "major depressive episode" within the previous 12 months—almost 1 in 10 of our teenagers with major depression![37] Here is Kenneth Silk, a psychiatrist with the University of Michigan Health Service, in 2006: "There is a big push now to identify depression on college campuses—MIT, NYU—and big Pharma is putting some $$$ support to these college campus-wide efforts—but some cynics wonder if big Pharma's enthusiasm for the project has to do with the idea that the more you can identify those students who are depressed, the more antidepressants get prescribed and certainly, having gone back to seeing students myself again (last time I did that was in 1974–1975 at Yale)—we are much more ready to write that Rx today than we were (myself included) 30 years ago."[38] Can anyone doubt that campus depression had vastly increased over those three decades?

It is not just among campus cut-ups but adolescents in general that the consumption of psychiatric drugs has risen so much. An analysis by Medco Health Solutions of prescriptions for psychotropic drugs for some 370,000 adolescents found that the prevalence of adolescent girls taking antipsychotic drugs grew 117% over the period from 2001 to 2006, "whereas boys that age had an increase of 71 percent." Girls increased their sleep medications by 80% over those years and their medications for hyperactivity by 74%.[39]

Do these vast increases in the consumption of psychotropic medications stem from a real increase in the incidence of melancholic and nonmelancholic depression? Or are they due to the willingness of doctors to confer the diagnosis or patients' ardor to demand it? Indeed, one study looking at the onset of depression by birth cohort found that in the younger cohorts, depression began at increasingly earlier ages. This study, however, called upon older adults to recall when their depressive illnesses first began, a chancy business, and later-born cohorts might have had their memories consolidated by the act of taking antidepressants. A meta-analysis of 26 studies of childhood depression by year of birth involving over 60,000 observations on children born between 1965 and 1996 found no increase in depression across birth cohorts. The authors concluded that "If more depressed children are being identified, or are receiving antidepressant medication, this is more likely to be the result of increased sensitivity to a long-standing problem..." than the result of a real, epidemic-style increase.[40] So it seems as though the diagnosis of depression is increasing but not the real illness.

But how many people with the diagnosis of depression are sad? This is the big question. How many of the supposedly depressed patients have a disorder of mood involving sadness, hopelessness, and the other emotions of despair? Raymond Battegay in Basel, one of the founders of psychopharmacology in Switzerland, told David Healy in an interview that "I don't agree that depressions are mainly mood disorders. Mood is concerned secondarily ... [Depression] is a disequilibrium of the limbic-hypothalamic-pituitary-adreno-cortical system and, secondarily in most cases, but not in all, mood is affected. What we call masked depressions seem to be the real depressions, since the mood is not visibly affected."[41] (There is more on this below at the discussion of Adalbert Kral and affective equivalents.) These patients are clearly suffering from some kind of nervous disorder, but why call them depressed?

Within an urban medical practice, as many as one patient in five has a diagnosis of major depression.[42] Yet in the American population as a whole, only 3.3% of people in a random-sample poll said they are sad "all or most of the time," according to data from the National Center for Health Statistics.[43] This presumably is the core of individuals with a depressive illness. This would be the reality.

But diagnosis is different from reality. Many of those with a diagnosis of depression do not have a low mood: 50% of the Philadelphia patients in the mid-1960s diagnosed with "mild depression" did not have a low mood nor did 25% of those with "moderate depression."[44] In research led by David Healy, a group of 39 patients with depression were given a Quality of Mood Questionnaire and Checklist, and asked to check off what they felt. (The term *sadness* was explicitly removed from the list.) The words the patients chose most frequently were dispirited (20); sluggish, wretched (19); empty, washed out, awful, bothered, dull (18); listless, tightened up (17); exhausted, gloomy (16); burdened (15); and desolate, powerless, purposeless (14). Healy comments that "It would certainly seem that the words endorsed most frequently in the survey are not the words that people who are simply miserable or unhappy would be likely to offer spontaneously. Dispirited, sluggish, empty, and washed out suggest a somewhat different state from the normal experience of sadness."[45] We are therefore inclined to ask the following: Does this kind of wretchedness really mean low mood? Sadness?

The question is important because sadness is a meaningful term to patients though no longer to clinicians. There was once a German-inspired tradition that sought to differentiate normal sadness from "the sadness of depression," finding the latter not really sad at all but tired, without hope, inexplicable in origin, and seemingly lasting in duration.[46] The following issue arises: Was this "special quality" of the sadness of depression really measuring depression or some other underlying entity?

But today, neither American nor French psychiatry recognizes sadness as a psychiatric concept, for it is not in the main psychiatric dictionaries of those countries.[47] Sadness, or Traurigkeit, remains, however, in the main German psychiatric dictionary,[48] which is revealing because it was the Germans who founded the field of psychopathology, the exact description of what patients feel and how they behave. The Germans had, therefore, the semantic tools for studying clinical sadness, yet there are no good data that they actually found much of it. "One cannot mistake the base note" in depression, Walter Schulte, director of a German provincial asylum, said in 1961. "It is not sad, but rigidly hard, empty, vacant, indifferent, non-vital, dead, and burned out." The patients were not sad but were incapable of feeling.[49] The bottom line is that when we try to break through the psychiatric short-hand about "depressed mood" and learn what it is that these millions of patients with the diagnosis of depression are actually feeling, we run into something of a semantic stonewall.[50]

So this is the problem: We have all these patients with the diagnosis of depression. But they are not particularly sad and they have all kinds of other symptoms. What is the point of calling them "depressed"?

It is also interesting that a number of patients who are on antidepressants do not have depression. According to data from the National Ambulatory Medical Care Surveys for 1996, at 59.5% of office visits at which antidepressants were prescribed, there was no psychiatric diagnosis. (This share had risen to 72.7% by 2007.)[51] Is this sloppy record-keeping? Among the almost 150,000 patients seen in 39 family medical practices in South Carolina in 1996, 9335 were prescribed antidepressants. Of these 9335, 4022, or 43%, *did not have a diagnosis of depression*. And a good share of them had already received antidepressants in the past, despite not being depressed.[52] Similarly, the Collaborative Psychiatric Epidemiologic Surveys, using national random-sample data, found for the years 2001–2003 that 52% of those taking antidepressants had not had any psychiatric disorder for the past 2 years, and that 26.3% had not had any psychiatric problem on a lifetime basis.[53] Such use of "antidepressants," a term that now belongs in ironic quotation marks, is explicable only as a consequence of the relentless promotion of pharmaceutical products: Whatever ails you must be a depression of some kind because you read it in the media—but the good news is you can be helped with antidepressants.

Lots of people, of course, do get the diagnosis of depression. How confident may we be of the diagnosis in them? The large international differences in the prevalence of depression are not encouraging. At a conference in 1974 Owen Wade, a pharmacologist at the University of Birmingham, said, partly in jest, "Speaking as somebody from a developing country—what is called depression in the United States, is referred to by the British as just 'a chap being under the weather.'" (Laughter).⁵⁴ An epidemiological comparison led by Myrna Weissman at Columbia University in 1996 found huge international differences in the lifetime rate of major depression per 100 population, ranging from 1.5% in Taiwan to 16.4% in Paris, France. (The rate in the United States was 5.2% of the population having major depression on a lifetime basis.) For separated and divorced women, the rates ranged from 3.0 per 100 population for Korea to 43.8 per 100 for Paris. (The United States rate of major depression per 100 separated or divorced women was 13.5.)⁵⁵ These figures demonstrate that in something like the occurrence of depression, culture and society play a large role.

Still, the figures make us wonder. Almost half of the formerly married Parisian women are so sad that they qualify for what, on the face of it, is a serious psychiatric diagnosis? And one American woman in seven who has left her husband behind qualifies? That all these women should be so fragile lacks face validity. Do they have something else?

Calling a depression nonmelancholic is not to trivialize it. Nonmelancholic depression can be a serious illness and can end in suicide. " . . . The functioning of depressed patients is comparable with or worse than that of patients with major chronic medical conditions," said a team from the RAND Corporation led by UCLA psychiatrist Kenneth Wells in 1989. "The only chronic conditions having associations with functioning comparable with those of depressive symptoms were current heart conditions."⁵⁶

But what kind of an illness is community depression, as opposed to melancholia? Mainly sadness? "I honestly think that depression is a disease of the whole body," said Columbia psychiatrist Alexander Glassman in an interview in 2003. "There is something going on that's affecting the whole body." He noted that depression tended to cause strokes, and that bone metabolism was affected by depression. Kicking off a huge subsequent literature about depression and heart disease, Glassman noted that cardiac mortality was higher. "I gave this lecture at medicine rounds," he said, "and some ophthalmologist came to me and said, you know, there's a literature about depression and vascular disease of the eye. I didn't know about that."[57] So, there is no doubt that depression is real. We are not talking about a latter day version of hysteria. These patients are not just victims of "medicalization," or the assigning of medical diagnoses to people who are not sick. But these patients with real depression, what do they actually have? If it is a disease of the whole body, maybe they have nervous disease?

Let us look at the components of the nervous syndrome and see how often they occur in patients diagnosed as depressed.

New York psychiatrist James Kocsis saw a number of them out of the corner of his eye as they trudged about the doctors' offices of Manhattan. We wanted "to show that antidepressant medications worked for these people," he said in an interview in 2005. "A lot of clinicians didn't believe they did. They didn't even believe these people had affective illnesses. They thought they had something else and the patients also believed that. They thought they were misdiagnosed and went to medical clinics and internists who ordered all kinds of X-rays and tests. After getting the results they'd say, 'I'm sorry there's nothing wrong with you, it must be in your head.'"[58] When such patients reached Kocsis, he put them on TCAs such as amitriptyline and many of them did get better (which demonstrates that not that all these nonsad patients had secret depressions but that tricyclic drugs are effective for the much wider range of illness we have been describing as nervous).

What symptoms do these nervous patients have? A cardinal symptom is fatigue, or weakness. In 1955 psychiatrist Mandel Cohen, a biologically oriented clinician at Harvard who had been exiled to the neurology department by his psychoanalytic colleagues, led a study of the symptoms of 100 manic-depressive patients (the term of the day for serious depression) versus medically-ill patients and healthy controls. What symptoms did they have? Of the depressives 54% reported "weakness," as opposed to 3% of the healthy controls.[59]

An analysis of the National Comorbidity Survey of 1990–1992 divided the respondents into subgroups of depression and anxiety and looked at the frequency of various symptoms in each. Here are the findings for "lack of energy": of those with mild psychological depression, 71.4% lacked energy; psychological anxious depression, 88.8%; somatic depressed anxiety 92.3%; restless somatic depression, 100.0%. ("Low distress," meaning normals, 22.8%.)[60] Thus the depressed population today is certainly fatigued and lacking in energy.

Somatic symptoms were part of the old nervous syndrome. Today, they abound in depression. The Cohen analysis of the manic-depressive patients in Boston found that 49% had headaches (versus 25% of the healthy controls), 77% dyspnea, or labored breathing (versus 3% of controls), and 53% reported paresthesias, or abnormal skin sensations (versus 5% of controls).[61] The National Comorbidity Survey did not focus so much upon the somatic side but did ask about "stomach problems," reported by 79.5% of those with restless somatic depression.[62] Again, it sounds as though little has changed since the olden days of nerves.

How about anxiety? Anxiety was certainly part of the nervous syndrome of yore, and flourished in the first half of the twentieth century in the diagnosis mixed anxiety-depression. Anxiety is definitely not lacking among the depressed of today. In the Cassidy study of Boston, 57% of the patients with manic-depressive illness experienced palpitation (versus 10% of healthy controls), or pounding of the heart; 33% had anxiety attacks (versus 5% of controls).[63] In a study of the patients with major depression about to enter a drug study at the Massachusetts General Hospital and the New York State Psychiatric Institute, 91% had psychic anxiety at baseline and 68% had somatic anxiety.[64] In a World Health Organization (WHO) study in 1996 of almost 5500 primary-care patients in 15 locations worldwide, "Nearly half of the cases of depression and anxiety appeared in the same patients and at the same time."[65] The WHO administrators chose to express the relationship rather oddly because they firmly believed in the doctrine of comorbidity, meaning two separate diseases that just happened to occur in the same patient, such as leukemia and mumps. But it is not surprising that just as in the past, many of their depression patients were also anxious (that half of them were apparently not anxious makes us question the thoroughness of the investigation). Another study of the primary-care patients without a formal psychiatric diagnosis organized by the World Health Organization went ever further: "These findings provide support for the existence of a mixed anxiety-depression category crossing the diagnostic boundaries of current anxiety and depression disorders."[66] To any student of the history of psychiatry this will not come as such big news!

Moreover, the family physicians participating in this WHO study prescribed exactly the same agents for depression and anxiety: Of the patients with recognized depression, 28% got sedatives and 22% got antidepressants; of the anxiety patients, 31% were treated with sedatives and 21% with antidepressant agents.[67] Thus, in terms of differential treatments, the doctors themselves saw no differences.

Statistical studies showing a great overlap between depression and anxiety could be recited many times over and it would be tedious to review a long list of them.[68]

What is interesting is that informal opinion in psychiatry confirms substantially that depression and anxiety are really a single disease. At a meeting of the Psychopharmacological Agents Advisory Committee of the Food and Drug Administration in 1977, under discussion were—what was called at the time—the minor and major tranquilizers. Harold Stevens, a psychiatrist of long experience at St. Elizabeths Hospital in Washington, DC, said, "We have talked glibly about using this for depression and that for anxiety. Actually, there is almost always an intermix, and it is very difficult to identify the purely depressed and the purely anxious."[69] He threw this off as a casual observation.

Just as a kind of post-holing in the great prairie of informal discussion in psychiatry over the decades: It is 1997 and Joseph Autry at the National Institute of Mental Health is being interviewed by Leo Hollister, a leading United States psychopharmacologist.

AUTRY: "In talking to my internist friends, they say that probably 40–50% of the patients that they see have some significant component of depression or anxiety disorder."

HOLLISTER: "It is interesting that you have mentioned the two together, because for many years John Overall and I were doing studies in depression, and we found that anxiety was just as frequent and just as severe in depressed patients as depression."

AUTRY: "I think that's absolutely correct. I think you also are seeing that many of the antidepressants that have been developed have in turn been used to treat anxiety disorders over the past several years."[70]

Here is one more example, from across the Atlantic, not just for the sake of accumulating examples but to show that most clinicians, in their heart of hearts, thought anxiety and depression were really the same illness: It was only the *DSM* drafters who wanted to keep them apart. At a conference in the United Kingdom in 1991, the subject was panic disorder. John Francis William ("Bill") Deakin, professor of psychiatry at Manchester University, said that "There is evidence that panic disorder is different from other forms of anxiety, although it does seem to emerge in the course of depressive illness. I don't think that other symptoms of anxiety are distinct from depressive symptoms. They are all symptoms of minor affective disturbance. Very few people have generalized anxiety without symptoms of depression, either at the same time or emerging during the course of their lifetime disturbance."[71]

Yes, indeed. Anxiety and depression are part of the same package, and it helps take the emphasis off mood and put it on the body as a whole if we refer to this package not as mixed anxiety-depression but with another term. I have proposed nerves, but am not entrenched on this, and a national discussion would be timely.

Postscript: Anxiety Today

It has not escaped many observers that today we are drenched in anxiety. As Francis P. Rhoades, a 64-year-old Detroit family doctor, said at an FDA hearing in 1966: "We live in a society that is characterized by anxiety. Practically everybody is anxious about something all the time."[72] Musing about the age of anxiety has become a talk show staple. Where did this come from?

It is not just depression that was extracted from nerves and made into a disorder of mood. The same fate happened to anxiety.[73] The disappearance of anxiety from the nervous diagnosis and its conversion into a mood disorder began in 1948 at the Boston Psychopathic Hospital with advocacy of methamphetamine for use in the treatment of tension (the "Pervitin interview").[74] (In 1947 methamphetamine was already being promoted for weight loss.[75]) Thus, a pharmacological torch was carving out tension. Then in the same year, 1948, T. M. Ling and Lloyd Davies at the new Roffey Park Rehabilitation Centre for "industrial neuroses" in Horsham, Sussex, administered methamphetamine to 140 patients with "chronic anxiety" and "acute posttraumatic anxieties." The drug was said to help the patients "relive their painful traumatic experiences with dramatic relief of tension, and a feeling of relaxation. In the cases that abreacted, the drug was of therapeutic value. In others, the use of the drug uncovered material available to the patient's consciousness for integration and assimilation."[76] So here we have anxiety hived off from everything else and made pharmacologically into a separate illness.

In 1955 the pharmaceutical industry moved into anxiety in a big way with the launch of meprobamate, promoted by Wallace Laboratories as Miltown and by Wyeth Laboratories as Equanil. Meprobamate was flogged not as a sedative (which would have made it appropriate for nervous conditions) but as a tranquilizer, a new term. Meprobamate was thought to share with chlorpromazine (which was later an antipsychotic) and reserpine (an antihypertensive drug that enjoyed a brief sojourn in the psychiatric tent) the quality of making anxious patients tranquil. Because there were no tranquilizers for the other components of the nervous syndrome—depression, fatigue, and somatic symptoms—labeling a drug a tranquilizer and indicating it for anxiety silenced the discussion of anxiety as a nervous symptom. Wyeth's ads stressed heavily that Equanil was an "antianxiety" drug and reduced muscular tension as well.[77] Nothing was said about sedation or nerves. Similarly, Wallace

Laboratories, which had originated the drug, billed Miltown as "an entirely new type of tranquilizer," indicating it for "anxiety, tension and mental stress."[78] All this reinforced the idea of anxiety as an independent illness.

Chlorpromazine, the first antipsychotic, reached French markets in 1953 as Largactil, billed by its original manufacturer Rhône-Poulenc as a "sedative," among other uses. But the term was soon downplayed for "anxious states, psychasthenias, and neurovegetative dystonias," a diagnosis popular in Europe for somatic anxiety that did not reach the trans-Atlantic world.[79] Smith Kline & French Laboratories brought out chlorpromazine in the United States in 1954 as Thorazine, indicating it as an antiemetic. Yet the company had bigger fish to fry than the vomiting of cancer chemotherapy, and from 1955 on they were selling it for pain, psychosis, and anxiety (chlorpromazine is in fact effective for all three).[80] An ad for Thorazine in "a child with a behavior disorder" in 1956 had every appearance of making the drug look like a sedative: "calming effect in seriously disturbed youngsters ... reduces hyperactivity and aggressiveness."[81] As for "anxiety, tension, and agitated depression" in the "menopausal patient," hey come on! Chlorpromazine is the drug of choice.[82] Throughout this barrage of mood indications Smith Kline did not use the term sedative, and insisted that chlorpromazine was a tranquilizer.

Thus, around 1955 two powerful new drugs were launched—meprobamate and chlorpromazine—that claimed to treat anxiety independently of other conditions. They were not thought of as sedatives, and the "n" word for nervous was never, ever used in promoting them to the profession. Pharmaceutical marketing thus completed the process psychoanalysis had begun of cutting loose anxiety from nerves and casting it adrift as an independent disease.

The anxiety picture came even more sharply into focus with the discovery, or the claim, that the new benzodiazepine drug class, introduced with Librium in 1960, treated anxiety specifically rather than just generally sedating. There was a certain logic to calling this drug class, effective in many disorders, antianxiety agents. As Chicago neurophysiologist Ralph Gerard, an early American leader in neuroscience, explained in 1957, 3 years before the launch of Librium, "If a given drug is called a tranquilizer, it is likely to be prescribed for disturbed psychotics, to be compared with chlorpromazine ... and to be regarded in the patient's milieu as a stigma on the taker; if it is called a hypnotic, it is likely to be used on a ten- or twentyfold larger scale, to be compared with barbiturates, and to be accepted as neutrally as is aspirin."[83] Roche was wise. They chose a name that would win a large and anxious public, without inviting invidious comparisons with other popular agents such as Miltown. The benzodiazepines were to be antianxiety drugs.

And the benzodiazepines did seem to have a specific antianxiety effect. In 1974 Malcolm Lader and colleagues at the Maudsley Hospital in a double blind trial put a barbiturate head to head against three benzodiazepines and a placebo in 20 outpatients with chronic anxiety. The three benzodiazepines beat the barbiturate and the placebo hands down.[84] The implication was clearly that anxiety was a disease of its own, miles away from whatever it was that the hoary old barbiturates had claimed to treat.

This new clinical focus on anxiety may have been responsible for some of the increase in anxiety—either as a subjective state or as a diagnosis—that seems to have occurred in the twentieth century. Fear has always existed, but anxiety does seem to be up. As journalist Patricia Pearson reminds us, "In these times we speak a great deal about fear, the politics of fear, the culture of fear … But fear and anxiety are vitally different experiences, and it is actually anxiety that characterizes our age. Fear is involved by an immediate threat, and galvanizes a response … The signature vexation of anxiety is that it is objectless. It washes over one in formless waves, pulls one under until the pressure and constriction are tangible and panic rears. 'I'm in deep. I'm going down.'"[85]

In an analysis of 5450 patient charts at seven different clinics, an outpatient service, and a private practice in the Netherlands for the years 1900 to 1985, Giel Hutschemaekers found "a clear overall increase in anxiety complaints." Before 1910, 41% of patients reported anxiety; in the early 1980s 72% did so. The incidence of anxiety had thus almost doubled, whether because of greater patient subjective complaints or increased physician sensitivity to anxiety, now that treatments for it were available[86] (but treatments had been available, notably the barbiturates, in the previous period as well).

Within the grab-bag of anxiety disorders that *DSM* created in 1980, one stands closest to the nervous breakdown, panic disorder. And it is the epidemic of panic that strides in the shadow of the epidemic of depression.

The symptoms of panic disorder are like a snapshot in time of a more general breakdown: the desperate feeling of being unable to catch one's breath, the pounding heart, the overwhelming anxiety about coping with this flood of symptoms cascading over the body. Within the panoply of anxiety symptoms, panic is not the most frequent: "Unspecified" anxiety disorders are by far the most common in office visits in the United States. Yet among the "specified" kinds of anxiety—phobia, obsessive-compulsive, posttraumatic—panic is in the lead, and has been sharply increasing in frequency.[87]

Panic disorder first surfaced late in the nineteenth century (see Chapter 5), then the paroxystic forms of anxiety languished in obscurity because patients with them had such an organic feeling that the psychoanalysts were not interested. The revival of interest in panic disorder began with the brilliant Harvard psychiatrist Mandel Cohen, arguably the founder of biological thinking in American psychiatry, in 1940, with his work on inducing panic chemically in patients who had an underlying anxiety disorder by having them rebreathe carbon dioxide (if you put a paper bag over your head and take and expel deep breaths for a few minutes you will do approximately the same experiment that Cohen did). His subjects began "clutching at throat, writhing and wringing hands," and "experienced feelings and sensations resembling or identical with their anxiety attacks."[88] He revisited the subject again in 1951 with Harvard cardiologist Paul Dudley White, who was President Eisenhower's physician after his heart attack in 1955—under the label "neurocirculatory asthenia": "The patients may have chief complaints of choking and smothering spells, rapid heart beat, pain in the chest, nervousness, 'get tired easily' …or 'I believe I have heart trouble.'" Neurocirculatory asthenia resembled the nervous syndrome in that 95% of the patients with it "tired easily." Eighty-eight percent reported "nervousness," and 50% reported "unhappiness," the contemporary equivalent of what we would call depression. The disorder had a chronic form and an acute form, which latter probably corresponds to a panic attack: "Choking and smothering feelings are prominent, especially in crowds; patients complain 'I have to open the windows' or 'leave the crowded bus.'" At the onset of symptoms, the patients dread having an "anxiety attack" and "may avoid church or the cinema, or if attending the latter, sit near the rear …in order to insure hasty egress, if necessary."[89] The term neurocirculatory asthenia, however, did not catch on.

In 1967 Ferris Pitts in the Department of Psychiatry at Washington University in St. Louis, prompted by the observation that anxious individuals tended to produce excess amounts of blood lactic acid during exercise, in a double-blind study undertook to administer infusions of lactate to patients with histories of anxiety and to controls. The anxiety patients responded to the lactate by developing anxiety attacks, but the controls on the whole did not. The investigators, who presumably did not know about Cohen's one-page article in 1940, said, "This is the first reported demonstration that anxiety attacks and anxiety symptoms can be produced predictably by a specific stimulus …"[90] The paper put the organicity of anxiety attacks back on the table for discussion: Did these patients have a separate chemistry, comparable perhaps to the imputed neurochemistry of depression ("serotonin deficiency")?

Meanwhile, events were on the move elsewhere. The terms "panic" and "anxiety attack" had been used sporadically in psychiatry for decades. Of 100 Boston patients with manic-depressive disease in 1957, 33% also had "anxiety attacks," as opposed to 4% of medically sick controls.[91] At the Second

International Congress of Psychiatry in Zurich in 1957, Douglas Goldman, a Cincinnati psychiatrist and one of the pioneers of psychopharmacology, said offhandedly, "We see many cases of acute panic reactions that are schizophrenic in form," as though the audience were perfectly familiar with the term.[92] In 1959, Martin Roth, a pioneering student of illness classification then at Newcastle upon Tyne, anticipated panic disorder with his diagnosis "the phobic anxiety-depersonalization syndrome": "There was a fearful aversion to leaving familiar surroundings, to walking in the streets and to entering shops, travelling in vehicles or visiting cinemas or theatres. Waiting or sitting still in such settings was prone to evoke a sense of impeding disaster, acute agitation and flight in panic."[93] Again, the diagnosis, perhaps because of its very clunkiness, did not catch on, but the term panic was certainly abroad.

It was therefore not such a stretch for Donald Klein and Max Fink to think about panic in the patients at Hillside Hospital in eastern Queens whom they started on the new TCA imipramine, once it became available for trials in the United States in the late 1950s. In one of the earliest double-blind studies in American psychopharmacology, discussed above, in 1962 Klein and Fink reported that anxious patients with symptoms of panic responded to imipramine whereas anxious patients with phobic symptoms did not. Klein and Fink had basically used a psychopharmacological torch to carve out panic from the great block of anxious illness and make it a separate disease. After 1962, Klein went on to differentiate panic as a separate illness while Fink turned to other subjects.[94] And panic disorder is indissolubly associated with Klein's work. Many authorities thought that panic was related to depression, but in 1982 Klein showed that imipramine had a specific effect on panic unrelated to depression.[95] In the 1970s panic with and without agoraphobia—the differentiation was somehow seen as important—boomed as a diagnosis and was incorporated into *DSM-III* in 1980[96] (see pp. 141–42).

Klein had experienced great success with imipramine (Tofranil)—and there is considerable evidence of the effectiveness of the tricyclics in panic[97]—but other drug classes seemed effective too. In 1967 Smith Kline & French Laboratories in Philadelphia began indicating their antipsychotic drug Stelazine (trifluoperazine) for "the panic-prone patient."[98] This was not illogical, as the antipsychotics had a long history of efficacy in anxiety disorders, to which panic indisputably belonged. The benzodiazepine lorazepam (Ativan) became advertised for panic in 1987 ("Documented efficacy in panic attacks").[99]

These were relatively uncontroversial developments. But the panic pool was poisoned by a debacle that occurred after the Upjohn Company, in

Kalamazoo, Michigan, sought systematically to expand the panic market with a lavish promotion of its benzodiazepine alprazolam (Xanax), which had been launched for anxiety in 1981. They asked Gerald Klerman, a senior figure, to lead an international trial to establish its efficacy, and the trials and its conclusions proved terribly controversial. English psychiatrist Peter Tyrer, later editor of the *British Journal of Psychiatry*, recalled the lavish marketing meeting at Key Biscayne, Florida, in 1982, "where for the first time I felt physically dirty after being tarnished by the broad sweep of the Upjohn brush into every part of 'agoraphobia with panic,' which I and others have named ADS (the alprazolam deficiency syndrome) ever since."[100] Upjohn launched Xanax for panic after FDA approval in 1990. These events led to an unpleasant exchange between Isaac Marks at the Maudsley and Klerman in the late 1980s, on the grounds that panic did not exist as a separate disease and the larger anxiety syndrome was readily responsive to psychotherapy rather than drugs (the Maudsley crowd had always been uneasy about psychopharmacology). At the time of Klerman's death in April 1992, his draft reply to Marks lay as yet unsent on his writing table, and his widow Myrna Weissman objected to Marks's actions.[101]

Yet despite these British reservations, panic disorder does seem to be a disease of its own. Whereas garden-variety anxiety has always been part of the nervous syndrome, paroxystic expressions of anxiety, now called panic, do appear to be a thing apart. And Donald Klein is correctly considered among the pioneers of psychopharmacology rather than the foremost advocate of a passing diagnostic fad. (On the specificity of alprazolam for panic there is, however, some dubiety. There is substantial agreement that the benzodiazepines as a whole, not just alprazolam, are effective in panic. Upjohn's marketing campaign deafened serious discussion of these issues for a long time.)

Panic disorder is of interest here because its symptoms often match those of the historic nervous breakdown. Just as the acute nervous breakdown was distinct from chronic expressions of the nervous syndrome, acute attacks of panic seem to be different from general chronic anxiety and mixed anxiety-depression.[102]

In sum, the years after 1960 saw the return of the true depression, melancholia, which had never really been a part of the nervous syndrome; those years saw the rise of the false depression, major depression, pieces of which had always been a part of the nervous syndrome. Finally, those years witnessed the rise of panic disorder, which had once been part of the nervous breakdown. Blinded by artifacts and stumbling about in a kind of nosological gloom, psychiatry lost track of the diseases that had once been its core diagnoses and substituted for them heterogeneous artifacts that were meaningful only to the pharmaceutical industry.

12

Nerves Redux

WE MIGHT HAVE thought that the concept of nerves ended in 1957 when the United States Post Office Department initiated a fraud proceeding against John Winters of New York City, who had been promoting a product called Orbacine containing bromide and niacin for "every-day nervousness and its symptoms."[1] Although Winters' claims went a bit beyond nerves, the Post Office wanted an end to the whole business and Orbacine disappeared.

But the concept of nerves had enemies other than the Post Office. Three in particular had tried to do away with it: psychoanalysis, psychopharmacology, and the *DSM* series. All failed to kill it completely, and the concept lingers on because of its obvious face value: Our patients clearly have a nervous illness or something resembling it. They do not have a "mood disorder."

A Rose by Another Other Name…

In medicine the nervous syndrome, the condition that dare not speak its name, has taken on various allures. Once upon a time, hysteria was the equivalent of a nervous diagnosis in women. There were physicians who had little patience with calling their former hysteric patients "depressed": They remained hysteric! Jacques Frei, a member of the department of psychiatry of the University of Lausanne in Switzerland, noted in 1984 "the importance that depressive symptomatology has taken today as a call for help among female hysterics.…It seems that the hysterical woman today has a better chance of a hearing if she presents with a depressive picture, even evoking suicidal ideas."[2] Although hysteria today is discredited as a diagnosis, it is interesting that older clinicians such as Frei saw it as a diagnosis that trumped depression; he even argued that his patients at Cery Hospital were modeling their symptoms to conform to the new diagnoses.

The 1950s and 1960s saw alternative diagnoses to the nervous syndrome come and go, fragments of clinical experience that seemed to make sense to individual physicians but were not more widely taken up because their originators did not have prestigious academic appointments. Take "the housewife syndrome" that Palma Formica proposed in 1962. (Formica, a young unknown family doctor in Old Bridge, New Jersey, was later celebrated as a female medical pioneer in New Jersey.) Just as soon as the patients entered her office, they began crying. Their chief complaint was fatigue. "Her commonest complaint—chronic tiredness—is largely ignored in the medical literature.... Her daily, mechanical repetition of monotonous, exhausting, routine duties that stretch endlessly into the future." The strain of making the family budget meet ends, the numerous obligations to school and church, "and still have energy left for companionship with her husband, contribute to constant weariness and a conviction of defeat." Are these patients depressed? No. They have insight. "Nor are they neurotic." How do they cope? First, they try "will power." "They do not seek medical help until they are completely miserable, and their irritability and inertia have nearly disrupted the family." The women are then embarrassed "to take up a physician's time" with what they presume to be trivia. The symptoms themselves of "the housewife syndrome" were various aches and pains, "an excessive desire for sleep but inability to sleep soundly," and "constant lassitude, uninterest in home duties and in the marital relation. They invariably end their recital with, 'Doctor, I am so tired: I never used to feel this way.'"[3] The housewife syndrome never caught on, but it clearly is a restatement of nerves, even though it is possible that Dr. Formica was unfamiliar with that ancient diagnosis.

That was suburban New Jersey in the early 1960s. Then came *DSM-III* in 1980, the ascent of psychopharmacology, the end of the dominance of psychoanalysis, and the triumph of major depression. What alternatives have more recently come along?

As one alternative to the major depression trap, the late twentieth century saw a revival in thinking about mixed anxiety-depression as a single disorder. There were voices from all about the vast psychiatric hall.

Edward Sachar, head of psychiatry at Columbia University, was a kind of Wunderkind of biological psychiatry, having begun with psychoanalysis and moved rapidly to heading teams of combined laboratory and clinical investigators on the biological side. It is therefore interesting that in 1979 he articulated the existence of a syndrome going beyond clinical depression (though he continued to call it depression) "From the welter of conditions involving unhappiness, misery, grief, disappointment, despair etc have emerged certain depressive syndromes that seem clearly to be 'somatic affections.'"[4] There would be no reason for naming these sprawling syndromes depression, since the patients did not necessarily seem depressed but expressed their distress on the somatic side. (see below on depressive equivalents).

Speculation continued to flow in the direction of nerves, without using that term. At the Food and Drug Administration—not exactly a bastion of innovative thinking about the classifying of illness—Paul Leber, head of the neuropharmacology section of the office that approves new drugs, mused casually in 1983 to an advisory committee: What came first in a given illness, the depression or the anxiety? The FDA had been in the past reluctant to grant labeling for both. "What do you think of the idea of outpatient dysphoria, the mixed state, as being real? One that responds in the first week to benzodiazepines and in the third week to classical antidepressants? You would have to rework the nosology of the field."[5] Indeed. Restoring mixed anxiety-depression would entail dethroning major depression. It would be a first tapping step toward nerves. Discussions of mixed anxiety-depression then surged in the 1990s and after.

Nerves as a Term Lingers on

The terms nervousness and nerves have now vanished from psychiatry, but elsewhere in medicine they remain current although not widely discussed concepts.

In 1955 Paul Hoch at the New York State Psychiatric Institute, one of the leaders of biological thinking in postwar American psychiatry, said rather contemptuously that the family doctors were indiscriminately diagnosing the new antipsychotic drug chlorpromazine (Thorazine) for "nerves" and the like. Of course, by then forward-thinking psychiatrists would never use such a term, but it remained, he believed, current among slow-lane types in family medicine.[6]

In 1968, at a conference at McGill University, Stephen Taylor, an important figure in English psychiatric epidemiology, was discussing a survey of neurotic disorders that he and Sidney Chave had undertaken earlier. What they essentially found was the nerve syndrome. "We found, among people who were *not* necessarily attending their doctors, a sub-clinical neurosis syndrome. The symptoms, which tend to cluster, are: mild depression; undue irritability; 'nerves' or excessive nervousness, and insomnia. This group constitutes about 30 percent of the population."[7] So nerves had not been entirely forgotten! Except that in the United States this syndrome would have been called "depression."

And was there a touch of nerves in the many anxiety diagnoses that *DSM* had created in 1980? Eugene Paykel and George Winokur, editors of a special issue on anxiety in 1986 of the *Journal of Affective Disorders*, said in their editors' preface, "Whether these classifications [agoraphobia, obsessional illness] are appropriate remains for further research. The distinction between generalized anxiety disorder and simple nervousness also needs to be evaluated." This is a circumspect way of saying that "We don't believe in generalized anxiety disorder and think that it is plain old nervousness."[8] But that these international leaders in 1986 would be discussing nervousness is an interesting testimonial to the staying power of the diagnosis, conceived in the eighteenth century and not struck entirely dead even by the potent *DSM*.

Wherever one looked, casual references to nerves leapt off the pages, as though it were something so natural it did not even have to be explained. At an FDA meeting in 1992 on side effects of Upjohn's hypnotic drug Halcion, generically named triazolam, Lawrence Olanoff, a physician and vice-president of clinical development of Upjohn, said in passing that they had evaluated the drug for "nervousness" and did not find any particular safety issues in that indication.[9]

These scattered references over the years and continents do not represent solid diagnoses but an almost subliminal current of thought that bubbled from below, fed by decades and centuries of experience, into the profession's consciousness. The word "nerves" was all of a sudden just there, part of a kind of unspoken agenda of diagnosis and treatment that was felt to be right but did not fit in with the official schemes at all.

"Depressive Equivalents"

There was as well the diagnosis of "depressive equivalents": illnesses in patients who do not look depressed, but in whom depression was assumed to exist as the real underlying problem. Since the patient does not actually appear depressed, we would agree to the notion of depressive-equivalents only if we thought that depression was some kind of master diagnosis, and that anyone with anxiety, somatic symptoms, obsessive thinking, and so forth must at bottom be depressed. Yet perhaps the whole concept of somatic symptoms supposedly caused by underlying mood and anxiety disorders is equivalent to the nervous syndrome rather than equivalating depression? Only because the attention of the profession was becoming increasingly riveted upon depression was depression sought out as the supposed puppeteer that caused everything else in the body to move.

The doctrine of depressive equivalents actually has quite a history. It had long been known that major psychiatric illnesses were often accompanied by changes in blood pressure and heart rate (vasomotor disturbances), indeed that psychiatric symptoms often seemed secondary to the headaches, irritable bowels, thyroid disturbances, and skin eruptions that psychiatrists observed in their in-patients. These were called "vasomotor neuroses," a term coined around 1900.[10]

The next step was asserting that such vasomotor changes could represent a "depressive equivalent," that the patients were depressed even though they did not seem to have mood symptoms. In 1929 Walter Cimbal, a national figure in German psychiatry who practiced in the Hamburg suburb of Altona, proposed the concept of "vegetative equivalents of depressive disorders." "Gentlemen," he told a medical meeting, "I want to convince you that neurotic disorders of the autonomic system are not only accompanying symptoms of a manic-depressive or a thyrogenic mood disorders, but that they might present even as equivalents in place of such an episode. Next to such an equivalent, the actual depressive mood change may recede to the point of being scarcely perceptible or it might be reduced to a slightly increased lability and irritability."[11] This opened the door to calling almost any autonomic dysregulation a "depressive equivalent."

In 1934 Berthold Wichmann, a young assistant at the university psychiatric clinic in Münster, decided that the autonomic changes were so impressive that their terminology should be unhitched entirely from psychiatric lingo, and he called them "vegetative dystonia," an independent disease entity (vegetative means autonomic nervous system; the other great nervous system in the body, the voluntary, controls movement and the muscles). He played down mental changes as secondary to these vast autonomic tides.[12]

Both "depressive equivalents" and "vegetative dystonia" went on to become major diagnoses in Europe after World War II. But vegetative dystonia remained unfamiliar in the Anglo-Saxon world. [George Beaumont of Geigy (later Novartis) said they were not able to conduct a clinical trial of opipramol (Insidon) in England for "psychovegetative dystonia" because nobody had ever heard of it.[13]] The doctrine of depressive equivalents, on the other hand—depression without depression—went on to enjoy epic success in Anglo-American psychiatry.

Under the influence of the doctrine that said "the overwhelming number of neurotic states are in reality mild or severe depressions,"[14] Adalbert Kral in Montreal—who had trained in Prague and needed no lessons in German psychiatry—proposed in 1958 the concept of "masked depression." At the Allan Memorial Institute, which was the department of psychiatry of McGill University, there had been a number of middle-aged men having a positive family history of depression with the following symptoms: "At first, the clinical picture was in all cases dominated by anxiety, tension and hypochondriacal ruminations. Depressive mood and psychomotor retardation were minimal." The patients had loads of somatic changes, such as insomnia, weight loss, and impotence. They were unresponsive to psychotherapy but did well on electroconvulsive therapy (ECT). Kral concluded that their underlying problem must be depression: "It would seem therefore that in the cases reported, anxiety and tension formed only part of the clinical picture and masked the underlying depression." Possibly so, but 50 years earlier the diagnosis would have been nerves, or "neurosis," and it is unclear why it must be concluded that the patients were depressed: Other illnesses as well respond to ECT.[15]

And so the concept of affective equivalents—depression without depression—diffused in the English-speaking world. But it spread with a kind of psychoanalytic overlay that brings the whole concept into question. After the work of psychoanalyst Franz Alexander in 1950, arthritis, asthma, peptic ulcer, and dermatitis were all seen as depressive equivalents because all were, following psychoanalytic theory, considered psychogenic.[16] In 1965, for example, Anthony Hordern, a psychiatrist at King's College Hospital in London, declared that "Depressive states are also encountered as affective equivalents—periodic, spontaneously remitting 'physical' illnesses, such as rheumatism, asthma, peptic ulcer and dermatitis."[17] But today we definitely do not see asthma, peptic ulcer, and arthritis as psychogenic! And dermatological conditions usually have organic not psychological causes.[18] So the whole notion that these were somehow the psychic equivalents of depression collapses. "I ask myself if it is really justified to utilize the term 'masked depression' in cases where there is no sign of depression," said Dutch psychiatrist Herman van Praag at a conference in 1973.[19] What can be said is that these "equivalence" patients may or may not have had a mood disorder, and that the concept of depression was being stretched to its outer limits.

The highpoint of the depressive equivalents doctrine was probably the declaration of Dietrich Blumer, a psychiatrist at the Henry Ford Hospital in Detroit, in 1982 that chronic pain could be an equivalent form of depression. He termed the syndrome "pain-prone disorder" and viewed it "as a variant of depressive disease."[20] The point is not that chronic pain patients might not also be depressed in their heart of hearts. It is that if these patients are also anxious, and fatigued, and have other somatic symptoms, and obsess about the whole business, then perhaps depression is too narrow a diagnosis. These are nervous patients who are also in pain.

The bottom line is that nerves still hover outside the profession, like windy drafts at night in a rickety house. The term has been so useful in the past that medicine's collective unconscious will not let it vanish. In recent decades, various templates, such as the housewife syndrome, have been adumbrated for understanding nervous illness as an illness of the entire body, not just the mind and brain. That depression continues to clasp the discipline of psychiatry in its clammy embrace is evidence of the failure of the scientific imagination.

13

Context

CONSIDER THE CURRENT landscape of depression. In an ABC poll in 2002, 15% of Americans said they felt "really depressed" once a week or more. Another 17% said once a month. That means that one-third of the American population believes itself to be depressed in a given month.[1] If you are riding on a subway train with a hundred other people, one-third of them will be currently depressed, or have just been, or are about to be. That is a lot.

In fact, it is way too many. We know that only 3% of the population is chronically sad. We know that the serious disease, melancholia, is only a fraction of the ranks of the depressed. Far too many people have received the diagnosis of depression.

Whose fault is this?

At the beginning of our story, psychiatry spoke German. From around 1870 to 1933, German-speaking Europe was the epicenter of world psychiatry. This was so for two reasons.

One, German, Swiss, and Austrian psychiatrists saw large numbers of very sick individuals because they practiced in mental hospitals, leaving outpatients to other practitioners. Of course this was true of alienists elsewhere, but there were more mental hospitals in Germany affiliated with universities because Germany had so many universities. Almost all had university psychiatric hospitals. This was not true elsewhere. So German psychiatry was oriented toward the academic study of large numbers of patients, and a genial figure such as Emil Kraepelin used these resources to make big strides.

Second, German psychiatrists had a thorough familiarity with internal medicine because they were also trained as neurologists. From the viewpoint of subject matter, neurology has always been treated as a subspecialty of internal medicine, even though in Central Europe it was hived off to the nerve specialists. In learning so much neurology, German psychiatrists acquired a feeling for brain illness as involving the entire body: They were indeed attuned to looking at the body as a whole, in contrast to Anglo-Saxon psychiatrists, who usually did not also train as internists. (In Toronto, where I live, neurology still is a subspecialty of internal medicine, and the psychiatrists have only a nodding familiarity with it.) This whole-body perspective is entirely salutary, for a disease such as melancholia has deep roots in the endocrine system, and reaches into the adrenal glands. Anxiety sets the entire body aflutter with palpations, gastrointestinal upset, and the like. Having a comprehensive knowledge of internal medicine can be very useful to a psychiatrist in sorting the wheat from the chaff.

The German psychiatrist-neurologists managed to codify and crystallize an enormous amount of information about basic diseases in psychiatry. They sought their main diagnostic implements in the toolbox of psychopathology: the close study of patients' signs and symptoms. By 1933 German-speaking psychiatry had individuated the main natural disease entities in psychiatry: Ewald Hecker had described hebephrenia (from which "schizophrenia" evolved) in 1871; his tutor Karl Kahlbaum described catatonia in 1874; and the Danish psychiatrist Carl Georg Lange, Denmark's "first neurologist" who to all intents and purposes might have been German, differentiated periodic depression from melancholia in 1886, thus putting the study of the two depressions on a scientific basis.[2] These remain important illness concepts, and Emil Kraepelin's separation in 1899 of dementia-praecox from manic-depressive illness is one of the cornerstones of psychiatry today. So the contributions of these skilled German-speaking psychopathologists with their deep backgrounds in internal medicine have been epochal.

Now we fast-forward to Freud's psychoanalysis in the 1920s. With one fell swoop, psychoanalysis managed to discard all of this carefully accumulated knowledge about psychopathology and disease classification and to divert the discipline of psychiatry to the study of what were essentially figments: unconscious conflict as the motor of symptom formation; early childhood socialization as the seedbed of illness in adults; dream analysis and free association as the basis of treatment. The painstakingly accumulated information about psychiatric genetics—some of which, it is true, leaped the rails of science in Hitler's Germany; the interest in brain anatomy as the seat of psychiatric illness; the fine differences in the presentations of various disease entities: All these were discarded as outmoded and uninteresting literally within the space of a decade! In the annals of modern science, I am unaware of any comparable wholesale demolition of a field of scientific knowledge and its replacement with a fairy castle of fantasies. It is as though the field of cardiology had suddenly been overtaken by a school of investigators who believed moonbeams the key to understanding cardiovascular illness, and the knowledge about coronary occlusions and electrocardiographic findings that had accumulated by 1930 was discarded in favor of a set of moonbeam doctrines.

The parable, though fanciful, is not far-fetched. By the time psychoanalysis began to collapse from sheer incredulity and lack of therapeutic results in the 1960s, psychiatry found itself with the cupboard bare. Little of the former knowledge base had survived. In any event, it was mostly in German, which nobody read anymore. The new sciences of psychopharmacology and neurophysiology confronted a tabula rasa. Moreover, the practitioners of psychiatry had lost that strong connection to neurology and the other subspecialties of internal medicine that had been such a motor of progress. As well, under the influence of psychoanalysis, the university departments of psychiatry were all chaired by analysts and future scientific developments in psychiatry—well into the 1970s and 1980s—would occur in what the English call the "red-bricks," secondary provincial academic centers rather than in the academic heartland.

Thus, when confronted with "depression," the new generation of nonanalyst psychiatrists, who were slowly tapping their way back toward biology, were left quite without critical scholarly tools. In the United States in the 1970s, psychopathology was a dead letter, and if treated at academic meetings it would be during the last session of the last day. The study of the major mental illnesses in seriously ill patients, such as melancholia and catatonia, had given way to analytic speculations in outpatients about the role of the patient's toilet training. And medical colleagues in other specialties sooner regarded psychiatry as an esoteric branch of social work rather than as a sister scientific discipline fast-charging its way forward.

It was from the work of Kraepelin and Freud that depression had become a familiar concept in psychiatry. But when *DSM-III* launched "major depression" in 1980, psychiatrists found themselves quite without defenses. Many sensed that there was a big problem in conflating endogenous depression and reactive unhappiness: We were told that breaking up with your boyfriend was on a par with lying curled into a fetal, melancholic ball. Both could be major depression as long as the "Chinese menu" of criteria was satisfied.

How do we fight back against something like this if we have lost all the skills of the psychopathologist, if we never absorbed enough internal medicine to say "Yoo hoo, there's something wrong with the endocrine system here," and if our main source of pharmaceutical knowledge is promotional material from the drug companies—companies that now see in major depression a lot of runway space. The answer is that individual psychiatrists who were uneasy about the depression epidemic exploding about them lacked the critical skills for arresting it. Their private reservations and personal eyebrow raisings were steamrollered by the wave of enthusiasm for depression in the 1980s and 1990s.

Psychiatry's inability to stop the depression epidemic is an appalling story of the collective failure of a scientific discipline to ward off a public-health disaster. The loss of the view of two depressions—melancholia and nonmelancholia—means that poorly diagnosed patients are denied the benefit of proper treatment while being exposed to all the side effects of classes of medication, such as the Prozac-style drugs, that are ineffective for serious illness.

It is time for a turn-around.

Coda

Is it all doom and gloom? I want to close on a positive note. There are lessons here both for doctors and patients that will improve the understanding of what has been called depression. Depressed mood is only a small corner of a much wider illness condition involving feelings of anxiety, fatigue, bodily aches and pains, and worried obsession about the whole thing. It is important to understand that people's symptoms are real signs of illness, not part of some process of medicalization in which normal worries and feelings somehow become objects of medical attention.

The first lesson is that we have got to get the emphasis off low mood, which is the essence of the concept of depression. People with the nerve syndrome are not necessarily sad, weepy, or down in the dumps any more than the population as a whole. They feel ill at ease in their bodies, preoccupied with their state of mind, and are unable to get their thoughts off their internal psychic condition. This book proposes nerves as a good label for what they have, given that I, as a historian, have a fondness for concepts that have stood the test of time. But this is not mandatory. We do not have to call what they are experiencing nerves. We can invent some other term. The main point is to move the discussion's center of gravity off the term depression.

Indeed, there is some evidence that this is happening already. In recent years scholars such as David Barlow, at the Center for Anxiety and Related Disorders at Boston University, have begun to signal the intrinsic connection between depression and anxiety.[3] Increasingly, depression is being conceived as a total body experience—an unwitting reversion to the nerves concept—rather than as a disorder of mood. There is evidence that pain, depression, and anxiety are all mediated via the γ-aminobutyric acid B (GABA-B) receptor; neuroscientist Salvatore Enna, for many years head of pharmacology at the University of Kansas, says, "In the long term I would hope that our work would reveal the role of the GABA-B receptor in mediating pain and the emotional response to it with the aim of developing drugs that could be used to ameliorate these conditions."[4]

The immune system is also pulled in. One team of researchers at Harvard University proposes "surrogate markers" for depression that include measures of immune function such as tumor necrosis factor-alpha levels.[5] Neurobiologist Paul Patterson at the California Institute of Technology wrote in 2011 that "There is now little doubt that the immune system and immune-related molecules are an integral part of the story of major depressive disorder."[6] At the National Institute for Mental Health, a group led by Thomas Insel and Bruce Cuthbert known as the Research Domain Criteria (RDoC) project sets out to identify the neural circuits responsible for behavioral domains. The range of the investigators is the entire body. They write, "In this manner, depression might be viewed akin to the way that a fever is viewed today, suggesting specific tests for a panel of potentially active diagnostic markers that will steer the clinician to the appropriate treatment among any number of possible disordered processes that might underlie the depression."[7] We are a long way from Prozac here.

The second lesson is for doctors. But I want to make it clear that I am speaking as a historian capable of identifying agents that in the past have a record of failure or success. We know that in recent history the current crop of drugs referred to as antidepressants are ineffective in real depressive illness, which is to say melancholia,[8] and somehow land wide of the mark in treating nervous illness. Innovation in psychopharmacology is desperately needed, given that no truly new drugs for patients who are agitated, upset, and preoccupied with their bodies have been developed in the past 30 years. My job is not to pioneer new trails in psychopharmacology. But I cannot help observing that in the past, effective agents for nervous illness did exist that today have been largely forgotten. Patients who are worn out and weary require stimulation; those who are agitated and preoccupied require sedation. And you know: Half a century ago the pharmaceutical industry marketed a highly successful combination of barbiturates and amphetamines—Smith Kline's version, called Dexamyl, hit the market in 1950—that treated both domains of illness at once. Until the Food and Drug Administration and the Drug Enforcement Agency swept this combination from the market in the 1970s, along with almost all other barbiturates and amphetamines (except for a few tightly controlled indications), Dexamyl was widely effective in treating nervous illness.[9] Today, of course, this has been forgotten, and one English psychiatrist told me that he simply would not be able to make his fingers move to write a prescription for either barbiturates or amphetamines. That is a cultural, not a scientific, reflex, born of decades of overwrought hype about the exceptional dangers of barbiturates and amphetamines.

All drugs are dangerous in that all have side effects, but the risks have to be weighed against the expected benefits, which in the case of the barbiturates and amphetamines in the treatment of mood disorders are considerable. This is not an argument for the revival of Dexamyl or of the amphetamines and barbiturates as drug classes, but a flare in the night to alert physicians that the treatment of nervous illness requires some combination of sedation and stimulation. It does not require "antidepressants."

The last lesson is for patients. Millions of people have been led to believe that they are depressed when in fact their illness involves much more than their mood—it involves their entire brain and body. It is the whole that has to be treated, not the mood as such—because their feelings might well reflect demoralization, discouragement, discomfort, or disarray, but not depression. These are separate concepts. A skilled psychopathologist can tease them out. (In a recent interview Richard Shader at Tufts University, one of the kingpins of U.S. psychopharmacology, deplored the ignorance of many younger clinicians, "who don't know the difference between being demoralized and being depressed."[10])

But the public is not interested in the technical issues of psychopathology: People simply want to feel better; they want relief. It is important to understand that what you are experiencing at the level of your whole body and the various sensations it sends to your brain and mind is not capable of being reduced to depression. It is a more general bodily illness. But it responds to exercise. It responds to the skills of psychotherapy. If you are so anxious that you need to be sedated, you must be aware that sedation is not a curse word (as most physicians see it, conditioned by decades of pharmaceutical advertising about "anxiolytics"), but a blessing that may be pharmaceutically achieved. If you are so leaden that you need to be stimulated, the same logic applies. Stimulants are not just for superenergetic young lads with supposed attention deficit disorder, but legitimate treatments to wrest adults as well from the slough of dysphoria.

There is help available. But physicians must be thoughtful in diagnosing their patients' problems, and the patients must be alert in making sure that the diagnosis and treatment they receive are appropriate to their needs and not the fruit of punchy pharmaceutical advertising.

Acknowledgments

IT IS MY privilege to work with a highly gifted little band of researchers and once again I have the opportunity to acknowledge their help. They have been led by Susan Bélanger, and include Esther Atkinson, Ellen Tulchinsky, and Kathryn Segesser. Beverly Slopen, my agent and dear friend, has been a font of wise advice. At Oxford University Press I am glad to thank editor David D'Addona and production editor Emily Perry, who made so many useful suggestions.

Earlier versions of this book were read by Max Fink, David Healy, Barney Carroll, Walter Vandereycken, and, on behalf of Oxford University Press, Clark Lawlor, all of whom made valuable suggestions for improvement.

Research in this volume was partially financed by grants from the Social Science and Humanities Research Council of Canada and the Canadian Institutes of Health Research.

Notes

ABBREVIATIONS USED IN THE NOTES

AJP	American Journal of Psychiatry
Annales MP	Annales Médico-Psychologiques
AZP	Allgemeine Zeitschrift für Psychiatrie
BJP	British Journal of Psychiatry
BMJ	British Medical Journal
JAMA	Journal of the American Medical Association
NEJM	New England Journal of Medicine

CHAPTER I

1. See the review of "depressive psychoses," meaning serious depression, in six epidemiological studies conducted between 1933 and 1960 in Charlotte Silverman, "The Epidemiology of Depression—A Review," *AJP*, 124 (1968), 883–891; the prevalence rates for minor depression were "generally two to three times greater than the rates for psychoses" (p. 889). M. Olfson, "Prevalence of Anxiety, Depression, and Substance Use Disorders in an Urban General Medicine Practice," *Archives of Family Medicine*, 9 (2000), 876–883; according to data from the National Institute of Mental Health, the rate of outpatient treatment for depression rose from 0.73 per 100 population in 1987 to 2.33 in 1997. Mark Olfson et al., "National Trends in the Outpatient Treatment of Depression," *JAMA*, 287 (Jan. 9, 2002), 203–209.

2. Dan G. Blazer et al., "The Prevalence and Distribution of Major Depression in a National Community Sample: The National Comorbidity Survey," *AJP*, 151 (1994), 979–986; 17.1% was the estimated lifetime risk for major depression.

3. Aug. 1, 2011.

4. Junko Kitanaka, *Depression in Japan: Psychiatric Cures for a Society in Distress* (Princeton: Princeton University Press, 2012), 78–79.

5. Laura A. Pratt et al., "Antidepressant Use in Persons Aged 12 and Over: United States, 2005–2008," National Center for Health Statistics, Data Brief, no. 76, Oct. 2011, 1.

6. Bernard Carroll, personal communication, Jan. 13, 2012.

7. James Sims, "Pathological Remarks upon Various Kinds of Alienation of Mind," *Memoirs of the Medical Society of London*, 5 (1799), 372–406, p. 406.

8. Joseph Zubin, discussion comment, in Lee N. Robins and James E. Barrett, Eds., *The Validity of Psychiatric Diagnosis* (New York: Raven, 1989), 244; the occasion was the 1988 meeting of the American Psychopathological Association.

CHAPTER 2

1. "Nervous Breakdowns by Any Name, Aren't What They Used to Be," *Wall Street Journal*, Dec. 3, 1996.

2. Richard Hunter, "Psychiatry and Neurology," *Proceedings of the Royal Society of Medicine*, 66 (1973), 359–364, p. 360; delivered as an address in Oct. 1972.

3. The term "symptom cluster" is currently fashionable; the symptoms that typically cluster are depression, anxiety, and fatigue. See, for example, Sergio Baldassin et al., "The Characteristics of Depressive Symptoms in Medical Students," *BMC Medical Education*, 8 (2008), 6.

4. Jules Falret, "Discussion sur la folie raisonnante," *Annales MP*, 4th ser., Vol. 1 (1866), 382–426, p. 407. "C'est là une maladie nerveuse et non une folie."

5. Maurice de Fleury, *Manuel pour l'étude des maladies du système nerveux* (Paris: Alcan, 1904), 836–839, 849–850, 852, 858.

6. Wellcome Library, London, England; Contemporary Medical Archives Centre; Frederick Parkes Weber Casebooks, 1906–1907, case of Marion D.

7. Angelo Hesnard, *Les syndromes névropathiques* (Paris: Doin, 1927), 1–8.

8. Joseph Collins, "The General Practitioner and the Functional Nervous Diseases," *JAMA*, 52 (Jan. 9, 1909), 87–92, p. 89.

9. Karl Jaspers, *Allgemeine Psychopathologie* (Berlin: Springer, 1913), 53.

10. "Mrs. Bloodgood Kills Herself," *New York Times*, Jan. 9, 1908, 6.

11. J. H. Blount, "Essay on the Classification of Mental Alienation," *Asylum Journal*, 1 (1854), 93–96, 137–141; quote 93–94.

12. Lothar Kalinowsky, in discussion of Kalinowsky, Eugene Barrera, and William A. Horwitz, "Electric Convulsive Therapy of the Psychoneuroses," *AMA Archives of Neurology and Psychiatry,* 52 (1944), 498–504, p. 504.

13. Angelo Hesnard, *Les syndromes névropathiques* (Paris: Doin, 1927), 1–8.

14. Oswald Bumke, *Lehrbuch der Geisteskrankheiten* (1919), 2nd ed. (Munich: Bergmann, 1924), 414; for neurasthenia, he drew upon the opinions of his psychiatrist colleague Paul Julius Möbius.

15. Joseph Zubin, "Perspectives on the Conference," in Martin M. Katz et al., Eds., *The Role and Methodology of Classification in Psychiatry and Psychopathology: Proceedings of a Conference held in Washington, DC, November, 1965* (Washington, DC: Public Health Service/National Institute of Mental Health, 1968), 556–559, p. 557.

16. Psychopharmacological Drugs Advisory Committee, FDA, Transcript of Proceedings, Mar. 21, 1977, 104; obtained from the Food and Drug Administration through the Freedom of Information Act.

17. Charles Beasley interview, in Thomas A. Ban, Ed., *An Oral History of Neuropsychopharmacology,* Vol. 8 (Brentwood, TN: American College of Neuropsychopharmacology, 2011), 22.

18. David Goldberg and Peter Huxley, *Mental Illness in the Community: The Pathway to Psychiatric Care* (London: Tavistock, 1980), 5, 83–84.

19. John P. Feighner, Eli Robins, Samuel B. Guze, Robert A .Woodruff, Jr., George Winokur, and Rodrigo Muñoz, "Diagnostic Criteria for Use in Psychiatric Research," *Archives of General Psychiatry*, 26 (1972), 57–63, p. 59; these became known as the "Feighner criteria."

20. Aaron T. Beck, *Depression: Clinical, Experimental, and Theoretical Aspects* (New York: Hoeber, 1967), 16, Tab. 2–3.

21. Max Hamilton, "Frequency of Symptoms in Melancholia (Depressive Illness)," *BJP*, 154 (1989), 201–206, p. 205.

22. Robert Musil, *Der Mann ohne Eigenschaften*, Vol. I. (1930) reprint (Hamburg: Rowohlt, 1978), 458.

23. Heinrich Schade, *Ergebnisse einer Bevölkerungsuntersuchung in der Schwalm [Hessen]* (Mainz: Verlag der Akademie der Wissenschaften/Franz Steiner, 1951), 442–443.

24. Erik Essen-Möller, *Individual Traits and Morbidity in a Swedish Rural Population* (Copenhagen: Munksgaard, 1956), 77.

25. College of General Practitioners, Research Committee, *Morbidity Statistics from General Practice*, Vol. 3 (*Disease in General Practice*) (London: HMSO, 1962), 51; General Register Office, Studies on Medical and Population Subjects, no. 14.

26. Conrad Rieger to Emil Kraepelin, June 23, 1882; in Wolfgang Burgmair et al., Eds., *Emil Kraepelin, Briefe I, 1868–1886* (Munich: Belleville, 2002), 238.

27. G. F. D. Heseltine, Ed., *Psychiatric Research in Our Changing World* (Amsterdam: Excerpta Medica, 1969), 42; the conference took place in 1968. Stephen [Lord] Taylor and Sidney Chave, *Mental Health and Environment* (London: Longmans, 1964).

28. Herbert Berger, "Management of Neuroses by the Internist and General Practitioner," *New York State Medical Journal*, 56 (1956), 1783–1788, pp. 1785–1786.

29. J. S. Schiller et al., "Summary Health Statistics for U. S. Adults." National Health Interview Survey, 2010. National Center for Health Statistics. *Vital Health Statistics*, 10 (252), 2012, Tab. 16, p. 61.

CHAPTER 3

1. John Purcell, *A Treatise of Vapours, or Hysterick Fits* (1702), 2nd ed. (London: Place, 1707), 13.

2. Robert Halsband, Ed., *The Complete Letters of Lady Wortley Montagu*, Vol. 2. (Oxford: Clarendon, 1966), 423.

3. [Louis Sébastien Mercier], *Tableau de Paris,* new ed. (Amsterdam: no publisher, 1782), Vol. 2, 88.

4. Étienne-Jean Georget, *De la physiologie du système nerveux*, Vol. 2 (Paris: Ballière, 1821), 250.

5. Günther Goldschmidt, edited and translated from Latin. *Felix Platter Observationes: Krankheitsbeobachtungen in drei Büchern* (Berne: Huber, 1963), 84; the three volumes are consecutively paginated in one; Vol. 1 appeared in 1602.

6. Thomas Willis, *An Essay of the Pathology of the Brain and Nervous Stock in Which Convulsive Diseases Are Treated of* (London: Dring, 1684), 8, 31, 69.

7. Charles F. Mullett, Ed., *The Letters of Doctor George Cheyne to Samuel Richardson (1733–1743)* (Columbia: University of Missouri Press, 1943), 50, 54, 61, 87, 104, 105.

8. Robert Whytt, *Observations on the Nature, Causes, and Cure of Those Disorders Which Have Been Commonly Called Nervous, Hypochondriac, or Hysteric: To which are prefixed some Remarks on the Sympathy of the Nerves,* 2nd ed. (Edinburgh: Becket, 1765), iv. The author's name is sometimes written Whyte. According to a personal communication from Walter Vandereycken, the first edition seems to have been printed in 1765 as well.

9. William Cullen, *First Lines of the Practice of Physic* (1769), new corrected ed., Vol. 3 (Edinburgh: Elliot, 1789), 249–250.

10. William Buchan, *Domestic Medicine: Or, A Treatise on the Prevention and Cure of Diseases,* 10th ed. (London: Cadell, 1788), 466–467. According to Christopher Lawrence, the text of *Domestic Medicine* changed little across the many editions, and presumably the quoted passages are close to what Buchan and Smellie wrote in 1769. Smellie's name was absent from later editions. C. J. Lawrence, "William Buchan: Medicine Laid Open," *Medical History,* 19 (1975), 20–35.

11. Ralph M. Wardle, Ed., *Collected Letters of Mary Wollstonecraft* (Ithaca, NY: Cornell University Press, 1979), 118, 126, 171.

12. Leslie A. Marchand, Ed., *Byron's Letters and Journals,* Vol. 2 (London: Murray, 1973), 111–112. Italics in original.

13. David Baumgardt, Ed., *Seele und Welt: Franz Baader's Jugendtagebücher, 1786–1792* (Berlin: Volksverband der Bücherfreunde [no date]), 14.

14. Annie Le Brun et al., Eds., *Oeuvres complètes du Marquis de Sade,* Vol. 8: *Histoire de Juliette, ou les Prosperités du vice* (Paris: Pauvert, 1987), 540.

15. Philippe Pinel, *Nosographie philosophique, ou la méthode de l'analyse appliquée à la médecine* (1798), 4th ed. (Paris: Brosson, 1810), Vol. 3, 1–2.

16. C-H. Machard, *Essai sur la topographie médicale de la ville de Dôle* (Dôle: Joly, 1823), 132.

17. Ernst von Feuchtersleben, *Lehrbuch der ärztlichen Seelenkunde* (Vienna: Gerold, 1845), 265.

18. Cullen, Vol. 3, 253.

19. Testimony of Dr. E. C. Texter, "In the Matter of: Depressant and Stimulant Drugs, Docket No. FDA-DAC-1," June 27–Sept. 16, 1966, Hearing of Aug. 11, 1966, 3221. U.S. Food and Drug Administration, Division of Dockets Management, Rockland, MD; obtained through the Freedom of Information Act.

20. Flavio Gregori, *Blackmore, Sir Richard (1654–1729), Oxford Dictionary of National Biography* (Oxford University Press, 2004); online ed. Jan. 2009. [http://www.oxforddnb.com.myaccess.library.utoronto.ca/view/article/2528, accessed 16 June 2011.]

21. Richard Blackmore, *A Treatise of the Spleen and Vapours: Or, Hypochondriacal and Hysterical Affections* (London: Pemberton, 1725), 17, 25–27.

22. Robert Whyte, *Observations on the Nature, Causes, and Cure of Those Disorders Which Have been Commonly Called Nervous, Hypochondriac, or Hysteric* (Edinburgh: Becket, 1765), 172, 312, 520. He spells his name "Whytt" in this edition and "Whyte" in later editions.

23. W. Buchan, *Domestic Medicine,* 10th ed., 500–501.

24. Leslie A. Marchand, Ed., *Byron's Letters and Journals,* Vol. 4 (London: Murray, 1975), 26.

25. Edward Bulwer Lytton, *Confessions of a Water-Patient* (London: Colburn, 1845), 14–15.

26. Louis Verhaeghe, *Du traitement des maladies nerveuses par les bains de mer* (Brussels: Tircher, 1850), 50–51.

27. Herbert F. H. Newington, "Some Incidents in the History and Practice of Ticehurst Asylum," *Journal of Mental Science,* 47 (1901), 62–72, p. 70.

28. Michael Garvey et al., "Frequency of Constipation in Major Depression: Relationship to Other Clinical Variables," *Psychosomatics,* 31 (1990), 204–206.

29. D. Kumar et al., "Role of Psychological Factors in the Irritable Bowel Syndrome," *Digestion,* 45 (1990), 80–87.

30. Willi Mayer-Gross comment in discussion, in E. Beresford Davies, Ed., *Depression: Proceedings of the Symposium, Held at Cambridge 22 to 26 September 1959* (Cambridge: Cambridge University Press, 1964), 68.

31. Wilhelm Griesinger, "Neue Beiträge zur Physiologie und Pathologie des Gehirns," *Archiv für physiologische Heilkunde,* 3 (1844), 69–98, p. 94.

32. Wilhelm Griesinger, *Die Pathologie und Therapie der psychischen Krankheiten* (Stuttgart: Krabbe, 1845); 2nd ed. Berlin, 1861.

33. Ewald Hecker, "Die Hebephrenie," *Archiv für pathologische Anatomie und Physiologie,* 52 (1871), 394–429.

34. Heinrich Laehr, *Die Heil- und Pflegeanstalten für Psychisch-Kranke des deutschen Sprachgebietes,* new ed. (Berlin: Reimer, 1882), 86–87.

35. Eugene Taylor, "On the First Use of 'Psychoanalysis' at the Massachusetts General Hospital, 1903 to 1905," *Journal of the History of Medicine,* 43 (1988), 447–471, p. 451.

36. Mary J. Serrano, translated from French, *Marie Bashkirtseff: The Journal of a Young Artist, 1860–1884* (New York: Cassell, 1889), 27, 35–36.

37. *Medical Directory,* 1908, ad page 1981.

38. W. G. Schauffler, "The Treatment of Chronic Nervous Conditions," *Journal of the Medical Society of New Jersey,* 3 (1907), 197–203, p. 197.

39. Alfred T. Schofield, *The Management of a Nerve Patient* (London: Churchill, 1906), 4, 184–185.

CHAPTER 4

1. Summarized in Simon Wessely, "Old Wine in New Bottles," *Psychological Medicine,* 20 (1990), 35–53.

2. Robert Halsband, Ed., *The Complete Letters of Lady Wortley Montagu* (Oxford: Clarendon, 1965), Vol. 1, 116–117; letter to Philippa Mundy of Feb. 11, 1712.

3. Adrien Proust and Gilbert Ballet, *L'hygiène du neurasthénique* (Paris: Masson, 1897).

4. Philip Kolb, Ed., *Marcel Proust Correspondence,* Vol. 9, 1909 (Paris: Plon, 1982), 219.

5. Li Fischer-Eckert, *Die wirtschaftliche und soziale Lage der Frauen in dem modernen Industrieort Hamborn im Rheinland* (Hagen: Carl Stracke, 1913), 91–92; Staatswiss Inaug. Dissertation University Tübingen.

6. Archibald J. Cronin, *Adventures in Two Worlds* (Toronto: Ryerson, 1952), 196–197.

7. George A. Waterman, "The Treatment of Fatigue States," *Journal of Abnormal Psychology,* 4 (1909), 128–139, p. 128.

8. Erik Essen-Möller, *Individual Traits and Morbidity in a Swedish Rural Population* (Copenhagen: Munksgaard, 1956), 63; *Acta Psychiatrica et Neurologica Scandinavica,* Suppl. No. 100.

9. Karl Jaspers, *Allgemeine Psychopathologie,* 9th ed. (Berlin: Springer, 1973), 132, 445; this is based unchanged on the 1942 edition.

10. Maria Bidlingmaier, *Die Bäuerin in zwei Gemeinden Württembergs,* Eberhard-Karls-Universität Tübingen, Staatswiss. doctoral dissertation (Stuttgart: Kohlhammer, 1918), 61.

11. I have located and perused more than a hundred of these, keenly searching for references to fatigue and the like.

12. Peter Voswinckel, "Das 'Tagebuch' eines Distrikt-Krankenhauses 1866/67 als Quelle der Sozialgeschichte," *Historia Hospitalium,* 17 (1986/88), 121–134.

13. See Edward Shorter, "The 'Hot-Fat' Line and the Medical History of Diet: The Consumption of Fatty Acids in Pre-Modern Europe," *Medicina & Storia,* 3 (Nov. 5, 2003), 69–83.

14. J. M. H. Campbell, "Chlorosis: A Study of Guy's Hospital Cases During the Last Thirty Years," *Guy's Hospital Reports,* 73 (1923), 247–297.

15. See, for example, Edwin Bramwell, "Discussion on the Mental Sequelae of Encephalitis Lethargica," *Proceedings of the Royal Society of Medicine,* 18 (1925), 17–39. For an overview of the epidemic see Joel A. Vilensky, *Encephalitis Lethargica: During and After the Epidemic* (New York: Oxford University Press, 2011).

16. James Crichton-Browne, *Victorian Jottings from an Old Commonplace Book* (London: Etchells, 1926), 244–245.

17. Anson Rabinbach, *The Human Motor: Energy, Fatigue, and the Origins of Modernity* (Berkeley: University of California Press, 1990), 39.

18. Anon. [Harriet Martineau], *Life in the Sick-Room, by an Invalid* (London: Moxon, 1844), 7, 167, 171.

19. Gaby Weiner, Ed., *Harriet Martineau's Autobiography,* 2 Vols. (London: Virago, 1983), Vol. 2, 172; the autobiography was written in 1855 and first published in 1877.

20. Ibid. Quotations are from Vol. 1, 75, 147, 193, 265; Vol. 2, 134, 430–431.

21. Silas Weir Mitchell, *Lectures on Diseases of the Nervous System, Especially in Women* (London: Churchill, 1881), 48.

22. Bäder-Almanach: *Mittheilungen aus den Bädern, Luftcurorten und Heilanstalten* (Frankfurt/M: Mosse, 1882), xv.

23. *Medical Directory for 1908* (London: Churchill, 1908), advertisement p. 1953.

24. D. Mabin, "Sommeil et automédication de Marcel Proust. Une analyse à partir de sa correspondance," *Journal of Clinical Neurophysiology,* 24 (1994), 63.

25. Maurice Craig, *Psychological Medicine: A Manual on Mental Disease for Practitioners and Students,* 3rd ed. (London: Churchill, 1917), 115.

26. Nortin M. Hadler, "Editorial: Labeling Woefulness: The Social Construction of Fibromyalgia," *Spine,* 30 (2004), 1–4.

27. James J. Putnam, "Not the Disease Only, But Also the Man," *Boston Medical and Surgical Journal,* 141 (July 27, 1899), 77–81, p. 80.

28. George Beard, "Neurasthenia, or Nervous Exhaustion," *Boston Medical and Surgical Journal,* 80 (Apr. 29, 1869), 217–221, pp. 217–218.

29. George M. Beard, *A Practical Treatise on Nervous Exhaustion (Neurasthenia)* (New York: Wood, 1880), quotes from "second and revised edition," also published in 1880, 32, 34, 44, 47, 53, 66, 76, 78.

30. Paul Hartenberg, *Traitement des neurasthéniques* (Paris: Alcan, 1912), 5–7.

31. Hermann Oppenheim, *Lehrbuch der Nervenkrankheiten,* 5th ed. (Berlin: Karger, 1908), Vol. 2, 1268.

32. For the initial description of Mitchell's rest cure see S. Weir Mitchell, "Rest in Nervous Disease," in Edouard C. Seguin, Ed., *A Series of American Clinical Lectures,* Vol. 1: Jan.–Dec. 1875 (New York: Putnam, 1876), 368–373. On the background of Mitchell's cure, see Edward Shorter, *A History of Psychiatry* (New York: Wiley, 1997), 130–135.

33. H. Neumann, *Handbuch der Heil-, Pflege- und Kuranstalten (Privat-Anstalten),* 1901 (Berlin: Leuchter, 1901), 10.

34. *American Medical Directory*, 1913, ad page 63.

35. Ibid., ad page 54.

36. Rev X's chart is in the Contemporary Medical Archives Centre in London, *Frederick Parkes Weber collection, case book 1906–1907,* at p. 337.

37. Simon Wessely, "History of Postviral Fatigue Syndrome," *British Medical Bulletin,* 47 (1991), 919–941, pp. 921–922.

38. Maurice Dide and Paul Guiraud, *Psychiatrie du médecin praticien* (Paris: Masson, 1922), 85–86.

39. Tom A. Williams, "The Bases of So-called Neurasthenic States" (1921), reprinted in *Practitioner*, 108 (1922), 220–222.

40. Kurt Schneider, *Psychiatrische Vorlesungen für Ärzte*, 2nd ed. (Leipzig: Thieme, 1936), 42; first published in 1933.

41. Ruth E. Taylor, "Death of Neurasthenia and Its Psychological Reincarnation," *BJP*, 179 (2001), 550–557.

42. E. Farquhar Buzzard, "The Dumping Ground of Neurasthenia," *Lancet*, 1 (Jan. 4, 1930), 1–4, p. 2.

43. See Sigmund Freud, "Über die Berechtigung von der Neurasthenie einen bestimmten Symptomenkomplex als 'Angstneurosen' abzutrennen" (1895), reprinted in Sigmund Freud, *Gesammelte Werke* (London: Imgo, 1952), 315–342; Freud, "Die Sexualität in der Ätiologie der Neurosen" (1898), reprinted in ibid., Vol. 1, 491–516.

44. See Wilhelm Stekel, *Nervöse Angstzustände und ihre Behandlung* (1908), 3rd ed. (Berlin: Urban, 1921), 600.

45. ICD-10: *The ICD-10 Classification of Mental and Behavioural Disorders* (Geneva: World Health Organization, 1992), Diagnostic code F48, p. 170.

46. *American Psychiatric Association, DSM-II: Diagnostic and Statistical Manual of Mental Disorders*, 2nd ed. (New York: APA, 1968), 40–41, p. 43.

47. *New York Times*, June 19, 1898, 22; I am indebted to Ellen Tulchinsky for conducting this computer search of the *New York Times* on-line database.

48. *New York Times*, Apr. 4, 1935, 23.

49. Cheryl Krasnick Warsh, *Moments of Unreason: The Practice of Canadian Psychiatry and the Homewood Retreat, 1883–1923* (Montreal: McGill-Queen's University Press, 1989), 69.

50. S. Weir Mitchell, "Clinical Lecture on Nervousness in the Male," *The Medical News and Library*, 35 (1877), 177–184, p. 181.

51. Angelo Mosso, *La fatigue intellectuelle et physique*, Fr trans (Paris: Alcan, 1894); first Italian ed. 1891.

52. Emil Kraepelin, *Psychiatrie: ein Lehrbuch für Studierende und Ärzte* (Leipzig: Barth, 1915), Vol. 4, 1407.

53. See, for example, Kraepelin, *Psychiatrie*, 5th ed. (Leipzig: Barth, 1896), 341–351.

54. Heinrich Averbeck, "Die akute Neurasthenie, die plötzliche Erschöpfung der nervösen Energie," *Deutsche Medizinal-Zeitung*, no. 30 [no Vol. given] (Apr. 12, 1886), 325–328, pp. 325, 327.

55. Charles L. Dana, "The Partial Passing of Neurasthenia," *Boston Medical and Surgical Journal*, 150 (Mar. 31, 1904), 339–344, p. 341.

56. Richard von Krafft-Ebing, *Lehrbuch der Psychiatrie*, 3rd ed. (Stuttgart: Enke, 1888), 517–518; the final edition, the 7th, appeared in 1903. See pp. 456–469 for the discussion of "insanity on the basis of neurasthenia" ("das Irresein auf neurasthenischer Grundlage").

57. Eduard Hirt, "Behandlung und Versorgung der rechtsgesetzlich versicherten Nervenkranken," *Allgemeine Zeitschrift für Psychiatrie*, 84 (1926), 217–236, p. 230.

58. Maximilian Laehr, "Die Heilstätte für Nervenkranke 'Haus Schönow' 1899 bis 1927," *Psychiatrisch-Neurologische Wochenschrift*, 30 (Jan. 28, 1928), 39–46. Laehr discussed

these conditions in the context of who might be admissible to the "Volksheilstätte für Nervenkranke" (Public Treatment Centers for Nervous Patients) that he envisioned.

59. Adolf Hoppe, "Gegenwartsaufgaben der Nervensanatorien," *Psychiatrisch-Neurologische Wochenschrift*, 34 (March 26, 1932), 157–160, pp. 158–159. The contrast was between the "Erschöpften" of yesteryear and the "Zermürbten" of today.

60. Philip Seymour-Price, discussion comment following a paper by Farquhar Buzzard, *BMJ*, 1 (May 2, 1931), 754.

61. "Ex-Official Kills Wife and Himself," *New York Times*, May 2, 1934, 16.

62. The asthenic personality disorder of *DSM-II* (1968) was, according to the index of *DSM-III*, collapsed into "dependent personality disorder." It was said to be "rarely used" (*DSM-III*, 1980), 379.

CHAPTER 5

1. Food and Drug Administration, Psychopharmacologic Drugs Advisory Committee Meeting, Nov. 6, 1980, 81; obtained through the Freedom of Information Act.

2. Aubrey Lewis, "The Ambiguous Word 'Anxiety,'" *International Journal of Psychiatry*, 9 (1970), 62–79, p. 68.

3. Augustin Jacob André-Beauvais, *Séméiotique ou traité des signes des maladies* (1809), 2nd ed. (Paris: Brosson, 1815), 327, 329.

4. William Sargant and Peter Dally, "Treatment of Anxiety States by Antidepressant Drugs," *BMJ*, 1 (Jan. 6, 1962), 6–9, p. 6.

5. George Beaumont, interview, "The Place of Clomipramine in Psychopharmacology," in David Healy, Ed., *The Psychopharmacologists* (London: Chapman & Hall, 1996), Vol. 1, 309–327, p. 325; based on an interview first published in 1993.

6. *American Psychiatric Association, DSM-II: Diagnostic and Statistical Manual of Mental Disorders,* 2nd ed. (Washington, DC: APA, 1968), 39.

7. Otto Fenichel, *The Psychoanalytic Theory of Neurosis* (New York: Norton, 1945), 193.

8. Edward Shorter and Max Fink interview with Robert Spitzer, Mar. 14, 2007, 12.

9. Fritz Freyhan, "The Evolution of Compensatory Therapy With Drugs in Modern Psychiatric Practice," in P. B. Bradley et al., Eds., Neuro-Psychopharmacology: Proceedings of the First International Congress of Neuro-Pharmacology (Amsterdam: Elsevier, 1959), 227–242, p. 239.

10. Alan Breier, Dennis S. Charney, and George R. Heninger, "The Diagnostic Validity of Anxiety Disorders and Their Relationship to Depressive Illness," *AJP*, 142 (1985), 787–797, p. 787.

11. Thomas Ban interview, Aug. 12, 2006, Toronto.

12. Harry S. Friedlander, "Anxiety, Tension and Emotional Stress: A Report on the Joint Use of Mephenesin and a Barbiturate in Their Treatment in General Practice," *Medical Times,* 81 (1953), 411–415, p. 411.

13. See the RCT that found mephenesin valueless in the treatment of hospital patients on a "neurosis unit" with anxiety. Edward H. Hare, "The Effects of Mephenesin in Neurotic Anxiety," *Journal of Mental Science*, 101 (1955), 172–174.

14. Serpasil advertisement, *New York State Journal of Medicine*, 54 (1954), 2137.

15. Suavitil advertisement, *New York State Journal of Medicine*, 58 (1958), 274–275.

16. *American Psychiatric Association, Diagnostic and Statistical Manual of Mental Disorders*, 4th ed. (Washington, DC: American Psychiatric Association, 1994), 436.

17. Centre for Contemporary Medical Archives, London, Parkes Weber collection, casebook for 1913 and after, at p. 198.

18. Jean Stoner, translator, Jerome Cardan, *The Book of My Life* (Latin 1575) (London: Dent, 1931), 25.

19. Günther Goldschmidt, editor and translator, *Felix Platter Observationes: Krankheitsbeobachtungen* (Vol. 1, 1602) (Berne: Huber, 1963), 76.

20. Vincenzo Chiarugi, *Della Pazzia*, Vol. 2 (Florence: Carlieri, 1794), 5.

21. Philippe Pinel, *Nosographie philosophique, ou la méthode de l'analyse appliquée à la médecine (1798)*, 4th ed. (Paris: Brosson, 1810), Vol. 3, 91.

22. John Haslam, *Observations on Madness and Melancholy,* 2nd enlarged ed. (London: Callow, 1809), 103.

23. Friedrich Christian August Heinroth, *Lehrbuch der Störungen des Seelenlebens* (Leipzig: Vogel, 1818), 359; I have translated "Gemüthsstörungen" as affective disorders, even though at the time the meaning was somewhat broader.

24. Soeren Kirkegaard, *The Concept of Anxiety* (Princeton: Princeton University Press, 1981).

25. German Berrios and C. Link, "Anxiety Disorders: Clinical Section," in German E. Berrios and Roy Porter, Eds., *A History of Clinical Psychiatry: The Origin and History of Psychiatric Disorders* (London: Athlone, 1995), 545–562.

26. Joseph Guislain, *Leçons orales sur les phrénopathies,* Vol. 1 (Ghent: Hebbelynck, 1852), 126–127.

27. Stuttgart: Krabbe, 1861.

28. Wilhelm Griesinger, *Die Pathologie und Therapie der psychischen Krankheiten,* 2nd ed. (1861) (reprinted Amsterdam: Bonset, 1964), 230.

29. Emil Kraepelin, *Psychiatrie: Ein Lehrbuch für Studierende und Ärzte,* 8th ed., Vol. 1 (Leipzig: Barth, 1909), 348–349.

30. William Murray, *A Treatise on Emotional Disorders of the Sympathetic System of Nerves* (London: Churchill, 1866), 18–19.

31. Centre for Contemporary Medical Archives, Wellcome MS 5162.

32. .Centre for Contemporary Medical Archives, Wellcome MS 5157

33. Lars E. Troide et al., Eds., *The Early Journals and Letters of Fanny Burney*, Vol. 3 (Oxford: Clarendon, 1994), 113, 118.

34. Joyce Hemlow, Ed., *The Journals and Letters of Fanny Burney (Madame D'Arblay),* Vol. 1 (Oxford: Clarendon, 1972), 160.

35. Anton Theobald Brück, *Das Bad Driburg in seinen Heilwirkungen dargestellt, für practische Ärzte* (Osnabrück: Rackhorst, 1844), 117.

36. Carl Friedrich Flemming, "Über Präcordialangst," *AZP,* 5 (1848), 341–361, pp. 342, 345, 356–357.

37. Hanns Kaan, *Der neurasthenische Angstaffect* (Vienna: Deuticke, 1892), 74.

38. Carl Friedrich Flemming, *Pathologie und Therapie der Psychosen* (Berlin: Hirschwald, 1859), 66, 68.

39. Jules Falret, "Discussion sur la folie raisonnante," *Annales MP*, 4th Ser., Vol. 1 (1866), 382–426, pp. 414–416.

40. Bénédict-Augustin Morel, "Du délire emotif: Névrose du système nerveux ganglionnaire visceral," *Archives Générales de Médecine*, Se.r 6, Vol. 7 (1866), 385–402, 530–551, 700–707. The term "délire" can be translated into English in several ways; in this sense, it means severe illness, not the disordered thought of formal "insanity." Morel did not believe his patients were incapable of rational thought. He reminded readers of the old saying in psychiatry, "Si toute folie est un délire, tout délire n'est pas une folie" (p. 386).

41. Wilhelm Griesinger, "Über einen wenig bekannten psychopathischen Zustand," *Archiv für Psychiatrie und Nervenkrankheiten*, 1 (1868), 626–635, p. 635.

42. Jacob M. DaCosta, "On Irritable Heart; a Clinical Study of a Form of Functional Cardiac Disorder and Its Consequences," *American Journal of the Medical Sciences*, NS, 61 (1871), 17–52, pp. 22, 32.

43. Thomas Lewis, *The Soldier's Heart and the Effort Syndrome* (London: Shaw and Sons [1918]), 47–48.

44. Carl Westphal, "Die Agoraphobie," *Archiv für Psychiatrie und Nervenkrankheiten*, 3 (1872), 138–161, pp. 139–140, 143–144, 160.

45. Carl Westphal, "Über Platzfurcht," *Archiv für Psychiatrie und Nervenkrankheiten*, 7 (1877), 377–383, see p. 379.

46. See Carl Flemming, "Über Schwindel-Angst," *AZP*, 29 (1873), 112–114.

47. Carl Westphal, "Über Zwangsvorstellungen," *Berliner Klinische Wochenschrift*, 14 (Nov. 12, 1877), 669–689, see p. 670. It is not my intention to lay bare the entire historical roots of obsessive-compulsive disorder, but Richard von Krafft-Ebing, then on staff at the Illenau Asylum, introduced the notion of obsession-compulsion, or Zwang, into German psychiatry in 1867, apropos "compulsive thoughts," Zwangsvorstellungen. Krafft-Ebing, *Beiträge zur Erkennung ... krankhafter Gemüthszustände* (Erlangen: Enke, 1867). In the context of "simple psychic depression," he spoke of "painful feelings of continuously present thoughts that stand in no relationship to awareness (Zwangsvorstellungen)" (p. 13). A whole debate about the nature of obsessive thoughts and compulsive actions then arose, well summarized in Oswald Bumke, "Die psychischen Zwangserscheinungen," *Allgemeine Zeitschrift für Psychiatrie*, 63 (1906), 138–146.

48. Henry Maudsley, *The Physiology and Pathology of the Mind* (New York: Appleton, 1867), 332.

49. Henri Legrand du Saulle, *La folie du doute (avec délire du toucher)* (Paris: Delahaye, 1875), 24, 28–29.

50. Édouard Brissaud, "De l'anxiété paroxystique," *La Semaine Médicale*, 9 (1890), 410–411.

51. Paul Hartenberg, *Les timides et la timidité (1901)*, 4th ed. (Paris: Alcan, 1921), 4–6.

52. Fulgence Raymond and Pierre Janet, *Les obsessions et la psychasthénie*, Vol. 2 (Paris: Alcan, 1903), 190–192.

53. Ibid., x–xi.

54. See, for example, Hugo Gugl, "Die Grenzformen schwerer cerebraler Neurasthenie," in Hugo Gugl and Anton Stichl, *Neuropathologische Studien* (Stuttgart: Enke, 1892), 124–151, who often uses the terms anxious (ängstlich) and anxiousness (Ängstlichkeit), as well as fear of death (Todesangst); Kaan, *Neurasthenische Angstaffect* (1892), passim.

55. Ewald Hecker, "Über larvirte und abortive Angstzustände bei Neurasthenie," *Centralblatt für Nervenheilkunde*, 16 (1893), 565–572, p. 567.

56. Sigmund Freud, "Über die Berechtigung von der Neurasthenie einen bestimmten Symptomenkomplex als 'Angstneurose' abzutrennen" (1895), reprinted in *Freud, Gesammelte Werke*, Vol. 1, 315–342, p. 316.

57. Sigmund Freud, "Die Sexualität in der Ätiologie der Neurosen" (1898), in *Gesammelte Werke*, Vol. 1, 491–516, see pp. 497–498. Freud was scarcely the first writer to have incriminated sexual practices in psychiatric illness. See Leopold Löwenfeld, *Die nervösen Störungen sexuellen Ursprungs* (Wiesbaden: Bergmann, 1891).

58. Smith Ely Jelliffe, "Nervous and Mental Disease Dispensary Work," *Post-Graduate*, 27 (1912), 467–482, 593–607, p. 595.

59. Ludwig Frank, *Affektstörungen: Studien über ihre Ätiologie und Therapie* (Berlin: Springer, 1913), 135–143.

60. Ludwig Frank, *Die psychokathartische Behandlung nervöser Störungen (Psychoneurosen—Thymopathien)* (Leipzig: Thieme, 1927), 17.

61. Paul Hartenberg, "La névrose d'angoisse," *Revue de médecine*, 21 (1901), 464–484, 612–631, 678–699.

62. Aubrey Lewis, "The Ambiguous Word 'Anxiety,'" *International Journal of Psychiatry*, 9 (1970), 62–79, p. 66. His argument obliged him, however, to considerably exaggerate the role of the diagnosis of Angst in pre-Freudian Central Europe.

63. Wilhelm Stekel, "Wandlungen der Psychotherapie," *Wiener Klinische Wochenschrift*, 49 (1936), 1071–1074, p. 1073.

64. Sigmund Freud, "Hemmung, Symptom und Angst" (1926), in *Gesammelte Werke*, 14, 111–205, pp. 115–117.

65. Freud, "Die gemeine Nervosität," 392–406, see p. 404; this is lecture 24 in the work "Vorlesungen zur Einführung in die Psychoanalyse" in *Gesammelte Werke*, 11.

66. Librium ad, *Diseases of the Nervous System*, 32 (1971); they were quoting psychoanalyst Joseph Wolpe in 1963; Wolpe, however, soon rebelled against analysis and became a pioneer of behavior therapy.

67. Thomas Gray to Richard West, May 27, 1742; in Paget Toynbee et al., Eds., *Correspondence of Thomas Gray*, Vol. 1 (Oxford: Clarendon, 1971), 209.

68. Edward Mapother, "Discussion on Manic-Depressive Psychosis," *BMJ*, 2 (Nov. 13, 1926), 872–876, p. 873; Gillespie discussion comment, p. 879.

69. Joseph Guislain, *Les Phrénopathies* (Brussels: Établissement Encyclographique,1852), 126–128.

70. Heinrich Schüle, *Handbuch der Geisteskrankheiten* (Leipzig: Vogel, 1878), 531–532.

71. Emil Kraepelin, *Psychiatrie: Ein Lehrbuch für Studirende und Aerzte,* 5th ed. (Leipzig: Barth, 1896), 571.

72. Carl Wernicke, *Grundriss der Psychiatrie in klinischen Vorlesungen (1900),* 2nd ed. (Leipzig: Thieme, 1906), 227–235.

73. See Karl Leonhard, "Die Angstpsychose in Wernickes und Kraepelins Betrachtungsweise" (1939), reprinted in *Internationale Wernicke-Kleist-Leonhard-Gesellschaft* e.V., ed. Karl Leonhard, *Das wissenschaftliche Werk,* Vol. 1 (Berlin: Ullstein, 1992), 296–297.

74. Paul Nitsche, [brief report] *AZP,* 62 (1905), 864. After World War II, Nitsche was convicted of participating in the Nazi euthanasia program and was executed.

75. Henry Maudsley, *The Pathology of Mind* (London: Macmillan, 1879), 365.

76. William James, *The Varieties of Religious Experience: A Study in Human Nature* (New York: Longmans, 1905), 160.

77. August Cramer, "Zur Symptomatologie und Therapie der Angst," *Deutsche Medizinische Wochenschrift,* 36 (Aug. 11, 1910), 1473–1478, p. 1476.

78. Harry A. Paskind, "Brief Attacks of Manic-Depressive Depression," *[AMA] Archives of Neurology and Psychiatry,* 22 (1929), 123–134, p. 124.

79. Oskar Diethelm, "Panic," *[AMA] Archives of Neurology and Psychiatry,* 28 (1932), 1153–1168, p. 1154. See also Diethelm, "Panikreaktion vom Standpunkt psychobiologischer Psychiatrie," in Hans Prinzhorn, Ed., *Die Wissenschaft am Scheidewege von Leben und Geist: Festschrift Ludwig Klages* (Leipzig: Barth, 1932), 58–64.

80. Josef Westermann, "Über die vitale Depression," *Zeitschrift für die gesamte Neurologie und Psychiatrie,* 77 (1922), 391–422, p. 421.

81. Kurt Schneider, "Die Schichtung des emotionalen Lebens und der Aufbau der Depressionszustände," *Zeitschrift für die gesamte Neurologie und Psychiatrie,* 59 (1920), 281–286.

82. Juan J. Lopez-Ibor, *La Angustia Vital* (Madrid: Montalvo, 1950).

83. Juan J. Lopez-Ibor, "Manic-Depressive Psychosis and Anxiety (The Timopathic Circle)," *Acta Psychiatrica Scandinavica,* 27 (1952), 269–286, p. 278.

CHAPTER 6

1. John S. Price, "Chronic Depressive Illness," *BMJ,* 1 (May 6, 1978), 1200–1201, p. 1200.

2. J. S. Schiller et al., Summary Health Statistics for U.S. Adults. National Health Interview Survey, 2010. National Center for Health Statistics. *Vital Health Statistics,* 10 (252), 2012, Tab. 14, p. 55.

3. Anne Olivier Bell, Ed., *The Diary of Virginia Woolf* (New York: Harcourt, 1982), Vol. 1, 66, 233; Vol. 3, 103; Vol. 4, 55, 181.

4. Ibid., Vol. 3, 111, 235.

5. Gordon Parker, "Melancholia," paper given to *Società Italiana di Psicopatologia*, Rome, 15 Feb. 2012.

6. *Diary of Virginia Woolf* (New York: Harcourt, 1982), Vol. 1, 223.

7. William Sargant, "The Physical Treatments of Depression: Their Indications and Proper Use," in E. Bereford Davies, Ed., *Depression: Proceedings of the Symposium Held at Cambridge 22 to 26 September 1959* (Cambridge: Cambridge University Press, 1964), 274–287, pp. 286–287.

8. Oswald Bumke, *Landläufige Irrtümer in der Beurteilung von Geisteskranken* (Wiesbaden: Bergmann, 1908), 33.

9. "Wife of Merchant Plunges to Death," *New York Times,* Mar. 2, 1934, 3.

10. Rachel Gittelman-Klein, interview in 1998, in Thomas G. Ban, Ed., *An Oral History of Neuropsychopharmacology: The First Fifty Years. Peer Interviews,* Vol. 7 (Brentwood, TN: ACNP, 2011), 306.

11. C. A. H. Watts, "The Mild Endogenous Depression," *BMJ,* 1 (Jan. 5, 1957), 4–8, p. 7.

12. James Crichton Browne, "Clinical Lectures, III: Simple Melancholia," *BMJ*, 2, (Oct. 12, 1872), 403–406, p. 403.

13. Jean Delay, *L'électro-choc et la psycho-physiologie* (Paris: Masson, 1946), 55.

14. Peter Berner, discussion, in Paul Kielholz, Ed., *États dépressifs: Dépistage, évaluation, traitement* (Berne: Huber, 1972), 205.

15. Randolph Swiller, letter, *Psychiatric News,* Apr. 6, 2007, 27.

16. Price, *BMJ* (1978), 1200.

17. "Suffering from Melancholia When He Made His Will," *New York Times*, Mar. 15, 1894, 9.

18. Among the first to describe psychomotor retardation in melancholia was Georges Dumas, *Les états intellectuels dans la mélancolie* (Paris: Baillière, 1895), 41–66, 90.

19. Gordon Parker and Dusan Hadzi-Pavlovic, *Melancholia: A Disorder of Movement and Mood* (Cambridge: Cambridge University Press, 1996).

20. George Riddoch, discussion, *Proceedings of the Royal Society of Medicine*, 23 (1930), 886.

21. Bumke, Landläufige Irrtümer (1908), 34–35.

22. "Doctor Cuts His Throat," *New York Times*, Mar. 21, 1911, 3.

23. B. J. Carroll, F. I. R. Martin, and Brian Davies, "Resistance to Suppression by Dexamethasone of Plasma 11-OHCS Levels in Severe Depressive Illness," *BMJ*, 2 (Aug. 3, 1968), 285–287. The story of hypercortisolemia, or endocrine involvement, in depression seems a bit more complicated than simple dysfunction of the hypothalamic-pituitary-adrenal (HPA) axis. Carroll and colleagues wrote in 2011, after extensive investigation, that "There was no evidence of excessive or irregular ACTH secretion in hypercortisolemic depressed patients at baseline or in the low-feedback condition. The classic theory of HPA axis overdrive by activated limbic-hypothalamic circuits was not supported." The authors speculated that sympathetic

input to the adrenal gland could be involved. B. J. Carroll et al., "Pathophysiology of Hypercortisolism in Depression: Pituitary and Adrenal Responses to Low Glucocorticoid Feedback," *Acta Psychiatrica Scandinavica* (2011), 1–14; DOI: 10.1111/j.1600-0447.2011.01821.x. Quotes from p. 1.

24. D. S. Goodin and M. J. Aminoff, "Does the Interictal EEG Have a Role in the Diagnosis of Epilepsy?" *Lancet*, 1 (1984), 837–839.

25. Edward Shorter and Max Fink, *Endocrine Psychiatry: Solving the Riddle of Melancholia* (New York: Oxford University Press, 2010).

26. On the DST today see Frederick Cassidy et al., "Dexamethasone Metabolism in Dexamethasone Suppression Test Suppressors and Nonsuppressors," *Biological Psychiatry*, 47 (2000), 677–680.

27. "Two Women Tell of Mrs. Rankine's Melancholia as Police Drag River for Her Body," *New York Times*, Apr. 7, 1921, 1.

28. *New York Times*, Aug. 14, 1884, 8. I am grateful to Ellen Tulchinsky for undertaking a computer search of the electronic database of *The New York Times*.

29. *New York Times*, Aug. 24, 1951, 22.

30. Robert Latham et al., Eds., *The Diary of Samuel Pepys*, Vol. 6 (Berkeley: University of California Press, 1974), 246.

31. See Stanley W. Jackson, *Melancholia and Depression: From Hippocratic Times to Modern Times* (New Haven: Yale University Press, 1996). Jackson stopped this admirable study just as he reached the nineteenth century; see further studies, Georges Minois, *Histoire du mal de vivre: de la mélancolie à la dépression.* (Paris: Editions de la Martinière, 2003); Hélène Prigent, *Mélancolie, les métamorphoses de la dépression* (Paris, Gallimard, 2005).

32. Ian Johnston, Ed., *Galen on Diseases and Symptoms* (Cambridge: Cambridge University Press, 2006).

33. Francesco Maria Guazzo, *Compendium Maleficarum (1608)* (reprinted London: Rodker, 1929), 170–171. He mentions the differential diagnosis of melancholia from demonic possession on p. 167.

34. [Margaret Cavendish] the Lady Marchioness of Newcastle, "A True Relation of my Birth, Breeding and Life" (1656), in Edward Jenkins, Ed., *The Cavalier and His Lady: Selections from the Works of the First Duke and Duchess of Newcastle* (London: Macmillan, 1872), 31f, 60, 70.

35. William N. Free, *William Cowper* (New York: Twayne, 1970), 35–41.

36. John D. Baird et al., Eds., *The Poems of William Cowper,* Vol. 1 (Oxford: Clarendon, 1980), 62; The poem dates from 1757.

37. Siegfried Scheibe, Ed., *Goethe: Aus meinem Leben: Dichtung und Wahrheit* (Berlin: Akademie-Verlag, 1970), 478.

38. Théodule-Armand Ribot, *La Psychologie des sentiments* (Paris: Alcan, 1896), 53.

39. Karl Jaspers, *Allgemeine Psychopathologie* (Berlin: Sprinter, 1913), 67.

40. Donald F. Klein, "Endogenomorphic Depression," *Archives of General Psychiatry,* 31 (1974), 447–454. In 1959 Leo Alexander and Austin Berkeley had a go at reviving it

using a pharmacological torch, yet their ideas were not widely taken up. "The Inert Psychasthenic Reaction (Anhedonia) as Differentiated from Classic Depression and Its Response to Iproniazid," *Annals of the New York Academy of Sciences,* 80 (1959), 669–679.

41. Philip Snaith, "Anhedonia: Exclusion from the Pleasure Dome," *BMJ,* 305 (July 18, 1992), 134.
42. *Fanny Burney Letters,* Vol. 11, 231.
43. P. Grof, J. Angst, and T. Haines, "The Clinical Course of Depression: Practical Issues," in Jules Angst, Ed., *Classification and Prediction of Outcome of Depression* (Stuttgart: Schattauer, 1974), 141–148, p. 144; the symposium took place in 1973.
44. Landon Carter Gray, "Three Diagnostic Signs of Melancholia," *Journal of Nervous and Mental Disease,* 17 (1890), 1–9, p. 8.
45. The Yates case is briefly discussed in Conrad M. Swartz and Edward Shorter, *Psychotic Depression* (New York: Cambridge University Press, 2007), 1–2.
46. Maurice Dide and Paul Guiraud, *Psychiatrie du médecin praticien* (Paris: Masson, 1922), 127.
47. Gaëtan Gatian de Clérambault, "L'homicide altruiste chez les mélancoliques," *Bulletin de la Société Clinique de Médecine Mentale,* 9 (1921), 83–92, pp. 83–84.
48. "Leila Herbert a Suicide," *New York Times,* Dec. 22, 1897, 1.
49. Monica Langley, "After Long Battle, A Wall Street Star Loses to Depression," *Wall Street Journal,* Jan. 17, 2006, A1.
50. Kenneth R. Conner, "A Call for Research on Planned vs. Unplanned Suicidal Behavior," *Suicide and Life-Threatening Behavior,* 34 (2004), 89–98. "Planned acts are associated with greater depression, hopelessness, and lethality" (p. 89).
51. John Scott Price, "Chronic Depressive Illness," *BMJ,* 1 (May 6, 1978), 1200–1201, p. 1201.
52. Holloway Sanatorium, case no. 380, closed women's service. *Centre for Contemporary Medical Archives,* Wellcome ms 5157.
53. Ibid., case no. 392.
54. Jane Hillyer, *Reluctantly Told (1926)* (New York: Macmillan, 1935), 42–44.
55. Holloway Sanatorium, case no. 421.
56. Günther Goldschmidt, editor and translator, *Felix Platter Observationes: Krankheitsbeobachtungen* (Vol. 1, 1602) (Berne: Huber, 1963), 72.
57. James Sims, "Pathological Remarks upon Various Kinds of Alienation of Mind," *Memoirs of the Medical Society of London,* 5 (1799), 372–406, pp. 378–381.
58. Leo Hollister, in discussion, Earl Usdin et al., Eds., *Neuroregulators and Psychiatric Disorders* (New York: Oxford University Press, 1976), 555–556.
59. John Ferriar, *Medical Histories and Reflections,* Vol. 2 (London: Cadell, 1819), 115–116.
60. Etienne Esquirol, "De la lypémanie ou mélancolie" (1820), reprinted in Esquirol, Ed., *Des maladies mentales,* Vol. 1 (Paris: Baillière, 1838), 398–481, see p. 406.

61. Joseph Guislain, *Leçons orales sur les phrénopathies,* Vol. 1 (Ghent: Hebbelynck, 1852), 103, 106.

62. Wilhelm Griesinger, *Die Pathologie und Therapie der psychischen Krankheiten* (Stuttgart: Krabbe, 1845), 40, 151–152. Griesinger does not use the term Einheitspsychose, although that is the sense of his views; nor does Heinrich Neumann, also often credited with coining the term, using instead the word "Irresein." Heinrich Neumann, *Lehrbuch der Psychiatrie* (Erlangen: Enke, 1859), 167. The originator of Einheitspsychose as a term has eluded the present author. On the inevitable progression from one of the primary disturbances [melancholia, mania or delusional disorder (Wahnsinn)] through total insanity (Verrrücktheit) to terminal dementia (Blödsinn), see Adolph Wachsmuth, *Allgemeine Pathologie der Seele* (Frankfurt/M: Meidinger, 1859), 326–346.

63. Karl Kahlbaum, *Die Katatonie oder das Spannungsirresein* (Berlin: Hirschwald, 1874).

64. Karl Kahlbaum, *Die Gruppirung der psychischen Krankheiten und die Eintheilung der Seelenstörungen* (Danzig: Kafemann, 1863); the classification of illness is found at pp. 133–136.

65. Richard von Krafft-Ebing, *Beiträge zur Erkennung und richtigen forensischen Beurtheilung krankhafter Gemüthszustände* (Erlangen: Enke, 1867), 12–13.

66. Theodor Tiling, "Über Dysthymia und die offenen Curanstalten," *Jahrbuch für Psychiatrie,* 3 (1879), 171–186.

67. Joseph J. Schildkraut, interview, "The Catecholamine Hypothesis," in David Healy, Ed., *The Psychopharmacologists,* Vol. 3 (London: Arnold, 2000), 111–134, p. 131.

68. Carl Georg Lange, *Om Periodiske Depressionstilstande* (Copenhagen: Lunds Forlag, 1886); I relied on the German translation, Lange, *Periodische Depressionszustände,* translated from the second Danish edition (Hamburg: Voss, 1896), 7, 9, 11–12, 15, 21–22. There was also a later English translation by Johan A. Schioldann, *The Lange Theory of "Periodical Depressions": A Landmark in the History of Lithium Therapy* (Adelaide: Adelaide Academic Press, 2001).

69. For convenience, the various editions of Emil Kraepelin's *Psychiatrie: Ein Lehrbuch für Studirende und Aerzte* appeared as follows: 1st, 1883; 2nd, 1887; 3rd, 1889; 4th, 1893; 5th, 1896; 6th, 1899; 7th, in 2 Vols. 1903–1904; 8th, in 4 Vols., 1909–1915. Abel in Leipzig published all editions up to the fourth, after which Barth in Leipzig became the publisher. Later editions substituted "Studierende" for "Studirende."

70. 5th ed., 578.

71. 5th ed., 561.

72. 6th ed., 359.

73. Georges L. Dreyfus, *Die Melancholie: ein Zustandsbild des manisch-depressiven Irreseins* (Jena: Fischer, 1907).

74. Eliot Slater, interview, in Greg Wilkinson, Ed., *Talking About Psychiatry* (London: Royal College of Psychiatrists, 1993), 1–12, p. 4.

75. Kraepelin, *Psychiatrie,* 8th ed., Vol. 3, 1265.

76. 8th ed., Vol. 3, 1350.

77. Alfred Erich Hoche, "Die Melancholiefrage," *Zentralblatt für Nervenheilkunde und Psychiatrie,* 33 (1910), 193–203, p. 193.

78. Adolf Meyer, discussion, *Journal of Nervous and Mental Disease,* 32 (1905), 114; the meeting was in 1904.

79. William Styron, *Darkness Visible: A Memoir of Madness* (New York: Random House, 1990), 37.

80. Henry Yellowlees, discussion, *Proceedings of the Royal Society of Medicine,* 23 (1930), 887.

81. Giovanni Mingazzini, "Die Modifikationen der klinischen Symptome, die einige Psychosen in den letzten Jahrzehnten erfahren haben," *Psychiatrisch-Neurologische Wochenschrift,* 28 (Feb. 6, 1926), 68–72, p. 71.

CHAPTER 7

1. Fred MacIsaac, "Nervous Breakdown," *Collier's,* Mar. 30, 1935, 10, 33, 48, quote on p. 48.

2. "Police Head Is Suicide," *New York Times,* Nov. 6, 1949, 29.

3. John E. Eichenlaub, "Joe's Nervous Breakdown," *Today's Health*, Nov. 1954, 18–19, p. 18.

4. There were a few exceptions to this rule. For an example of physicians using the term "nervous breakdown" in a professional publication, see Jurgen Ruesch et al., "The Acute Nervous Breakdown," *Archives of General Psychiatry,* 8 (1963), 197–207; yet as far as I can tell, these clinicians in the department of psychiatry of the San Francisco campus of the University of California School of Medicine, and the affiliated Langley Porter Neuropsychiatric Institute, did not enter the term in patients' charts but rather used it as a synonym for "acute illness." The article is a virtual singleton in the medical literature.

5. Thomas A. Ross, *The Common Neuroses: Their Treatment by Psychotherapy* (1923), 2nd ed. (London: Arnold 1937), 86.

6. Jacob Markowitz, "Nervousness and Nervous Breakdown," *Canadian Forum,* 16 (Apr. 1936), 13–17, p. 13.

7. See Edward Shorter, *Partnership for Excellence: Medicine at the University of Toronto and Academic Hospitals* (Toronto: University of Toronto Press, 2013).

8. Samuel Henry Kraines, *The Therapy of the Neuroses and Psychoses,* 2nd ed. (London: Kimpton, 1943), 503.

9. Etienne Esquirol, "De la folie" (1816), reprinted in *Esquirol, Des maladies mentales,* Vol. 1 (Paris: Baillière, 1838), 81.

10. Bénédict Augustin Morel, *Traité des maladies mentales* (Paris: Masson, 1860), 774.

11. See, for example, Jean-Martin Charcot, *Leçons du mardi à la Salpêtrière, Policlinique, 1888–1889* (Paris: Lecrosnier, 1889), 271–276; "la dormeuse."

12. Maurice Dide and Paul Guiraud, *Psychiatrie Clinique* (Paris: Librairie Le François, 1956), 91.

13. Megan Barke, Rebecca Fribush, and Peter N. Stearns attribute somewhat more importance to the concept in medicine, while admitting it never became an official diagnosis, "Nervous Breakdown in 20th-Century American Culture," *Journal of Social History*, 33 (2000), 565–584.
14. Ella Adelia Fletcher, *The Woman Beautiful* (New York: Brentano's, 1900), 527.
15. J. J. Putnam, "The Nervous Breakdown," *Good Housekeeping,* 49 (Nov. 1909), 595–598.
16. "Why the Jew is too neurotic," *Current Opinion*, 65 (Sep. 1918), 173–174.
17. *New York Times*, June 19, 1905, 1. Ellen Tulchinsky conducted the computer search on which this tabulation is based.
18. *New York Times*, Aug. 11, 1961, 2.
19. *New York Times*, May 14, 1909, 7.
20. *New York Times*, Feb. 16, 1941, 43.
21. *New York Times*, Jan. 3, 1947, 8.
22. Julian Huxley, *Memories* (London: Allen & Unwin, 1970), 97.
23. Peter M. Braunwarth et al., Eds., *Arthur Schnitzler Tagebuch,* Vol. 7, 1920–1922 (Vienna: Verlag der Österreichischen Akademie der Wissenschaften, 1981), 70–73, 108.
24. Edmund Wilson, Ed., *F. Scott Fitzgerald, The Crack-Up* (New York: New Directions, 1945), 71–72, 75, 80–81. Karl Jaspers, *Allgemeine Psychopathologie* (Berlin: Springer, 1913), 67.
25. Katharine Bement Davis, *Factors in the Sex Life of Twenty-Two Hundred Women* (New York: Harper & Brothers, 1929), 214.
26. See Edward Shorter, *A History of Psychiatry from the Era of the Asylum to the Age of Prozac* (New York: John Wiley & Sons, 1997), 113–144.
27. T. Seymour Tuke, "The Modern Treatment of the Insane," *BMJ*, 2 (Oct. 26, 1901), 1249–1251, p. 1250.
28. Ad for La Soldanelle, *Schweizerisches Medizinisches Jahrbuch 1940* (Basel: Schwabe, 1940), 327.
29. Margaret Case Harriman, "Are You Walking Around With a Nervous Breakdown?" *Ladies Home Journal*, 58 (1941), 16–17, quote p. 17.
30. Ralph Swindle, Jr., et al. "Responses to Nervous Breakdowns in America Over a 40-Year Period," *American Psychologist*, 55 (2000), 740–749, p. 744.
31. Lisa J. Rapport et al., "The Diagnostic Meaning of 'Nervous Breakdown' Among Lay Populations," *Journal of Personality Assessment*, 7 (1998), 242–252, p. 244.
32. "The Truth about Nervous Breakdowns," *Good Housekeeping*, 150 (1960), 151.

CHAPTER 8

1. Oswald Bumke, *Landläufige Irrtümer in der Beurteilung von Geisteskranken* (Wiesbaden: Bergmann, 1908), 37.
2. Joyce Hemlow, Ed., *The Journals and Letters of Fanny Burney*, Vol. 1 (Oxford: Clarendon, 1972), 115.

3. M. R. D. Foot, Ed., *The Gladstone Diaries*, Vol. 2 (Oxford: Clarendon, 1968), 358, 375.

4. J. H. Blount, "Essay on the Classification of Mental Alienation by Dr. M. Baillarger," *Asylum Journal of Mental Science*, 1 (1854), 137–141, p. 137.

5. I consulted Auguste Axenfeld and Henri Huchard, *Traité des névroses (1863)*, 2nd ed. (Paris: Baillière, 1883); on pp. viii–ix Huchard explains Axenfeld's original conceptions. Axenfeld died in 1876.

6. The quotation is from Richard von Krafft-Ebing, *Lehrbuch der Psychiatrie*, Vol. 2 (Stuttgart: Enke, 1879), 3.

7. Emil Kraepelin, *Psychiatrie: Ein Lehrbuch für Studierende und Aerzte* (Leipzig: Barth, 1915), Vol. 4, 1813.

8. Karl Jaspers, *Allgemeine Psychopathologie* (Berlin: Springer, 1913), 163.

9. Kurt Schneider, "Die Schichtung des emotionalen Lebens und der Aufbau der Depressionszustände," *Zeitschrift für die gesamte Neurologie und Psychiatrie*, 59 (1920), 281–286.

10. Josef Westermann, "Über die vitale Depression," *Zeitschrift für die gesamte Neurologie und Psychiatrie*, 77 (1922), 391–422.

11. E. S. Paykel, "Classification of Depressed Patients: A Cluster Analysis Derived Grouping," *BJP*, 118 (1971), 275–288; Kay C. Thomson and Hugh C. Hendrie, "Environmental Stress in Primary Depressive Illness," *Archives of General Psychiatry*, 26 (1972), 130–132. Later, see also E. S. Paykel, "The Evolution of Life Events Research in Psychiatry," *Journal of Affective Disorders*, 62 (2001), 141–149.

12. Joseph Zubin, discussion, in J. Zubin et al., Eds., *Disorders of Mood* (Baltimore: Johns Hopkins University Press, 1972), 30; the meeting took place in 1971.

13. Sigmund Freud, "Trauer und Melancholie" (1916), in *Freud, Gesammelte Werke* (London: Imago, 1946), Vol. 10, 428–446, p. 430.

14. Sigmund Freud, "Die Frage der Laienanalyse" (1926), in *Freud, Gesammelte Werke* (London: Imago, 1948), Vol. 14, 209–286, pp. 262–263.

15. Sigmund Freud, "Bemerkungen über die Übertragungsliebe" (1915), in *Freud, Gesammelte Werke* (London: Imago, 1946), Vol. 10, 306–321, pp. 312–313.

16. Karl Abraham, "Ansätze zur psychoanalytischen Erforschung und Behandlung des manisch-depressiven Irreseins und verwandter Zustände," *Zentralblatt für Psychoanalyse*, 2 (1912), 302–315, p. 302; paper given at a conference in 1911.

17. E. Farquhar Buzzard, "Discussion on the Diagnosis and Treatment of the Milder Forms of the Manic-Depressive Psychosis," *Proceedings of the Royal Society of Medicine*, 23 (1930), 881–883, p. 881.

18. Sandor Rado, "The Problem of Melancholia," *International Journal for Psychoanalysis*, 9 (1928), 420–438, p. 437; the conference was held in 1927.

19. Sandor Rado, "Psychodynamics of Depression from the Etiologic Point of View," *Psychosomatic Medicine*, 13 (1951), 51–55, p. 51. By this time Rado had abandoned the Hungarian accents on his name.

20. Otto Fenichel, *Outline of Clinical Psychoanalysis* (New York: The Psychoanalytic Quarterly Press and W. W. Norton Company, 1934), 395.

21. Otto Fenichel, *The Psychoanalytic Theory of Neurosis* (New York: W. W. Norton, 1945), 389, 391.

22. War Department Technical Bulletin, Medical 203. Reprinted as "Nomenclature of Psychiatric Disorders and Reactions," *Journal of Clinical Psychology*, 2 (1946), 289–296, p. 292.

23. *Diagnostic and Statistical Manual of Mental Disorders* (Washington, DC: American Psychiatric Association, 1952), 33–34.

24. *DSM-II. Diagnostic and Statistical Manual of Mental Disorders*, 2nd ed. (Washington, DC: American Psychiatric Association, 1968), 40.

25. Walter Bonime, "The Psychodynamics of Neurotic Depression," in Silvano Arieti, Ed., *American Handbook of Psychiatry*, Vol. 3 (New York: Basic, 1966), 239–255, p. 244.

26. Gershwin's sister-in-law apparently viewed his symptoms as part of "his relentless quest to call attention to himself," a psychoanalytic interpretation. Joan Peyser, *The Memory of All That: The Life of George Gershwin* (New York: Simon & Schuster, 1993), 217. See also Joan Peyser, letter, *New York Times*, Oct. 4, 1998, 2–4.

27. Robert Cancro, "The Uncompleted Task of Psychiatry," in Thomas Ban et al., Eds., *From Psychopharmacology to Neuropsychopharmacology in the 1980s* (Budapest: Animula, 2002), 237–244, p. 237.

28. Nathan Kline, discussion, in J. Angst, Ed., *Classification of Depression* (Zurich, Switzerland: Psychiatric University Hospital, 1974), 138.

29. Group for the Advancement of Psychiatry, *Trends and Issues in Psychiatric Residency Programs* (Topeka: GAP, 1955), 13; report no. 31, March 1955.

30. David Goldberg, "A Dimensional Model for Common Medical Disorders," *BJP*, 168 (Suppl. 30) (1996), 44–49, p. 48.

31. United Kingdom, Office for National Statistics, *Social Trends*, no. 33 (2003), Fig. 7.8, 134.

32. Food and Drug Administration, Psychopharmacological Drugs Advisory Committee, meeting of Dec. 4, 1981, Vol. 2, 178–179; obtained through the Freedom of Information Act.

33. Alan F. Schatzberg et al., "Depression Secondary to Anxiety: Findings from the McLean Hospital Depression Research Facility," *Psychiatric Clinics of North America*, 13 (1990), 633–649, p. 645.

34. David Goldberg and Peter Huxley, *Mental Illness in the Community: The Pathway to Psychiatric Care* (London: Tavistock, 1980), 83–84.

35. Goldberg, *BJP*, (1996), 48.

36. In a careful study of bipolar and unipolar depressives, Philip Mitchell and collaborators in the depression unit of the University of New South Wales write that "Overall, the findings are consistent with bipolar disorder being characterized by both melancholia and psychotic features." Philip B. Mitchell et al., "Comparison

of Depressive Episodes in Bipolar Disorder and in Major Depressive Disorder within Bipolar Disorder Pedigrees," *British Journal of Psychiatry*, 199 (2011), 303–309, p. 307.

37. Paula J. Clayton, "Depression Subtyping: Treatment Implications," *Journal of Clinical Psychiatry*, 59 (Suppl. 16) (1998), 5–12, Figs. 2, 8.

38. Kenneth S. Kendler et al., "The Identification and Validation of Distinct Depressive Syndromes in a Population-Based Sample of Female Twins," *Archives of General Psychiatry*, 53 (1996), 391–399, p. 397. Kendler, "Major Depression and Generalized Anxiety Disorder: Same Genes, (Partly) Different Environments—Revisited," *BJP*, 168 (Suppl. 30) (1996), 68–75.

39. Gavin Andrews et al., "The Genetics of Six Neurotic Disorders: A Twin Study," *Journal of Affective Disorders*, 19 (1990), 23–29.

40. Gavin Andrews, "Comorbidity and the General Neurotic Syndrome," *BJP*, 168, (Suppl. 30) (1996), 76–84.

41. Assen Jablensky and Robert E. Kendell, "Criteria for Assessing a Classification in Psychiatry," in Mario Maj et al., Eds., *Psychiatric Diagnosis and Classification* (Chichester: Wiley, 2002), 1–24, p. 11.

42. Marilyn K. Nations et al., "'Nerves': Folk Idiom for Anxiety and Depression?" *Social Science Medicine*, 26 (1988), 1245–1259.

43. Emil Kraepelin, *Psychiatrie: Ein Lehrbuch für Studierende und Ärzte*, 8th ed., Vol. 1 (Leipzig: Barth 1909), 349.

44. Edward Mapother, "Discussion on Manic-Depressive Psychosis," *BMJ*, 2 (Nov. 13, 1926), 872–876, p. 873.

45. J. W. Astley Cooper, "Rest in the Treatment of Neuroses," *BMJ*, 2 (Dec. 30, 1933), 1231–1232.

46. Thomas Arthur Ross, *An Enquiry into Prognosis in the Neuroses* (Cambridge: Cambridge University Press, 1936), calculated on the basis on cases on pp. 146–160.

47. Aubrey J. Lewis, "Melancholia: A Clinical Study of Depressive States," *Journal of Mental Science*, 80 (1934), 277–378, p. 355.

48. Fridolin Sulser, discussion, in Merton Sandler et al., Eds., *5-Hydroxytryptamine in Psychiatry: A Spectrum of Ideas* (Oxford: Oxford University Press, 1991), 191.

49. Jacques Launay, "Thérapeutique séméiologique des états dépressifs," *Annales Moreau de Tours*, 2 (1965), 74–78, p. 74.

50. Max Hamilton, discussion, in J. Angst, *Classification of Depression* (Zurich: Psychiatric University Hospital, 1974), 286.

51. John Overall and Sidney Zisook, "Diagnosis and the Phenomenology of Depressive Disorders," *Journal of Consulting and Clinical Psychology*, 48 (1980), 626–634, p. 632.

52. See Martin Roth and J. D. Morrissey, "Problems in the Diagnosis and Classification of Mental Disorder in Old Age: With a Study of Case Material," *Journal of Mental Science*, 98 (1952), 66–80.

53. Martin Roth, "The Phobic Anxiety-Depersonalization Syndrome," *Proceedings of the Royal Society of Medicine*, 52 (1959), 587–596.

54. M. W. P. Carney, M. Roth, and R. F. Garside, "The Diagnosis of Depressive Syndromes and the Prediction of E.C.T. Response," *BJP*, 111 (1965), 659–674, p. 669.

55. Martin Roth et al., "Studies in the Classification of Affective Disorders: The Relationship between Anxiety States and Depressive Illnesses—I," *BJP*, 121 (1972), 147–161, p. 158.

56. Akiskal, *Archives of General Psychiatry* (1978), 765.

57. Frank Fish, discussion, in F. A. Jenner, Ed., *Proceedings of the Leeds Symposium on Behavioural Disorders, 25–27 March 1965* (Dagenham: May & Baker, April 1965), 198.

58. R. E. Kendell, "The Classification of Depressions: A Review of Contemporary Confusion," *BJP*, 129 (1976), 15–28.

59. Ross Baldessarini interview with Edward Shorter and Max Fink, at McLean Hospital, Feb. 17, 2006, 18.

60. See Bernard Carroll to Donald Green (Hoffmann-La Roche), Sept. 28, 1982: re "well controlled inpatient studies": "This was the main reason why the FDA Advisory Committee did not approve the Upjohn compound, alprazolam, recently as an antidepressant. The only evidence Upjohn had for antidepressant efficacy was obtained among outpatients." Carroll Papers, *International Neuropsychopharmacology Archives*, University of California, Los Angeles.

61. Peter Tyrer, "The Case for Cothymia: Mixed Anxiety and Depression as a Single Diagnosis," *BJP*, 179 (2001), 191–193.

62. Benedict Carey, "Psychiatry Manual Drafters Back Down on Diagnoses," *New York Times*, May 8, 2012.

63. Raymond Battegay interview, "Forty-Four Years of Psychiatry and Psychopharmacology," in David Healy, Ed., *The Psychopharmacologists*, Vol. 3 (London: Arnold, 2000), 371–394, p. 383.

64. Gerald L. Klerman, "Evidence for Increase in Rates of Depression in North America and Western Europe in Recent Decades," in Hanns Hippius, Ed., *New Results in Depression Research* (Heidelberg: Springer, 1986), 7–15. Based on their study of North Wales, David Healy and co-workers have argued that the incidence of melancholia, especially the nonpsychotic version, has risen over the past hundred years. It remains to be seen whether these findings are generalizable. Margaret Harris, Fiona Farquhar, David Healy et al., "The Incidence and Prevalence of Admissions for Melancholia in Two Cohorts (1875–1924 and 1995–2005)," *Journal of Affective Disorders* (2011), DOI: 10.1016/j.jad.2011.06.015, 3, Tab. 1.

65. "Prof R. H. Syms Dead," *New York Times*, Dec. 9, 1912, 11.

66. Farquhar Buzzard, in "Discussion on Manic-Depressive Psychosis," British Medical Association meeting, *BMJ*, 1 (Nov. 13, 1926), 877.

67. Edgar Jones and Shahina Rahman, "Framing Mental Illness, 1923–1939: The Maudsley Hospital and Its Patients," *Social History of Medicine*, advance access published Mar. 5, 2008, p. 9 of 19, Tab. 3; DOI: 10.1093/shm/hkm115.

68. Paul Kielholz, "Drug Treatment of Depressive States," *Canadian Psychiatric Association Journal,* (1959), S129–S137, pp. S129–S130.

69. Linda Hilles, "Changing Trends in the Application of Psychoanalytic Principles to a Psychiatric Hospital," *Bulletin of the Menninger Clinic*, 32 (1968), 203–218, Tab. 3, p. 208.

70. Saul H. Rosenthal, "Changes in a Population of Hospitalized Patients with Affective Disorders, 1945–1965," *AJP*, 123 (1966), 671–681, p. 674. Tab. 2, p. 680.

71. Willi Mayer-Gross, discussion, in E. Beresford Davies, Ed., *Depression: Proceedings of the Symposium Held at Cambridge 22 to 26 September 1959* (Cambridge: Cambridge University Press, 1964), 57.

72. John G. Dewan, "Mild Depressions," *Medical Clinics of North America*, 36 (1952), 527–537, pp. 529–530.

73. William P. D. Logan et al., *Morbidity Statistics from General Practice*, Vol. 1 (London: HMSO, 1958; General Register Office, Studies on Medical and Population Subjects, no. 14), Tab. 9, 88–89.

74. The data on major depression, dysthymic disorder, and bipolar I disorder were reported in P. Waraich et al., "Prevalence and Incidence Studies of Mood Disorders: A Systematic Review of the Literature," *Canadian Journal of Psychiatry*, 49 (2004), 124–138.

75. A. M. W. Porter, discussion, in "The Medical Use of Psychotropic Drugs: A Report of a Symposium, Sponsored by the Department of Health and Social Security and Held at University College Swansea on 1–2 July, 1972," *Journal of the Royal College of General Practitioners*, 23, (Suppl. 2) (June, 1973), 14.

76. John Marks, discussion, in Hugh Freeman et al., Eds., *The Benzodiazepines in Current Clinical Practice* (London: Royal Society of Medicine Services, 1987), 32.

77. Myrna Weissman and Gerald L. Klerman, "The Chronic Depressive in the Community; Unrecognized and Poorly Treated," *Comprehensive Psychiatry*, 18 (1977), 523–532.

78. See Martin M. Katz and Gerald L. Klerman, "Introduction: Overview of the Clinical Studies Program," *AJP*, 136 (1979), 49–51, p. 51.

79. Martin B. Keller and Robert W. Shapiro, "'Double Depression': Superimposition of Acute Depressive Episodes on Chronic Depressive Disorders," *AJP*, 139 (1982), 438–442.

80. See Alison Bass, *Side Effects: A Prosecutor, a Whistleblower, and a Bestselling Antidepressant on Trial* (Chapel Hill, NC: Algonquin, 2008), 66–67.

81. Myrna Weissman, "Gerald Klerman and Psychopharmacology," in David Healy, Ed., *The Psychopharmacologists*, Vol. 2 (London: Chapman & Hall, 1998), 521–542, p. 530.

CHAPTER 9

1. For APA's initial conception of the limited nature of the revision see Walter Barton to Sidney Malitz, Mar. 20, 1973; APA Archives, Professional Affairs, box 17, folder 188.

2. See "Overview of Actions of the Board re DSM-III," undated document [1978]; APA Archives, Project Affairs, box 17, folder 188; Walter E. Barton, Medical Director to Sidney Malitz, Chairman, APA Council on Research and Development, Mar. 20, 1973; APA Archives, Project Affairs, box 17, folder 188.

3. Samuel Guze interview, "The Neo-Kraepelinian Revolution," in David Healy, Ed., *The Psychopharmacologists,* Vol. 3 (London: Arnold, 2000), 395–414, p. 404.

4. Sources for this paragraph included Robert Spitzer interview by Edward Shorter and Max Fink, Mar. 14, 2007, and the entry for Spitzer in Edward Shorter, *Historical Dictionary of Psychiatry* (New York: Oxford University Press, 2005), 284–285.

5. Name withheld, personal communication to author, Jan. 27, 2006.

6. Carolyn B. Robinowitz to Melvin Sabshin, memo of June 7, 1979; APA Archives, Education, box 16, folder 200.

7. Robert Spitzer interview with Edward Shorter and Max Fink, Irvington, NY, Mar. 14, 2007.

8. Donald Klein to Robert Spitzer, memo of April 24, 1978; APA Archives, Janet Williams Papers, Research, DSM-III-R, box 1, DSM-III files, folder "misc. affective."

9. APA Archives, Prof. Affairs, box 17, folder 188, date Sept. 4, 1974.

10. Robert Spitzer, discussion, in Abraham Sudilovsky et al., Eds., *Predictability in Psychopharmacology* (New York: Raven, 1975), 46.

11. Minutes. Task Force on Nomenclature and Statistics, meeting of September 4, 5 in New York. APA Archives, Professional Affairs, box 17, folder 188.

12. Donald Klein, personal communication, Apr. 30, 2006.

13. Robert L. Spitzer, Jean Endicott, and Eli Robins, "Research Diagnostic Criteria," *Archives of General Psychiatry,* 35 (1978), 773–782.

14. Michael Shepherd, "Evaluation of Drugs in the Treatment of Depression," *Canadian Psychiatric Association Journal,* 4, (Suppl.) (1959), S120–S128, p. S124.

15. "Initial Draft Version of DSM-III Classification of August 1, 1975," attached to Jarvik to Stetsky, Nov. 8, 1976; APA Archives, Paula Clayton Papers, box 30, folder 13. The Clayton Papers are now in the International Neuropsychopharmacology Archives, University of California, Los Angeles.

16. "Draft Version of DSM-III Classification as of March 1, 1976," attached to Task Force on Nomenclature and Statistics of the American Psychiatric Association, "Progress Report on the Preparation of DSM-III," March 1976; APA Archives, Professional Affairs, box 17, folder 193 (70 #3).

17. Memorandum, from The Chairman of the Assembly DSM III Task Force (Howard Berk) to District Branch Representatives and Alternate Representatives. Apr. 4, 1977; APA Archives, Assembly, box 18, folder 274.

18. APA Archives, Williams Papers, Research DSM-III-R, box 1. Misc DSM-III files [owing to inadequate labeling on the author's part, it is possible that this note comes from box 3].

19. Kay C. Thomson and Hugh C. Hendrie, "Environmental Stress in Primary Depressive Illness," *Archives of General Psychiatry*, 26 (1972), 130–132.

20. Lyman C. Wynne to "Affective Disorders Advisory Committee," Feb. 13, 1978; Clayton Papers, box 31.

21. Paula Clayton memo to Spitzer and "other members of the Major Affective Disorder Committee," Feb. 22, 1979; Clayton Papers, box 31.

22. Memo, Donald Klein to Robert Spitzer, Apr. 26, 1978; APA Archives, Williams Papers, Research, DSM-III-R, box 1; DSM-III files, "misc affective."

23. Donald F. Klein, "Endogenomorphic Depression," *Archives of General Psychiatry*, 31 (1974), 447–454.

24. Memo from Spitzer to Donald Klein, Nancy Andreasen, Rachel Gittelman, Michael Sheehy, Edward Sachar, and Arthur Rifkin, Mar. 29, 1979; APA Archives, Williams Papers, Research—DSM-III-R, box 2. The distribution shows the inner circle of the *DSM* drafters. Sachar, head of psychiatry at Columbia, was not even a member of the Task Force!

25. Robert Spitzer and Michael Sheehy to Klein, Andreasen, Sachar, Wynne, Endicott, Arthur Rifkin, Frederic Quitkin, and Sandy Glassman. These were mainly Spitzer's colleagues at PI and the New York area.

26. Memo, Robert L. Spitzer and Jean Endicott to Task Force, May 3, 1978; APA Archives, Williams Papers. Research, DSM-III-R, box 1, DSM-III, "misc affective."

27. Robert L. Spitzer to "Affective Disorder Mavens," July 10, 1978; APA Archives, Williams Papers. Research, DSM-III-R; DSM-III files, "misc affective."

28. Offerto F. Bertolini, "Cloropromazina e reserpina nel trattamento delle psichopatie," *Archivio di Psicologia, Neurologia, et Psichiatria*, 17 (1956), 623–627, p. 626.

29. Thomas Ban, interview, in Thomas Ban, Ed., *An Oral History of Neuropsychopharmacology: The First Fifty Years. Peer Interviews,* Vol. 4 (Brentwood, TN: ACNP, 2011), 20.

30. Roger Peele to Robert Spitzer, Mar. 12, 1979; Clayton Papers, box 31.

31. Robert Spitzer to Assembly Liaison, Joint American Psychoanalytic Association and American Academy of Psychoanalysis Committees, Mar. 27, 1979; APA Archives, Williams Papers, Research, DSM-III-R, box 3. Misc DSM-III files.

32. Donald Klein to Robert Spitzer, Mar. 30, 1979; Clayton Papers, box 31.

33. See Spitzer to Hector Jaso, Chair, DSM-III Assembly Liaison Committee, Apr. 18, 1979; APA Archives, Williams Papers, Research, DSM-III-R. Loose DSM-III files, Neurosis folder.

34. "Possible revision 4/25/79," APA, Williams Papers, Research, DSM-III-R, loose DSM-III files, Neurosis folder.

35. Bernard Carroll to Robert Spitzer, Feb. 19, 1979; APA Archives, Williams Papers, DSM-III-R, box 1, DSM-III Files, Major depressive disorder.

36. Robert Spitzer to Bernard Carroll, Mar. 2, 1979; APA Archives, Williams Papers, Research, DSM-III-R, box 1, DSM-III files. "Dear Barney, where have you been all this time?"

37. Michael Feinberg, Bernard Carroll, Meir Steiner, and Anne J. Commorato, letter, "Misdiagnosis of Endogenous Depression with Research Diagnostic Criteria," *Lancet*, 1 (Feb. 3, 1979), 267.

38. Memo, from Robert Spitzer and Janet B. W. Forman, to the Task Force, Affective Mavens, Assembly Liaison Committee, Mar. 15, 1979; APA Archives, Williams Papers, Research, DSM-III-R, box 1, DSM-III files; major depressive disorder. The Task Force *voted* on which of these choices they endorsed, as well as on matters such as whether unipolar mania should be part of Bipolar Affective Disorder. This is an astonishing comment on how science was once conducted in psychiatry. Scientists do not normally vote on matters such as the speed of light.

39. DSM-III (1980), 215.

40. Thomas A. Ban ms, "From Melancholia to Depression: A History of Diagnosis and Treatment," 34, Tab. 10.

41. Such loose criteria lead to an overdiagnosis of melancholia in research studies, although not in the community, where patients feared the term. In a study led by Pierre Blier of 105 patients with major depressive disorder, 80 qualified for the melancholic subtype. Pierre Blier et al., "Combination of Antidepressant Medications from Treatment Initiation for Major Depressive Disorder: A Double-Blind Randomized Study," *AJP*, 167 (2010), 281–288.

42. Bernard Carroll interview by Edward Shorter and Max Fink, Oct. 17, 2005.

43. See his account of this discovery in Donald F. Klein, "Anxiety Reconceptualized," *Modern Problems of Pharmacopsychiatry*, 22 (1987), 1–35, pp. 1–6.

44. Donald Klein and Max Fink, "Psychiatric Reaction Patterns to Imipramine," *AJP*, 119 (1962), 432–438.

45. Donald F. Klein, "Delineation of Two Drug-Responsive Anxiety Syndromes," *Psychopharmacologia*, 5 (1964), 397–408, p. 407.

46. Donald F. Klein, "Treatment of Phobias Characterized by Separation Anxiety," *International Drug Therapy Newsletter*, 2 (1967), 16; see also Julius J. C. Mendel and Donald F. Klein, "Anxiety Attacks with Subsequent Agoraphobia," *Comprehensive Psychiatry*, 10 (1969), 190–195.

47. DSM-II, 39–40.

48. I relied on the manuscript text of Sheehan's interview with David Healy, which Dr. Healy was kind enough to show me. The published version is slightly different. See James Sheehan, interview, "Angles on Panic," in David Healy, Ed., *The Psychopharmacologists*, Vol. 3 (London: Arnold, 2000), 479–503, p. 481.

49. Paula Clayton interview with Edward Shorter and Max Fink, Dec. 4, 2006.

50. Donald Klein to Robert Spitzer, June 1, 1978; APA Archives, Williams Papers. Research, DSM-III-R, box 1; DSM-III files, "misc affective."

51. Isaac Marks to Robert Spitzer, June 28, 1977; APA Archives, Williams Papers, Research. DSM-III-R, box 3, DSM-III files, misc. My own notes sourcing this document are incomplete, but I believe this is the correct citation.

52. Michael Gelder to Robert Spitzer, June 28, 1977; APA Archives, Williams Papers, Research. DSM-III-R, box 1. Klein's undated response is attached.

53. "Draft ... as of March 30, 1977," attached to APA Archives, Professional affairs, box 16, folder 177, DSM-III draft (2), Apr. 15, 1977. See Klein to Spitzer, Aug. 3, 1979 re "agoraphobia without panic attacks": "I think that category is not likely to be used much anyway, since such people are extremely rare." APA Archives, Williams Papers. Research, DSM-III-R, box 3; misc DSM-III files.

54. "Draft Version of DSM-III Classification as of March 1, 1976," attached to "Progress Report on the Preparation of DSM-III," March 1976; APA, Professional Affairs, box 17, folder 193 (70 #3).

55. "Draft of DSM-III Classification as of December 21, 1976," Clayton Papers, box 30, folder 11, attached to Spitzer to Task Force, Dec. 20, 1976.

56. "Annotated Classification of DSM-III," Nov. 15, 1979; Clayton Papers, box 30, folder 16.

57. "DSM-III Draft, first printing, 1/15/78"; foreword, ix; source: www.pmdocs.com, doc nos. 1000216651, 1000216662.

58. David V. Sheehan et al., "The Classification of Anxiety and Hysterical States. Part I. Historical Review and Empirical Delineation," *Journal of Clinical Psychopharmacology*, 2 (1982), 235–244, p. 242.

59. Juan Lopez Ibor, in Merton Sandler et al., Eds., *5-Hydroxytryptamine in Psychiatry: A Spectrum of Ideas* (Oxford: Oxford University Press, 1991), discussion, 193. 5-Hydroxytryptamine is serotonin.

60. Robert Spitzer interview, "A Manual for Diagnosis and Statistics," in David Healy, Ed., *The Psychopharmacologists*, Vol. 3 (London: Arnold, 2000), 415–430, p. 427.

61. Interview with George Arana by Max Fink, Charleston, South Carolina, Jan. 4, 2006, 12.

CHAPTER 10

1. "Primum non nocere," *Lancet*, 1 (Feb. 10, 1940), 275.

2. Francis D. Boyd, "Discussion on the Artificially Prepared Hypnotics, Their Use and Possible Abuse," *Edinburgh Medical Journal*, NS 5 (1910), 7–18, p. 9.

3. N. Mutch, "Proprietary Remedies, with Special Reference to Hypnotics," *BMJ*, 1 (Feb. 24, 1934), 319–322, p. 322.

4. Veronal-Natrium advertisement, *Wiener Medizinische Wochenschrift*, 63 (May 24, 1913), 1338.

5. Louis Vidal, *Dictionnaire de spécialités pharmaceutiques* (Brussels: Office de

Vulgarisation Pharmaceutique, 1931), 808, 997.

6. Nigel Nicolson et al., Eds., *The Letters of Virginia Woolf, 1929–1931*, Vol. 4 (London: Harcourt, 1978), 13; Virginia Woolf to Vita Sackville-West, Feb. 4, 1929.

7. See, for example, Philip Kolb, Ed., *Marcel Proust Correspondence*, Vol. 5, 1905 (Paris: Plon, 1979), passim; on Proust and Veronal see D. Mabin, "Sommeil et automédication de Marcel-Proust," *Neurophysiologie Clinique*, 24 (1994), 61–74, p. 66.

8. W. E. Hambourger, "A Study of the Promiscuous Use of the Barbiturates," *JAMA*, 112 (Apr. 8, 1939), 1340–1343.

9. See L. I. M. Castleden, "Hypnotic Drugs," *Practitioner*, 137 (1936), 358–368, p. 365.

10. Arthur N. Foxe, "On Sedativism," *Medical Record*, 156 (1943), 665–666, p. 665.

11. Louis Lasagna, "The Newer Hypnotics," *Medical Clinics of North America*, 41 (1957), 359–368, p. 366.

12. See Heinz Lehmann and Thomas Ban, *Pharmacotherapy of Tension and Anxiety* (Springfield: Charles C Thomas, 1970), 1–13.

13. Ian Tait, discussion, in E. M. Tansey et al., Eds., *Wellcome Witnesses to Twentieth Century Medicine*, Vol. 2 (London: Wellcome Institute for the History of Medicine, 1998), 169.

14. W. J. Bleckwenn, "Sodium Amytal in Certain Nervous and Mental Conditions," *Wisconsin Medical Journal*, 29 (1930), 693–696, pp. 693, 694.

15. Jacques S. Gottlieb, "The Use of Sodium Amytal and Benzedrine Sulfate in the Symptomatic Treatment of Depressions," *Diseases of the Nervous System*, 10 (1949), 50–52, p. 50.

16. *Research in Psychopharmacology: Report of a WHO Scientific Group* (Geneva: WHO, 1967; WHO Technical Report Series, no. 371), 10, Tab. 2.

17. Donald F. Klein and John M. Davis, *Diagnosis and Drug Treatment of Psychiatric Disorders* (Baltimore: Williams & Wilkins, 1969), 410.

18. Heinz Lehmann, discussion, in Jonathan O. Cole and Ralph W. Gerard, Eds., *Psychopharmacology: Problems in Evaluation* (Washington, DC: National Academy of Sciences—National Research Council, 1959), 602–603.

19. State of New York. *Nineteenth Annual Report of the Director of the New York State Psychiatric Institute for the Fiscal Year Ended March 31, 1948* (Utica: State Hospitals Press, 1948), 13.

20. See Edward Shorter, *From Paralysis to Fatigue: A History of Psychosomatic Illness in the Modern Era* (New York: Free Press, 1992).

21. Matthias M. Weber, *Die Entwicklung der Psychopharmakologie im Zeitalter der naturwissenschaftlichen Medizin* (Munich: Urban & Vogel, 1999), 45–47.

22. On the amphetamines in the treatment of nonmelancholic depression, see Edward Shorter, *Before Prozac: The Troubled History of Mood Disorders in Psychiatry* (New York: Oxford University Press, 2009), 24–33. On methylene blue in mood disorders see Pietro Bodoni, "Dell'azione sedativa del bleu di metilene in varie forme di psicosi," *Clinica Medica Italiana*, 38 (1899), 217–222; G. J. Naylor et al., "A Two-Year Double-Blind Crossover Trial of the Prophylactic

Effect of Methylene Blue in Manic-Depressive Psychosis," *Biological Psychiatry*, 21 (1986), 915–920; Maike J. Ohlow et al., "Phenothiazine: The Seven Lives of Pharmacology's First Lead Structure," *Drug Discovery Today*, 16 (2011), 119–131.

23. Joseph J. Schildkraut, "The Catecholamine Hypothesis of Affective Disorders: A Review of Supporting Evidence," *AJP*, 122 (1965), 509–522.

24. J. H. Gaddum, "Drugs Antagonistic to 5-Hydroxytryptamine," in E. W. Wolstenholme et al., Eds., *Ciba Foundation Symposium on Hypertension: Humoral and Neurogenic Factors* (London: Churchill, 1954), 75–77.

25. Arvid Carlsson et al., "On the Biochemistry and Possible Functions of Dopamine and Noradrenaline in Brain," in J. R. Vane et al., Eds., *Ciba Foundation Symposium on Adrenergic Mechanisms* (Boston: Little Brown, 1960), 432–439.

26. Carlsson recounted his humiliation and subsequent triumph in an interview with Edward Shorter and David Healy in Gothenburg, Feb. 27–28, 2007.

27. Arvid Carlsson, "Physiological and Pharmacological Release of Monoamines in the Central Nervous System," in U. S. von Euler et al., Eds., *Mechanisms of Release of Biogenic Amines* (Oxford: Pergamon Press, 1966), 331–346.

28. Alec Coppen et al., "Potentiation of the Antidepressive Effect of a Monoamine-Oxidase Inhibitor by Tryptophan," *Lancet*, 1 (Jan. 12, 1963), 79–81.

29. See D. L. Murphy at al., "Current Status of the Indoleamine Hypothesis of the Affective Disorders," in Morris A. Lipton et al., Eds., *Psychopharmacology: A Generation of Progress* (New York: Raven Press, 1978), 1235–1247, p. 1238.

30. Merton Sandler interview, in Thomas A. Ban, Ed., *An Oral History of Neuropsychopharmacology: The First Fifty Years. Peer Interviews,* Vol. 3 (Brentwood, TN: ACNP, 2011), 468.

31. Alec Coppen, "The Biochemistry of Affective Disorders," *BJP*, 113 (1967), 1237–1264, p. 1258.

32. Alvan Feinstein, discussion, in Joseph D. Cooper, Ed., *The Efficacy of Self-Medication* (Washington, DC: Interdisciplinary Communication Associates, 1973), 18; *Philosophy and Technology of Drug Assessment*, Vol. 4, of the Interdisciplinary Communications Program of the Smithsonian Institution (Washington, DC: Smithsonian Institution).

33. Marie Asberg et al., "'Serotonin Depression'—A Biochemical Subgroup within the Affective Disorders," *Science,* 191 (Feb. 6, 1976), 478–480, p. 478.

34. Thomas Ban, interview by Edward Shorter, July 11, 2002.

35. Peter Waldmeier interview, "From Mental Illness to Neurodegeneration," in David Healy, Ed., *The Psychopharmacologists*, Vol. 1 (London: Chapman & Hall, 1996), 565–586, p. 567.

36. G. W. Ashcroft et al., "Changes on Recovery in the Concentrations of Tryptophan and the Biogenic Amine Metabolites in the Cerebrospinal Fluid of Patients with Affective Illness," *Psychological Medicine*, 3 (1973), 319–325, p. 319.

37. George Ashcroft, interview, "The Receptor Enters Psychiatry," in David Healy Ed., *The Psychopharmacologists,* Vol. 3 (London: Arnold, 2000), 189–200, p. 192.

38. Alec Coppen, discussion, in B. I. Hoffbrand et al., Eds., "Biological Aspects of Clomipramine," *Postgraduate Medical Journal*, 52 (Suppl. 3) (1976), 16–17.

39. William Z. Potter et al., "Selective Antidepressants and Cerebrospinal Fluid: Lack of Specificity on Norepinephrine and Serotonin Metabolites," *Archives of General Psychiatry*, 42 (1985), 1171–1177.

40. William Z. Potter, interview, in Ban, *Oral History of Neuropsychopharmacology,* Vol. 5, 265–267.

41. Ross Baldessarini interview in Ban, *Oral History of Neuropsychopharmacology,* Vol. 5, 25.

42. Irving Kirsch, *The Emperor's New Drugs: Exploding the Antidepressant Myth* (New York: Basic Books, 2010).

43. Archibald Todrick et al., "The Inhibition of Human Platelet 5HT Uptake by Tricyclic Antidepressant Drugs," *Journal of Pharmacy and Pharmacology*, 21 (1969), 751–762.

44. Desipramine advertisement, *Diseases of the Nervous System*, 26 (1965), ad page.

45. Desipramine (Pertofrane) advertisement, *AJP*, 131 (1974).

46. Desyrel ad, *AJP*, 139 (1982).

47. Maprotiline ad, *AJP*, 140 (1983).

48. Edward J. Sachar and Miron Baron, "The Biology of Affective Disorders," *Annual Review of Neuroscience*, 2 (1979), 505–518, p. 514.

49. Seymour S. Kety, "Strategies of Basic Research," in Morris A. Lipton et al., Eds., *Psychopharmacology: A Generation of Progress* (New York: Raven Press, 1978), 7–11, p. 10.

50. Laurent Maitre, discussion, in "Biogenic Amines and Affective Disorders: Proceedings of a Symposium held in London 18–21 January 1979," in T. H. Svensson and A. Carlsson, Eds., *Acta Psychiatrica Scandinavica,* 61 (Suppl. 280) (1980), 19.

51. A. J. Puech, discussion, in "Colloque international sur l'approche moderne des désordres de l'humeur, Monte-Carlo, 3–5 Mai 1979," in P. Deniker, Ed., *L'Encéphale, ns 5* (1979), Suppl. 581.

52. Neil Risch et al., "Interaction Between the Serotonin Transporter Gene (*5-HT-TLPR*), Stressful Life Events, and Risk of Depression," *JAMA*, 301 (June 17, 2009), 2462–2471.

53. ProQuest Historical Newspapers: *The New York Times,* accessed September 8, 2011.

54. Eugene Paykel, discussion, in Ruth Porter, Ed., *Antidepressants and Receptor Function* (Chichester: Wiley, 1986), 164.

55. Prozac advertisement, *JAMA*, 259 (June 3, 1988), 3092 a-c.

56. Gavin Andrews et al. argue "that close to half the population can expect one or more episodes of depression in their lifetime." "Lifetime Risk of Depression: Restricted to a Minority or Waiting for Most?" *BJP*, 187 (2005), 495–496, p. 495.

CHAPTER 11

1. Of course *DSM-III* did create two depressions (aside from dysthymia): the depression of unipolar disorder, called "major depression" and usually nonmelancholic in nature, and the depression of bipolar disorder, which frequently is melancholia. Since then, bipolar disorder has been widely, but not universally, seen as distinct from major depression. I myself am quite skeptical of the supposed difference between these two depressions in any way other than melancholia versus nonmelancholia, but have decided not to take on the whole issue in the current volume, which is really axised along the demonstration of major depression as an inadequate shadow of the nerve syndrome. Readers wishing to learn more about the bipolar–unipolar similarity might consult Michael Alan Taylor and Nutan Atre Vaidya, *Descriptive Psychopathology: The Signs and Symptoms of Behavioral Disorders* (New York: Cambridge University Press, 2009), 380–383.

2. Michael Alan Taylor, *The Fundamentals of Clinical Neuropsychiatry* (New York: Oxford University Press, 1999), 167.

3. W. Mayer-Gross, Eliot Slater, and Martin Roth, *Clinical Psychiatry* (London: Cassell, 1954), 204–205.

4. Alfred M. Freedman, Harold I. Kaplan, and Benjamin J. Sadock, *Comprehensive Textbook of Psychiatry*, 2nd ed. (Baltimore: Williams & Wilkins, 1975), 2595. Freedman himself had ceased to be involved with the subsequent editions of the textbook that he began.

5. Thomas Ban, personal communication, Apr. 10, 2007.

6. Pierre Pichot, *Les voies nouvelles de la dépression* (Paris: Masson, 1978), 2.

7. Roland Kuhn, "Corrections of Statements in the Publication by David Healy on the History of the Discovery of Modern Antidepressants," in Thomas A. Ban et al., Eds., *From Psychopharmacology to Neuropsychopharmacology in the 1980s* (Budapest: Animula, 2002), 301–352, p. 318; Vol. 3 in the series *The History of Psychopharmacology and the CINP, As Told in Autobiography*.

8. Ibid., 334–335.

9. Bernard J. Carroll et al., "Resistance to Suppression by Dexamethasone of Plasma 11-O.H.C.S. Levels in Severe Depressive Illness," *BMJ*, 2 (Aug. 3, 1968), 285–287.

10. Bernard Carroll et al., "A Specific Laboratory Test for the Diagnosis of Melancholia," *Archives of General Psychiatry*, 38 (1981), 15–22.

11. Edward Shorter and Max Fink, *Endocrine Psychiatry: Solving the Riddle of Melancholia* (New York: Oxford University Press, 2010), 85–102.

12. Robin G. Priest, "A Patient Who Changed My Practice," *International Journal of Psychiatry in Clinical Practice*, 1 (1997), 221–222.

13. J. Craig Nelson, Dennis S. Charney, and Donald M. Quinlan, "Evaluation of the DSM-III Criteria for Melancholia," *Archives of General Psychiatry*, 38 (1981), 555–559.

14. T. Hallström, "Point Prevalence of Major Depressive Disorder in a Swedish Urban Female Population," *Acta Psychiatrica Scandinavica*, 69 (1984), 52–59.

15. Gordon Parker, personal communication to David Healy, copied to Edward Shorter, May 20, 2010. Parker emphasized that this was a "real guess," but said he knew "of no firm data as the definitions are either imprecise or useless." Healy himself estimates the community prevalence as about 1 per 1000 population, and adds, "It depends on what you think the gearing is between detected and undetected cases—how many go undiagnosed?" Healy to Shorter, Sept. 11, 2011.

16. Henry Yellowlees, discussion, following paper of E. Farquhar Buzzard on "The Diagnosis and Treatment of the Milder Forms of the Manic-Depressive Psychosis," *Proceedings of the Royal Society of Medicine*, 23 (1930), 888.

17. Duane G. Spiker and David J. Kupfer, "Placebo Response Rates in Psychotic and Nonpsychotic Depression," *Journal of Affective Disorders*, 14 (1988), 21–23.

18. Max Fink, *Convulsive Therapy: Theory and Practice* (New York: Raven Press, 1979); Max Hamilton, "The Effect of Treatment on the Melancholias (Depressions)," *BJP*, 40 (1982), 223–230; Michael E. Thase and A. John Rush, "Treatment-Resistant Depression," in Floyd E. Bloom and David J. Kupfer, Eds., *Psychopharmacology: The Fourth Generation of Progress* (New York: Raven Press, 1995), 1081–1097. On the revival of ECT, see Edward Shorter and David Healy, *Shock Therapy: A History of Electroconvulsive Treatment in Mental Illness* (New Brunswick: Rutgers University Press, 2007), 219–252.

19. Paul J. Perry, "Pharmacotherapy for Major Depression with Melancholic Features: Relative Efficacy of Tricyclic Versus Selective Serotonin Reuptake Inhibitor Antidepressants," *Journal of Affective Disorders*, 39 (1996), 1–6, p. 1.

20. Per Bech and Ole J. Rafaelsen, "The Use of Rating Scales Exemplified by a Comparison of the Hamilton and the Bech-Rafaelsen Melancholia Scale," *Acta Psychiatrica Scandinavica*, 62 (1980) (Suppl. 285), 128–132.

21. Per Bech, "A Review of the Antidepressant Properties of Serotonin Reuptake Inhibitors," *Advances in Biological Psychiatry*, 17 (1988), 58–69, p. 60.

22. Thomas Ban, personal communication, Jan. 26, 2006.

23. Robert D. Gibbons, David C. Clark, and John M. Davis, "A Statistical Model for the Classification of Imipramine Response to Depressed Inpatients," *Psychopharmacology*, 78 (1982), 185–189. These data were originally reported in Niels S. Reisby et al., "Imipramine: Clinical Effects and Pharmacokinetic Variability," *Psychopharmacology*, 54 (1977), 263–272.

24. Gordon Parker et al., "Sub-Typing Depression: Is Psychomotor Disturbance Necessary and Sufficient to the Definition of Melancholia?" *Psychological Medicine*, 25 (1995), 815–823.

25. Gordon Parker et al., Eds., *Melancholia: A Disorder of Movement and Mood* (Cambridge: Cambridge University Press, 1996), 4.

26. Daniel J. Widlöcher, "Psychomotor Retardation: Clinical, Theoretical, and Psychometric Aspects," *Psychiatric Clinics of North America*, 6 (1983), 27–40, p. 28.

27. Walter A. Brown, "Are Antidepressants as Ineffective as They Look?" *Prevention & Treatment*, article 25, posted July 15, 2002; journals.apa.org/prevention/volume5/pre0050026c.html.

28. Bernard J. Carroll, "Neurobiologic Dimensions of Depression and Mania," in Jules Angst, Ed., *The Origins of Depression: Current Concepts and Approaches* (Berlin: Springer, 1983), 163–186, p. 166.

29. Michael Alan Taylor and Max Fink, *Melancholia: The Diagnosis, Pathophysiology, and Treatment of Depressive Illness* (Cambridge: Cambridge University Press, 2006), xii–xiii.

30. Tom Bolwig et al., Eds., "Melancholia: Beyond DSM, Beyond Neurotransmitters," *Acta Psychiatrica Scandinavica*, 115 (2007) (Suppl. 433), 1–183.

31. Mark Olfson et al., "Trends in Office-Based Psychiatric Practice," *AJP*, 156 (1999), 451–457, p. 453 Tab. 1.

32. Anthony J. Marsella, Robert M. A. Hirschfeld, and Martin M. Katz, *The Measurement of Depression* (New York: Guilford Press, 1987), ix.

33. Wilson M. Compton et al., "Changes in the Prevalence of Major Depression and Comorbid Substance Use Disorder in the United States Between 1991–1992 and 2001–2002," *AJP*, 163 (2006), 2141–2147.

34. Ronald C. Kessler et al., "The Prevalence and Correlates of Serious Mental Illness (SMI) in the National Comorbidity Survey Replications (NCS-R)," 134–148, in Substance Abuse and Mental Health Services Administration. (2006). *Mental Health, United States, 2004* (Rockville, MD: Center for Mental Health Services).

35. Substance Abuse and Mental Health Services Administration. (2010). *Mental Health, United States, 2008*. HHS Pub. No. (SMA) 10-4590 (Rockville, MD: Center for Mental Health Services, SAMHSA, 164, Tab.11.15).

36. Laura A. Pratt et al., "Antidepressant Use in Persons Aged 12 and Over: United States, 2005–2008," National Center for Health Statistics, Data Brief, no. 76, Oct. 2011, 1.

37. "Substance Abuse" (2010), 85, Tab. 1.1.

38. Kenneth Silk, personal communication, May 18, 2006.

39. Medco "Latest News" of May 16, 2007, attached to an email press release from the Alliance for Human Research Protection of July 6, 2007.

40. E. Jane Costello et al., "Is There an Epidemic of Child or Adolescent Depression?" *Journal of Child Psychology and Psychiatry*, 47 (2006), 1263–1271, p. 1268.

41. Raymond Battegay, interview, "Forty-Four Years of Psychiatry and Psychopharmacology," in David Healy, Ed., *The Psychopharmacologists*, Vol. 3 (London: Arnold, 2000), 379.

42. M. Olfson et al., "Prevalence of Anxiety, Depression, and Substance Use Disorders in an Urban General Medical Practice," *Archives of Family Medicine*, 9 (2000), 876–883; the exact figure was 18.9%.

43. M. Lethbridge-Cejku et al., Summary health statistics for U.S. adults: National Health Interview Survey, 2004. National Center for Health Statistics. *Vital Health Statistics,* 10 (228), 2006, 42, Tab. 14; survey in 2004.

44. Aaron T. Beck, *Depression: Clinical, Experimental, and Theoretical Aspects* (New York: Hoeber, 1967), 16, Tab. 2–3.

45. David Healy, "Dysphoria," in Charles G. Costello, Ed., *Symptoms of Depression* (New York: Wiley, 1993), 23–42, pp. 26–27.

46. J. A. Ramos-Brieva et al., "Distinct Quality of Depressed Mood: An Attempt to Develop an Objective Measure," *Journal of Affective Disorders,* 13 (1987), 241–248.

47. Leland Hinsie and Jacob Shatzky, *Psychiatric Dictionary* (London: Oxford University Press, 1940); Robert Jean Campbell, *Psychiatric Dictionary*, 7th ed. (New York: Oxford University Press, 1996); Antoine Porot, *Manuel alphabétique de psychiatrie,* 7th ed. (Paris: Presses Universitaires de France, 1996).

48. Uwe Henrik Peters, *Wörterbuch der Psychiatrie und medizinischen Psychologie,* 4th ed. (Munich: Urban & Schwarzenberg, 1990), 539.

49. W. Schulte, "Nichttraurigseinkönnen im Kern melancholischen Erlebens," *Nervenarzt,* 32 (1961), 314–320, p. 315.

50. Allan V. Horwitz and Jerome C. Wakefield, *The Loss of Sadness: How Psychiatry Transformed Normal Sorrow into Depressive Disorder* (New York: Oxford University Press, 2007). The authors make a number of excellent points but they do not understand that sadness has never been an important concept in Anglo-American psychiatry. Moreover, in melancholia the primary affect is not sadness but pain, and the inability to feel.

51. Ramin Mojtabal and Mark Olfson, "Proportion of Antidepressants Prescribed without a Psychiatric Diagnosis Is Growing," *Health Affairs,* 30 (2011), 1434–1442.

52. Steven Ornstein et al., "Depression Diagnoses and Antidepressant Use in Primary Care Practices," *Journal of Family Practice,* 49 (2000), 68–72, p. 71.

53. Jina Pagura et al., "Antidepressant Use in the Absence of Common Mental Disorders in the General Population," *Journal of Clinical Psychiatry,* 72 (2011), 494–501.

54. Owen Wade, discussion, in Craig D. Burrell, Ed., *Drug Assessment in Ferment: Multinational Comparisons* (Washington, DC: Interdisciplinary Communication Associates, 1976), 8; Vol. 6 in the Philosophy and Technology of Drug Assessment series of the Interdisciplinary Communications Program of the Smithsonian Institution.

55. Myrna Weissman et al., "Cross-National Epidemiology of Major Depression and Bipolar Disorder," *JAMA,* 276 (July 24, 1996), 293–299, Tabs. 2, 8.

56. Kenneth B. Wells et al., "The Functioning and Well-being of Depressed Patients: Results from the Medical Outcomes Study," *JAMA,* 262 (Aug. 18, 1989), 914–919, p. 918.

57. Alexander Glassman, interview, in Thomas A. Ban, Ed., *An Oral History of Neuropsychopharmacology: The First Fifty Years. Peer Interviews,* Vol. 7 (Brentwood, TN: ACNP, 2011), 239–246, p. 246; some material in the manuscript of the interview was omitted from the published version.

58. James Kocsis, interview, in Thomas A. Ban, Ed., *The Oral History of Psychopharmacology: The First Fifty Years. Peer Interviews,* Vol. 4 (Brentwood, TN: ACNP, 2011), 215–225, p. 219.

59. Walter L. Cassidy, Mandel E. Cohen et al., "Clinical Observations in Manic-Depressive Disease," *JAMA,* 164 (Aug. 3, 1957), 1535–1546; the findings were first reported at a conference in 1955.

60. George J. Unick et al., "Heterogeneity in Comorbidity Between Major Depressive Disorder and Generalized Anxiety Disorder and Its Clinical Consequences," *Journal of Nervous and Mental Disease,* 197 (2009), 215–224, p. 218, Tab. 3. Similar results were obtained for "feeling fatigued," with the exception that those with mild psychological depression were no more fatigued than the normals.

61. Cassidy, Cohen et al. (1957), 1539, Tab. 4.

62. Unick (2009), 218, Tab. 3. Stomach complaints tend to be associated more with anxiety than depression. And these data sets show several depression categories as low in stomach problems. Yet if the mixed anxiety-depression form is the commonest presentation, then the lump in the stomach etc. would become depressive symptoms as well.

63. Cassidy, Cohen et al. (1957), 1539, Tab. 4.

64. Nadia Iovieno et al., "Residual Symptoms After Remission of Major Depressive Disorder with Fluoxetine and Risk of Relapse," *Depression and Anxiety,* 28 (2011), 137–144, p. 141, Tab. 3.

65. Norman Sartorius et al., "Depression Comorbid with Anxiety: Results from the WHO Study on Psychological Disorders in Primary Health Care," *BJP,* 168 (Suppl. 30) (1996), 38–43, p. 40.

66. M. Piccinelli et al., "Typologies of Anxiety, Depression and Somatization Symptoms among Primary Care Attenders with no Formal Mental Disorder," *Psychological Medicine,* 29 (1999), 677–688, p. 677.

67. T. B. Ustun and Norman Sartorius, *Mental Illness in General Health Care: An International Study* (Chichester; Wiley, 1995), 358, Tab. 6.

68. See Jack D. Maser and C. Robert Cloninger, Eds., *Comorbidity of Mood and Anxiety Disorders* (Washington, DC: American Psychiatric Press, 1990).

69. Transcript of Proceedings, Department of Health, Education, and Welfare, Psychopharmacological Agents Advisory Committee, Mar. 21, 1977, 91; obtained from the FDA through the Freedom of Information Act.

70. Transcript of interview of Joseph Autry by Leo Hollister, Apr. 15, 1997, in Thomas A. Ban, Ed., *An Oral History of Neuropsychopharmacology: The First Fifty Years. Peer Interviews* (Brentwood, TN: ACNP, 2011), Vols. 4, 6. Autry probably had the SSRI drug class in mind when he spoke of antidepressants used to treat anxiety. For Hollister and Overall's work on mixed anxiety-depression, see John E. Overall, Leo E. Hollister, Merlin Johnson, and Veronica Pennington, "Nosology of Depression and Differential Response to Drugs," *JAMA,* 195 (Mar. 14, 1966), 162–164.

71. Bill Deakin, discussion, in Merton Sandler et al., Eds., *5-Hydroxytryptamine in Psychiatry: A Spectrum of Ideas,* (Oxford: Oxford University Press, 1991), 195.

72. Francis P. Rhoades testimony, "In the Matter of Depressant and Stimulant Drugs, Docket no. FDA-DAC-1," Aug. 12, 1966, p. 3291; U.S. Food and Drug Administration, Division of Dockets Management, Rockland, MD; obtained through the Freedom of Information Act.

73. I am indebted to an article by David Healy for insight into this shift. David Healy, "Some Continuities and Discontinuities in the Pharmacotherapy of Nervous Conditions before and after Chlorpromazine and Imipramine," *History of Psychiatry,* 11 (2000), 393–412.

74. Julius Levine, Max Rinkel, and Milton Greenblatt, "Psychological and Physiological Effects of Intravenous Pervitin," *AJP,* 105 (1948), 429–434.

75. The first advertisement for methamphetamine of which I am aware was Abbott Laboratories' publicity for its Desoxyn brand in the treatment of obesity. See *New York State Journal of Medicine,* 47 (1947), 1473.

76. T. M. Ling and L. S. Davies, "The Use of Methedrine in the Diagnosis and Treatment of the Psychoneuroses," *AJP,* 109 (1952), 38–39.

77. Equanil ad, *Diseases of the Nervous System,* 17 (1956), 36.

78. Miltown ad, *New York State Journal of Medicine,* 56 (1956), 5.

79. See chlorpromazine ads in *Semaine des Hôpitaux,* 29 (1953), 1502; 80 (1954), 1555.

80. The first ad for Thorazine, "to relieve anxiety" appeared in the *New York State Journal of Medicine,* 55 (1955), 1833.

81. Thorazine ad, *Diseases of the Nervous System,* 17 (1956), 148.

82. Thorazine ad, *New York State Journal of Medicine,* 56 (1956), 781.

83. Ralph W. Gerard, "Drugs for the Soul: The Rise of Psychopharmacology," *Science,* 125 (Feb. 1, 1957), 201–203, p. 201.

84. Malcolm H. Lader et al., "Clinical Comparison of Anxiolytic Drug Therapy," *Psychological Medicine,* 4 (1974), 381–387.

85. Patricia Pearson, *A Brief History of Anxiety: Yours and Mine* (New York: Bloomsbury USA, 2008), 8–9.

86. Giel J. M. Hutschemaekers, "The Historical-Contextualist Approach: The Case of Neurotic Anxiety," in J. R. van de Vijver and Giel J. M. Hutschemaekers, Eds., *The Investigation of Culture: Current Issues in Cultural Psychology* (Tilburg: Tilburg University Press, 1990), 133–152, pp. 134–135.

87. Jeffrey S. Harman et al., "Physician Office Visits of Adults for Anxiety Disorders in the United States, 1985–1998," *Journal of General Internal Medicine,* 17 (2002), 165–172, p. 169, Fig. 1.

88. Stanley Cobb and Mandel E. Cohen, "Experimental Production During Rebreathing of Sighing Respiration and Symptoms Resembling Those in Anxiety Attacks in Patients with Anxiety Neurosis," *Journal of Clinical Investigation,* 19 (1940), 789.

89. Mandel E. Cohen and Paul D. White, "Life Situations, Emotions, and Neurocirculatory Asthenia (Anxiety Neurosis, Neurasthenia, Effort Syndrome)," *Psychosomatic Medicine,* 13 (1951), 335–357, p. 337

90. Ferris N. Pitts, Jr. and James N. McClure, Jr., "Lactate Metabolism in Anxiety

Neurosis," *NEJM*, 277 (Dec. 21, 1967), 1329–1336, p. 1334.

91. Cassidy, *JAMA* (1957), 1538, Tab. 3.

92. Douglas Goldman, discussion, in Nathan S. Kline, Ed., *Psychopharmacology Frontiers: Second International Congress of Psychiatry: Proceedings of the Psychopharmacology Symposium* [Boston: Little Brown, (1957)], 469.

93. Martin Roth, "The Phobic Anxiety-Depersonalization Syndrome," *Proceedings of the Royal Society of Medicine*, 52 (1959), 587–596, p. 590.

94. Donald F. Klein, "Delineation of Two Drug-Responsive Anxiety Syndromes," *Psychopharmacologia*, 5 (1964), 397–408.

95. Donald F. Klein, "Medication in the Treatment of Panic Attacks and Phobic States," *Psychopharmacology Bulletin*, 18 (1982), 85–90.

96. Panic was mentioned in *DSM-II* in 1968 as an extreme form of anxiety neurosis but not given independent diagnostic status. *American Psychiatric Association, DSM-II: Diagnostic and Statistical Manual of Mental Disorders,* 2nd ed. (Washington, DC: American Psychiatric Association, 1968), 9.

97. See Kjell Modigh, "Antidepressant Drugs in Anxiety Disorders," *Acta Psychiatrica Scandinavica*, 76 (Suppl. 335) (1987), 57–71.

98. Stelazine ad, *Diseases of the Nervous System*, 28 (1967).

99. Ativan (lorazepam) ad, *AJP*, 144 (1987).

100. Peter Tyrer, personal communication, Oct. 22, 2001.

101. On these events see Myrna Weissman, interview, "Gerald Klerman and Psychopharmacology," in David Healy, Ed., *The Psychopharmacologists,* Vol. 2 (London: Altman, 1998), 521–542, pp. 534–535. The Healy volume also contains an interview of Marks (pp. 543–560).

102. On increased anxiety about "unpredictable aversive events" as a marker for panic disorder, see Christian Grillon et al., "Increased Anxiety During Anticipation of Unpredictable But Not Predictable Aversive Stimuli as a Psychophysiologic Marker of Panic Disorder," *AJP*, 165 (2008), 898–899.

CHAPTER 12

1. F-D-C Reports/Pink Sheet, Feb. 25, 1957, 11–12.

2. J. Frei, "Contribution à l'étude de l'hystérie: Problèmes de définition et évolution de la symptomatologie," *Archives Suisses de Neurologie, Neurochirurgie et de Psychiatrie*, 134 (1984), 93–129, pp. 123–124.

3. Palma E. Formica, "The Housewife Syndrome: Treatment with the Potassium and Magnesium Salts of Aspartic Acid," *Current Therapeutic Research*, 4 (1962), 98–106, pp. 98–99.

4. Edward Sachar and Miron Baron, "The Biology of Affective Disorders," *Annual Review of Neuroscience*, 2 (1979), 505–518, p. 505.

5. Paul Leber, in discussion. Food and Drug Administration, Psychopharmacologic Drugs Advisory Committee, transcript of meeting of Feb. 24, 1983, Vol. 1, 155–156;

obtained from the FDA through the Freedom of Information Act.

6. Paul Hoch, "The Effect of Chlorpromazine on Moderate and Mild Mental and Emotional Disturbances," in *Chlorpromazine and Mental Health: Proceedings of the Symposium Held Under the Auspices of Smith, Kline & French Laboratories, June 6, 1955* (Philadelphia: Lea & Febiger, 1955), 99–111, p. 103.

7. The Lord [Stephen] Taylor, "The Role of Environment in Psychopathy, Psychosis and Neurosis," in *Psychiatric Research in Our Changing World: Proceedings of the International Symposium to Commemorate the 25th Anniversary of the Founding of the Department of Psychiatry of McGill University, Montreal, 3–5 October 1968* (Amsterdam: Excerpta Medica, 1969), 41–49, p. 42.

8. Eugene S. Paykel and George Winokur, "Editorial," *Journal of Affective Disorders,* 10 (1986), 1.

9. Department of Health and Human Services, Public Health Service, Food and Drug Administration, Psychopharmacologic Drugs Advisory Committee, meeting transcript May 18, 1992, 259–260. Obtained from the Food and Drug Administration with the Freedom of Information Act.

10. See Richard Cassirer, "Die vasomotorisch-trophischen Neurosen," *Zentralblatt für Nervenheilkunde, NF* 11 (1900), 591–598; Max Rosenfeld, "Zur Kasuistik der vasomotorischen-trophischen Neurose," *Centralblatt für Nervenheilkunde und Psychiatrie, NF* 17 (1906), 665–680.

11. Walter Cimbal, "Vegetative Äquivalente der Depressionszustände," *Deutsche Zeitschrift für Nervenheilkunde,* 107 (1928), 36–41, p. 36.

12. Bernhard Wichmann, "Das vegetative Syndrom und seine Behandlung," *Deutsche Medizinische Wochenschrift,* 68 (Oct. 5, 1934), 1500–1504.

13. George Beaumont, interview, "The Place of Clomipramine in Psychopharmacology," in David Healy, Ed., *The Psychopharmacologists,* Vol. 1 (London: Chapman & Hall, 1996), 309–327, p. 327

14. On the "overwhelming number of neurotic states [that] are in reality mild or severe depressions," see Leslie Hohman, "Some Facts That the Internist Should Know About Depressions," *Diseases of the Nervous System,* 1 (1940), 7–10, p. 9.

15. V. A. Kral, "Masked Depression in Middle Aged Men," *Canadian Medical Association Journal,* 79 (1958), 1–5. Kral believed that the "low sedation threshold" of the patients differentiated them from neurotic anxiety reactions.

16. Franz Alexander, *Psychosomatic Medicine* (New York: Norton, 1950).

17. Anthony Hordern, "The Antidepressant Drugs," *NEJM,* 272 (June 3, 1965), 1159–1169, p. 1160.

18. The index of Harrison's *Principles of Internal Medicine,* which is the standard work, does not contain the term "psychosomatic." And we can search the extensive dermatology chapters in vain for any references to the work of Franz Alexander. Dennis L. Kasper et al., Eds., *Harrison's Principles of Internal Medicine,* 16th ed. (New York: McGraw Hill, 2005).

19. Herman van Praag, discussion, in Paul Kielholz, Ed., *La dépression masquée* (Bern: Huber, 1973), 28; the conference, given over to the proposition that "masked depression" constituted an important but hitherto poorly recognized clinical entity, was sponsored by Ciba-Geigy and turned out to be a kind of infomercial for the company's antidepressant drug Ludiomil (maprotiline) that, strangely enough, was being indicated for what was called "depressio sine depressione." The conference dwelled long upon varying somatic symptoms as underlying depressive "equivalents." Yet the real point would have been the following: To what extent are somatic symptoms and nonmelancholic depression both manifestations of a deeper underlying illness, called here the nervous syndrome?

20. Dietrich Blumer and Mary Heilbronn, "Chronic Pain as a Variant of Depressive Disease: The Pain-Prone Disorder," *Journal of Nervous and Mental Disease*, 170 (1982), 381–406. In fact, on the basis of Blumer's clinical criteria, these patients did tend to fulfill the criteria for the nervous syndrome.

CHAPTER 13

1. Gary Langer, "On Air: Use of Anti-Depressants Is a Long-Term Practice," ABC News.com, http://abcnews.go.com/onair/WorldNewsTonight/poll00410.html, Apr. 10, 2002.

2. Details may be found in Edward Shorter, *Historical Dictionary of Psychiatry* (New York: Oxford University Press, 2005), passim.

3. David H. Barlow and Laura A. Campbell, "Mixed Anxiety-Depression and Its Implications for Models of Mood and Anxiety Disorders," *Comprehensive Psychiatry*, 41 (Suppl. 1) (2000), 55–60. This was the first of a number of contributions by Barlow on this theme.

4. Salvatore J. Enna, interview, in Thomas A. Ban, Ed., *An Oral History of Neuropsychopharmacology: The First Fifty Years. Peer Interviews,* Vol. 3 (Brentwood, TN: ACNP, 2011), 135–157, p. 151.

5. George I. Papakostas, "Surrogate Markers of Treatment Outcome in Major Depressive Disorder," *International Journal of Neuropsychopharmacology*, 2011. DOI: 10.1017/S1461145711001246.

6. Paul H. Patterson, *Infectious Behavior: Brain-Immune Connections in Autism, Schizophrenia, and Depression* (Cambridge, MA: MIT Press, 2011), 112.

7. Charles A. Sanislow, Bruce N. Cuthbert et al., "Developing Constructs for Psychopathology Research: Research Domain Criteria," *Journal of Abnormal Psychology,* 119 (2010), 631–639, pp. 637–638.

8. Michael Alan Taylor and Max Fink, *Melancholia: The Diagnosis, Pathophysiology, and Treatment of Depressive Illness* (New York: Cambridge University Press, 2006), 220–231.

9. See Edward Shorter, *Before Prozac: The Troubled History of Mood Disorders in*

Psychiatry (New York: Oxford University Press, 2009), 33. Today, Seroquel (quetiapine), initially launched as an antipsychotic in 1997, is occasionally referred to as "an all-purpose nerve tonic."

10. Richard Shader interview, in Thomas A. Ban, Ed., *An Oral History of Neuropsychopharmacology,* Vol. 8 (Brentwood, TN: American College of Neuropsychopharmacology, 2011), 326.

Index

abdominal symptoms. *See* gastrointestinal tract

Abraham, Karl, 114, 117

adolescents, and depression, 172

adrenal gland, 2, 81, 85, 166, 214*n*23

agoraphobia
    and imipramine, 142
    introduction and description, 61, 65, 129
    and panic, 67, 141, 142, 143, 183, 184

Akiskal, Hagop, 123

Alexander, Franz, 190

American Psychiatric Association, and *DSM*, 4, 44, 54, 129, 135, 138

amitriptyline, 156

amphetamines, 151, 152, 179, 197–98

Anafranil. *See* clomipramine

Andreasen, Nancy, 134

Andrews, Gavin, 120

Angelini Company, trazodone, 158

Angst, Jules, 89

anhedonia, 72, 89, 94, 107, 140

anorexia nervosa, 85

antidepressants
    effectiveness for depression, 2, 151, 197
    increase in prescriptions, 171–72
    taken by people without depression, 174–75
    See also selective serotonin reuptake inhibitors (SSRIs); tetracyclic antidepressants; tricyclic antidepressants (TCAs)

anxiety
    atypical, 69, 143
    drug treatments, 13, 53–54, 55, 179–81
    in drug trials, 52
    increases in, 14, 179, 181
    links with tension, 54
    as marker for larger disorders, 13–14, 53
    multiple meanings of, 51, 52–53, 52–54
    in nervous breakdowns, 62, 65, 69, 77
    and panic disorder, 51, 52, 60–62
    as part of nervous syndrome, x, 11, 14, 51, 52, 53, 56–60, 77, 141, 177, 179
    and psychoanalysis, 52–53, 69–71
    separation from depression by *DSM-III*, 54, 119, 121, 123–24, 129, 132–33, 144, 178, 179
    as stand-alone illness, 52, 53–54, 62–69, 179
    See also anxiety neurosis; mixed anxiety-depression; nervous syndrome; panic disorder/panic attacks; psychotic anxiety

anxiety hysteria, 53

anxiety neurosis, 43, 51, 52, 67–68, 69–70, 71–72, 114

anxiety psychosis, 73

anxiolytics, 54, 198

anxious melancholia, 51, 58, 73–74

Arieti, Silvano, 117

Asberg, Marie, 155

Ashcroft, George, 156